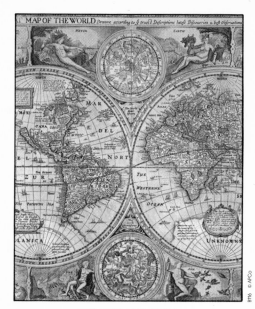

FROM THE LIBRARY OF

The Monoclonal Gammopathies

MULTIPLE MYELOMA AND
RELATED PLASMA-CELL DISORDERS

Publication Number 995
AMERICAN LECTURE SERIES®

A Monograph in
The BANNERSTONE DIVISION *of*
AMERICAN LECTURES IN LIVING CHEMISTRY

Edited by
I. Newton Kugelmass, M.D., Ph.D., Sc.D.
Consultant to the Departments of Health and Hospitals
New York City

THE
Monoclonal Gammopathies

MULTIPLE MYELOMA AND
RELATED PLASMA-CELL DISORDERS

By

ROBERT A. KYLE, M.D., M.S. (Internal Medicine)
Consultant, Division of Hematology and Internal Medicine,
Mayo Clinic and Mayo Foundation;
Professor of Medicine, Mayo Medical School; Rochester, Minnesota

and

EDWIN D. BAYRD, M.D., M.S. (Internal Medicine)
Senior Consultant, Division of Hematology and Internal Medicine,
Mayo Clinic and Mayo Foundation;
Professor of Medicine, Mayo Medical School; Rochester, Minnesota

With a Foreword by
I. Newton Kugelmass, M.D., Ph.D., Sc.D.
Consultant to the Departments of Health and Hospitals
New York City

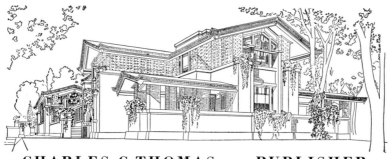

CHARLES C THOMAS · PUBLISHER
Springfield · Illinois · U.S.A.

Published and Distributed Throughout the World by
CHARLES C THOMAS • PUBLISHER
Bannerstone House
301-327 East Lawrence Avenue, Springfield, Illinois, U.S.A.

© *1976 by* CHARLES C THOMAS • PUBLISHER
ISBN 0-398-03545-8
Library of Congress Catalog Card Number: 75-44293

Library of Congress Cataloging in Publication Data

Kyle, Robert A.   1928-
  The monoclonal gammopathies.

  (American lecture series; publication no. 995)
  Bibliography: p.
  Includes index.
    1. Gammopathies, Monoclonal. 2. Multiple
  myeloma. I. Bayrd, Edwin A., joint author.
  II. Title. [DNLM: 1. Multiple myeloma. 2. Blood
  protein disorders. WH540 K99m]
  RC647.H9K9   616.9'94'71   75-44293
  ISBN 0-398-03545-8

Printed in the United States of America
C-1

The investigations presented in this book were supported in part by Research Grants CA-11911 F, G, H, DD and CA-16835 from the National Institutes of Health, Public Health Service.

Foreword

Our Living Chemistry Series was conceived by the editor and publisher to advance the newer knowledge of chemical medicine in the cause of clinical practice. The interdependence of chemistry and medicine is so great that physicians are turning to chemistry and to medicine in order to understand the underlying basis of life processes in health and disease. Once chemical truths, proofs, and convictions become sound foundations for clinical phenomena, key cross-disciplinary investigators clarify the bewildering panorama of biochemical progress for application in everyday practice, stimulation of experimental research, and extension of postgraduate instruction. Each of our monographs thus unravels the chemical mechanisms and clinical management of many diseases that have remained relatively static in the minds of medical men for thousands of years. Our new series is charged with the *nisus élan* of chemical wisdom, supreme in choice of international authors, optimal in standards of chemical scholarship, provocative in imagination for experimental research, comprehensive in discussions of scientific medicine, and authoritative in discussions of chemical perspective of human disorders.

The Foreword is written last, placed first, and read least. It is a subjective introduction to the objective matter that follows— excitement consequent on the transition from the bare facts to the first realization of the import of their unexplored relationships. Then comes the precision wherein width of relation is subordinated to exactness of formulation with new facts added to fit into the field, propounded with fruition. Immunology is a house of many mansions. It is built of facts the way a house is built of bricks. But an accumulation of facts is no more immunology than a pile of bricks is a house. Thus Doctor Kyle and Doctor Bayrd built this mansion by integrating our newer knowledge of immunoglobulins with identity amidst diversity. Its value lies not only in specific guidance but in the insight we gain while pursuing the factors that make up these ever-changing dynamic systems.

Since 1960 the term gamma globulin gave way to immunoglobulin and to gammopathies. A single clone of plasma cells proliferates, producing a homogeneous monoclonal (M) protein, regarded as a normal immunoglobulin to elucidate fundamental questions concerning the structure of antibodies ever present in the germ-line cell. Immunoglobulins G, A, M, D, E, and their subclasses are heterogeneous vertebrate proteins with antibody activity, synthesized by the lymphocyte-plasma cell series. Monoclonal immunoglobulins are associated with monoclonal gammopathies of indeterminate significance, multiple myeloma, macroglobulinemia, amyloidosis, lymphocytic leukemia, and lymphomas. Clinicians confronted with gammopathies will no longer be bewildered by diversity of concepts because all available data are crystallized for neoplasms of antibody-forming cells. Gammopathies are considered as a whole in order to be understood in detail.

"Newer knowledge is more than equivalent to clinical power."

I. NEWTON KUGELMASS, M.D., Ph.D., Sc.D.
Editor

Contents

ix

The Monoclonal Gammopathies

MULTIPLE MYELOMA AND
RELATED PLASMA-CELL DISORDERS

CHAPTER I

Introduction

M ONOCLONAL GAMMOPATHIES are synonymous with plasma-cell dyscrasias (Osserman and Isobe, 1972), immunoglobulin-opathies (Engle and Wallis, 1969), gammopathies (Waldenström, 1961), and dysproteinemias.

They are a group of disorders characterized by proliferation of a single clone of plasma cells that produce a homogenous, monoclonal (M) protein. A monoclonal immunoglobulin increase consists of two heavy polypeptide chains of a single class and subclass and two light polypeptide chains of a single type (Table 1). Thus it contrasts with a polyclonal immunoglobulin increase, which consists of one or more heavy-chain classes and both light-chain types.

The different kinds of monoclonal immunoglobulins are designated by capital letters that correspond to the class of their

TABLE 1

CLASSIFICATION OF IMMUNOGLOBULINS OF NORMAL HUMAN SERUM

Immunoglobulin	IgG	IgA	IgM	IgD	IgE
Synonyms	γ, 7Sγ, γ_2, γG	βx, β_2A, γ_1A, γA	γ_1, 19Sγ, β_2M, γ_1M, γM	γD	γE
Heavy-chain					
Classes	Gamma, γ	Alpha, α	Mu, μ	Delta, δ	Epsilon, ϵ
Subclasses	IgG1, IgG2, IgG3, IgG4	IgA1, IgA2	...	Ja, La	...
Light-chain types	Kappa, κ Lambda, λ	κ λ	κ λ	κ λ	κ λ
Molecular formula	$\gamma_2\kappa_2$ $\gamma_2\lambda_2$	$\alpha_2\kappa_2$* $\alpha_2\lambda_2$*	$(\mu_2\kappa_2)$ 5 $(\mu_2\lambda_2)$ 5	$\delta_2\kappa_2$ $\delta_2\lambda_2$	$\epsilon_2\kappa_2$ $\epsilon_2\lambda_2$
Designation	IgGκ IgG λ	IgA κ IgA λ	IgM κ IgM λ	IgD κ IgD λ	IgE κ IgE λ

* May form polymers.

3

heavy chains, which are designated by Greek letters: γ in IgG, α in IgA, μ in IgM, δ in IgD, and ϵ in IgE. Their subclasses are IgG1, etc., and their light-chain types are kappa or κ, and lambda or λ (because L and H are used for light and heavy chains).

The immunoglobulins in serum—and in urine—are detected and distinguished chiefly by electrophoresis and immunoelectrophoresis. The tall, narrow-based electrophoretic pattern of a homogenous monoclonal protein suggests benign monoclonal gammopathy, multiple myeloma, Waldenström's macroglobulinemia, amyloidosis, lymphoma, or the rare heavy-chain diseases. Occasionally immunoelectrophoresis proves that a broad protein peak contains only one heavy-chain class and one light-chain type and hence is monoclonal. Such a broad peak may result from polymer formation. Broad-based peaks of heterogenous polyclonal immunoglobulins often are associated with chronic infections, disorders of connective tissue, and chronic liver diseases; but they will not be included in this review (Waldenström, 1968).

CLASSIFICATION OF MONOCLONAL GAMMOPATHIES

I. Malignant monoclonal gammopathies

A. Multiple myeloma (IgG, IgA, IgD, IgE, and free light chains)
   1. Solitary plasmacytoma of bone
   2. Extramedullary plasmacytoma, solitary and multiple
   3. Plasma-cell leukemia
   4. Nonsecretory myeloma

B. Waldenström's macroglobulinemia (primary macroglobulinemia) (IgM)

C. Heavy-chain diseases (HCD)
   1. γ (gamma) HCD
   2. α (alpha) HCD
   3. μ (mu) HCD

D. Amyloidosis
   1. Primary
   2. With myeloma
   3. Secondary

4. Localized

5. Familial

II. Monoclonal gammopathies of unknown significance

A. Benign (IgG, IgA, IgD, IgM, and—rarely—free light chains)

B. Associated with malignant lymphoma

C. Associated with neoplasms of cell types not known to produce monoclonal proteins

We shall prepare for understanding of the monoclonal gammopathies by reviewing the structure, function, and synthesis of immunoglobulins: relating normal immunoglobulins to myeloma and macroglobulinemia; discussing the nature of monoclonal proteins; and then describing laboratory methods for the recognition and study of monoclonal proteins.

CHAPTER II

Immunoglobulin Groups: Structure, Function, and Synthesis

In 1937, Tiselius used electrophoretic techniques for separating serum globulins into three components, which he designated a, β, and γ. Two years later, Tiselius and Kabat (1939) localized antibody activity in the gamma globulin fraction of the plasma proteins. They noted that antibodies to egg albumin or to pneumococcus type I were found in the area of gamma mobility in rabbit serum, while antibodies to pneumococcal organisms migrated between beta and gamma in horse serum. Later it was recognized that some antibodies migrate in the fast gamma region and others in the slow, and some sediment in the ultracentrifuge as 7S and others as 19S; but the concept of a family of proteins with antibody activity was not proposed until the late 1950s (Heremans, 1959).

Prior to 1960, the term "gamma globulin" was used for any protein that migrated in the gamma mobility region (toward the cathode) of the electrophoretic pattern. Now these proteins are referred to as "immunoglobulins," and the five groups presently recognized and their properties are listed in Table 2. Comprehensive reviews have been published by Porter, 1967, 1973; Waldmann, 1969; Kyle et al., 1970a; Milstein and Pink, 1970; Hopper and Nisonoff, 1971; Kyle and Gleich, 1972; Edelman, 1973; Natvig and Kunkel, 1973; Solomon and McLaughlin, 1973; Park and Good, 1974.

IMMUNOGLOBULIN G (IgG)

Three-fourths of the immunoglobulin in normal serum is of the IgG type, and this is the type most thoroughly investigated. It has a molecular weight of 150,000 and a sedimentation coeffi-

TABLE 2

PROPERTIES OF IMMUNOGLOBULINS OF NORMAL HUMAN SERUM

	IgG	IgA	IgM	IgD	IgE
Electrophoretic mobility	Gamma to alpha-2	Gamma to beta	Gamma to gamma-2	Gamma to beta	Gamma to beta
Sedimentation coefficient	6.7S	7-15S*	19S	7S	8S
Molecular weight	150,000	170,000-500,000*	900,000	180,000	200,000
Carbohydrate, %	2.6	5-10	9.8	10-12	11
T½, days	23	5.8	5.1	2.8	2.3
Serum concentration, mean mg/ml	11.4	1.8	1.0	0.03	0.0003
Total serum immunoglobulin, %	74	21	5	0.2	0.002
Total body pool in intravascular space, %	45	42	76	75	51
Intravascular pool catabolized per day, % (normal)	6.7	25	18	37	89
Normal synthetic rate, mg/kg/day	33	24	6.7	0.4	0.02
Fixes complement	Yes	Alternate pathway	Yes	No	No
Crosses placenta	Yes	No	No	No	No

* Tends to form polymer of the monomer form.

Modified from Kyle, R. A., Bieger, R. C., and Gleich, G. J.: Diagnosis of syndromes associated with hyperglobulinemia. *Med Clin North Am, 54*:917-938, 1970. By permission of W. B. Saunders Company.

cient of 6.7S. Its electrophoretic mobility ranges from slow gamma to alpha-2. Many antibodies to both bacteria and viruses are of the IgG class. Unlike other immunoglobulins, IgG is transported selectively across the trophoblastic cells of the placenta by virtue of its Fc piece (Brambell, 1966). IgG levels fall during the first few months of life, because maternal IgG is catabolized; and then the serum content gradually increases to reach adult levels by age 5. IgG is readily purified from human serum by Cohn fractionation and can be obtained in sizeable quantities for structural studies.

Structure and Function: A reducing agent such as mercaptoethanol disrupts the disulfide bonds linking the polypeptide chains of the IgG molecule. And if the reduced protein is alkylated with iodoacetamide and fractionated in the presence of a solvent (such as guanidine or urea) capable of dissociating noncovalent bonds, two kinds of polypeptide chains can be recovered: heavy (H) and light (L) (Nomenclature Committee of the IUIS, 1972).

Both heavy chains of the IgG molecule are of the γ class; the two light chains are alike—both kappa or both lambda. The γ heavy chains have a molecular weight of approximately 55,000, and their structure comprises 440 to 450 amino acids. The light chains have a molecular weight of 22,500 and contain approximately 214 amino acids (Table 3).

TABLE 3

PROPERTIES OF IgG LIGHT AND HEAVY CHAINS

Property	Light	Heavy
Molecular weight	22,500	55,000
Carbohydrate	None	Yes
Major antigenic classes	Two major: κ, λ	Four known: IgG1, IgG2, IgG3, IgG4
Specificity		
Inv genotypic	Present (κ)	Absent
Oz	Present (λ)	Absent
Kern	Present (λ)	Absent
Gm genotypic	Absent	Present
Relation to Bence Jones protein	Same	Not related

The carbohydrate moiety of IgG is associated with the heavy chain.

Relation of Components: The relation of these chains in the structure of the immunoglobulin molecule is inferred from the effect of certain proteolytic enzymes (Figs. 1 and 2). Papain, by breaking the heavy chains, cleaves the molecule into three pieces: an Fc fragment (so named because in certain species it can be crystallized) and two Fab fragments (so named because they have antibody activity and combine with antigen).

The Fc fragment comprises the C-terminal portion of both heavy chains, still linked to each other by disulfide bonds. (Other

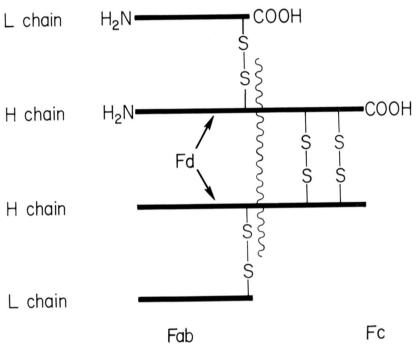

Figure 1. Representation of IgG molecule, with cleavage by papain into Fab and Fc fragments (Fab including Fd piece). (Modified from Kyle, R. A., Bieger, R. C., and Gleich, G. J.: Diagnosis of syndromes associated with hyperglobulinemia. *Med Clin North Am*, *54*:917-938, 1970. By permission of W. B. Saunders Company.)

IgG – Papain Digestion

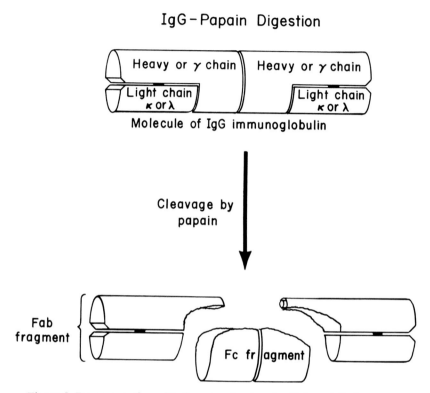

Figure 2. Representation of IgG molecule, showing Fab and Fc fragments.

designations of this fragment are fast, B, and III; and its molecular weight is 48,000.) Biologic activities of the Fc fragment include fixation of complement, PCA, binding with rheumatoid factors, binding with receptors on macrophages and lymphocytes, reaction with staphylococcal A protein, and transfer across the placenta. Specificity—that is γ (IgG), α (IgA), μ (IgM), δ (IgD), or ϵ (IgE)—resides in the Fc fragment. The Fc piece does not combine with antigen and is devoid of antibody activity.

Each Fab fragment is the N-terminal portion of a heavy chain and the light chain still bonded to it. (Other designations are slow, A, C, I, or II; molecular weight 52,000.) The antigen-combining site of the Fab is composed of perhaps 15 to 20 amino acid residues, some of which are in the heavy-chain portion and others in the light chain. The portion of the heavy chain in Fab is called the "Fd piece."

The part of the molecule where the disulfide bonds link the two heavy chains to each other is called the "hinge region"; and as indicated, papain cleavage leaves this part in the Fc fragment. Cleavage by pepsin, however, breaks the heavy chains on the other side of the hinge region. Its result is the somewhat shortened C-terminal portions of the two heavy chains, without bonds, and a single F(ab')₂ fragment corresponding to both Fab fragments plus the hinge region linking them together.

Subclasses of IgG: Immunologic analysis of myeloma proteins has disclosed four distinct subclasses of IgG heavy chains (Grey and Kunkel, 1964; Terry and Fahey, 1964): IgG1, IgG2, IgG3, and IgG4 (Nomenclature Committee of the IUIS, 1966) (Table 4). Two types of IgG4 proteins have been described, IgG4a and IgG4b (Kunkel et al., 1970). The IgG1 subclass constitutes 64 to 70% of normal IgG molecules, IgG2 23 to 28%, IgG3 4 to 7%, and IgG4 3 to 4% (Schur, 1972). A fifth IgG subclass (IgG5) has been reported, but it appears to be a variant of IgG2. Normal serum pools contain the following concentrations of IgG subclasses (mg/dl): IgG1, 5.1 to 8.1; IgG2, 2.5 to 3.6; IgG3, 0.55 to 0.70; and IgG4, 0.35 to 0.40 (Morell et al., 1972). Immunofluorescence studies demonstrated IgG subclasses in individual plasma cells in the same proportion as in the serum, except that IgG3 plasma cells were increased. This is consistent with the short T$\frac{1}{2}$ of IgG3 (Morell et al., 1975).

Among 900 patients with monoclonal protein, Schur et al. (1974) identified IgG1 in 77%, IgG2 in 14%, IgG3 in 6%, and IgG4 in 3%. In another study, Skvaril et al. (1972) found that

TABLE 4

NOMENCLATURE OF IgG SUBCLASSES

Terry	γ2b	γ2a	γ2c	γ2d
Kunkel	We	Ne	Vi	Ge
WHO	IgG1	IgG2	IgG3	IgG4
% of normal IgG	64-70	23-28	4-7	3-4
Serum concentration, mg/ml	8.1	3.6	0.7	0.4

IgG1 constituted 80% of 659 IgG myeloma proteins, IgG2 10%, IgG3 6.4%, and IgG4 3.6%. In both of these studies IgG1 components were seen more frequently and IgG2 subclasses less frequently than one would expect from the distribution of subclasses in normal serum. Skvaril and associates (1972) found that the kappa and lambda ratios in the four subclasses were not significantly different and were in the range that one would expect normally. Schur and associates (1974), from analysis of 339 of their cases of proved myeloma, stated that hypercalcemia and anemia tended to develop more frequently with IgG2 myeloma than with IgG1 or IgG4 myeloma, and anemia tended to develop more frequently with IgG3 myeloma than with IgG1 or IgG4 myeloma. Although the initial blood urea nitrogen (BUN) value tended to be higher in myeloma cases of the IgG3 type, azotemia developed with about the same frequency in all four subclasses. These findings are only suggestive and not statistically significant.

Immunologic Features: The IgG subclasses differ in the antigenicity of their Fc fragments. IgG3 is the most immunogenic in rabbits, so potent monospecific antisera to IgG3 can be made most readily. Monospecific antisera to the other three subclasses can be prepared in animals by first making them tolerant to a different IgG subclass and then immunizing with the desired IgG subclass protein (Spiegelberg and Weigle, 1968). It should be pointed out that the antigenic determinants of IgG3 are present in the Fd piece as well as the Fc fragment, so immunization with the Fc fragment is not sufficient for developing an adequate monospecific antiserum to IgG3.

The difficulties in obtaining monospecific antisera to the subclasses have turned interest to chemical typing of the immunoglobulins. After the monoclonal protein has been isolated, reduced, and alkylated with ^{14}C-iodoacetate, it is digested with pepsin and trypsin and then subjected to high-voltage electrophoresis. Peptides containing carboxymethylcysteine, detected by autoradiography, made it possible to distinguish the IgG subclasses (Frangione et al., 1969a; Kochwa et al., 1975). The inter H chain disulfide bridges and the amino acid residues around them were found to vary: two disulfide bridges in IgG1 and IgG4, four in IgG2, and five in IgG3 (Frangione et al., 1969b) (Table 5).

TABLE 5

DISULFIDE BONDS OF IgG SUBCLASSES

	No.	*Inter H Chain* *Position*	*Inter HL* *Position*
IgG1	2	226, 229	220
IgG2	4	226, 229, 219, 220	131
IgG3	5	226, 229, 210, 214, 220	131
IgG4	2	226, 229	131

Although many antigens evoke an antibody response within the IgG subclasses proportional to their distribution in normal serum, others produce antibodies mainly within one subclass (Tables 6 and 7). For example, almost all antibodies to Factor VIII (found in hemophiliacs, postpartum women, and elderly patients) are of the IgG4 subclass (Andersen and Terry, 1968; Robboy et al., 1970; Ali and Blajchman, 1972; Shapiro, 1975). Without predilection, only 3 to 4% of the antibodies would be of this subclass. An antibody to Factor IX of the IgG4 subclass has been found in one case (Pike et al., 1972) and an IgM λ

TABLE 6

ANTIBODY ACTIVITY OF IgG SUBCLASSES

	Thyroglobulin *Ab*	*ANA*	*Factor VIII*
IgG1	Yes	Yes	No
IgG2	Yes	Yes	No
IgG3	Yes	Yes	Rare
IgG4	Few	Yes	Yes

TABLE 7

ANTIBODY ACTIVITY OF IgG SUBCLASSES

	Diphtheria *and Tetanus*	*Dextran, Teichoic* *Acid, and Levan*	*Anti-Rh*
IgG1	Yes	No	Yes
IgG2	Some	Yes	No
IgG3	Some	No	Yes
IgG4	Few	No	Rare

antibody that inhibited Factor VIII in another (McKelvey and Kwaan, 1972).

A high proportion of antibodies to dextran, levan, and teichoic acid are limited to the IgG2 subclass (Yount et al., 1968). The majority of IgG antibodies in idiopathic thrombocytopenic purpura have been found to be of the IgG3 subclass, as has the anti-platelet antibody in a patient with post-transfusion purpura (Eisenberg et al., 1973), whereas one would expect only 4 to 7% of the antibodies to be of this class. In contrast, another study disclosed that all four subclasses of IgG aggregated platelets and released serotonin (Henson and Spiegelberg, 1973). These biologic functions are associated with the Fc portion of the molecule.

Physicochemical: The molecular weight of IgG1, IgG2, and IgG4 heavy chains (γ) are 54,200; that of IgG3 is 60,950 (Virella and Parkhouse, 1972). IgG2 and IgG4 tend to be anodal on electrophoresis and IgG1 and IgG3 are cathodal, with IgG1 constituting most of the monoclonal protein of very slow (cathodal) electrophoretic mobility (Table 8). Isoelectric focusing of IgG1 protein reveals considerable variation, but IgG2 and IgG3 are more restricted. No significant difference in the carbohydrate content of the four IgG subclasses has been demonstrated. However, there are differences in their digestion by proteolytic enzymes. For example, IgG3 proteins and most IgG1 proteins are very sensitive to papain digestion; but IgG2, IgG4, and a few IgG1 proteins resist papain digestion. IgG3 and IgG4 are sensitive to pepsin digestion, but the other two subclasses are resistant to it (Table 9).

TABLE 8

PHYSICOCHEMICAL DIFFERENCES OF IgG SUBCLASSES

	Molecular Weight	Electrophoretic Mobility	Isoelectric Focusing
IgG1	54,200	Cathodal	8.3-9.5 (widespread)
IgG2	54,200	Anodal	7-7.3
IgG3	60,950	Cathodal	8.4-8.9
IgG4	54,200	Anodal	

TABLE 9

ENZYME DIGESTION OF IgG SUBCLASSES

	Papain	*Pepsin*
IgG1	Sensitive (a few resist)	Very resistant
IgG2	Resistant	Resistant
IgG3	Very sensitive	Very sensitive
IgG4	Resistant	Sensitive

Biologic: The subclasses also have different biologic properties. IgG1 and IgG3 fix complement readily; IgG2 does so less well. It has been shown that aggregates of IgG4b, but not IgG4a, fix complement via the alternate pathway (Götze and Müller-Eberhard, 1971). Fixation of IgG to heterologous skin—passive cutaneous anaphylaxis (PCA)—occurs with IgG1, IgG3, and IgG4; monocyte-binding (macrophage receptor) occurs with IgG1 and IgG3. Rosette formation or monocytic-binding appears to be directly proportional to the quantity of IgG1 present on the red blood cells (Abramson and Schur, 1972). All subclasses except IgG3 react with staphylococcal A protein (Table 10). Lymphocytes, monocytes, and neutrophils bind unaggregated IgG1 and IgG3; monocytes and neutrophils also bind IgG4 (Lawrence et al., 1975).

In one study, the average biologic half-life of IgG1, IgG2, and IgG4 myeloma proteins injected into patients with malignancies was 21 days, whereas IgG3 had a half-life of 7 to 8 days (Morell et al., 1970) (Table 11). Another study showed the half-life of

TABLE 10

BIOLOGIC PROPERTIES OF IgG SUBCLASSES

	Fix C'	PCA	Monocyte Binding	React With Staph. A Protein	Placental Transfer
IgG1	Yes	Yes	Yes	Yes	Yes
IgG2	Yes	No	No	Yes	Yes
IgG3	Yes	Yes	Yes	No	Yes
IgG4	No	Yes	No	Yes	Yes

TABLE 11

METABOLISM OF IgG SUBCLASSES

	$T\frac{1}{2}$, Days	Catabolized, % of Pool/Day	Synthesis, mg/kg/Day
IgG1	21	6.9-9.0	25.4
IgG2	21	6.9-9.0	
IgG3	8	16.8	3.4
IgG4	21	6.9-9.0	

IgG1, IgG2, and IgG4 was 11 to 12 days while that of IgG3 was 8 days (Spiegelberg et al., 1968). In a third, utilizing a normal volunteer, the half-life of IgG2 was 24 days and that of IgG1 was 15 to 19 days, suggesting two or more forms of IgG1 (Watkins and Tee, 1970). Why the results of these studies differ is not apparent; but the methods used—as well as the types of subjects (normal volunteers or those with malignant disease)—might account for some of the differences. It is noteworthy that IgG3 has a significantly shorter half-life than the other subclasses. Its tendency to form aggregates may contribute to its rapid catabolism.

Genetic markers are present in most persons. The genetic factors that are associated with IgG and are present on the γ chain are referred to as "Gm factors" or "determinants" (Grubb, 1956; Muir and Steinberg, 1967; Steinberg, 1969). If one coats an Rh-positive red cell with an incomplete Rh antibody, the addition of rheumatoid serum (anti-gamma globulin) produces agglutination. Serum that prevents agglutination is called Gm+. By altering the coating of the red cell and the agglutinating sera, more than 20 Gm factors can be distinguished. Individual Gm factors are associated with individual subclasses of IgG; there are numerous Gm determinants on IgG1 and IgG3 but few on the other two subclasses (Table 12).

TABLE 12

Gm SPECIFICITY OF IgG SUBCLASSES

IgG1	1, 2, 3, 4, 17
IgG2	23, non-g
IgG3	RY (+ numerous others)
IgG4	γ_4 non-a

Analysis of Chains: Many of the initial studies of immunoglobulin structure were performed on rabbit IgG, but the large quantities of protein available in the serum and urine of patients with multiple myeloma attracted investigators to analyze these immunoglobulins.

Light Chains: In 1962, Edelman and Gally demonstrated that light chains prepared from a serum IgG myeloma protein and the *Bence Jones protein* in the same patient's urine behaved identically; that is, they precipitated when heated to between 40 and 60°C, dissolved on boiling, and reprecipitated when cooled to between 40 and 60°C.

Analysis of Bence Jones proteins (urinary light chains) and light chains prepared from myeloma proteins revealed the two antigenic types. Approximately 70% of serum IgG myeloma immunoglobulins are of the kappa type and about 30% lambda; and the proportion among light chains of normal IgG is similar.

Bence Jones proteins are synthesized de novo and are not degradation products (Putnam and Hardy, 1955). They are catabolized by the renal tubular cells (Wochner et al., 1967) or, when present in excess, excreted promptly in the urine.

Amino acid *sequence analyses* of individual light chains of each type have disclosed a remarkable fact: although the region of the chain from approximately position 107 to the carboxy terminus at position 214 is virtually identical in light chains of the same type (κ or λ), the region from the amino (NH_2) terminus (position 1) to position 107 has been different in every light chain thus far analyzed. Consequently, these are termed the *constant (C)* and *variable (V) portions* of the light (L) chains: C_L and V_L. Both constant and variable portions contain a loop consisting of approximately 60 amino acid residues (Putnam, 1969) (Figs. 3 and 4). In the variable portion there are many amino acid differences, whereas in the constant portion differences exist at one or two sites only. Three regions of "hypervariability" have been identified in V_L: positions 24 to 34, 50 to 56, and 89 to 97 (Wu and Kabat, 1970). This hypervariability and the existence of similar hypervariable regions on the variable portion of the heavy chain (V_H) at positions 31 to 37, 51 to 68,

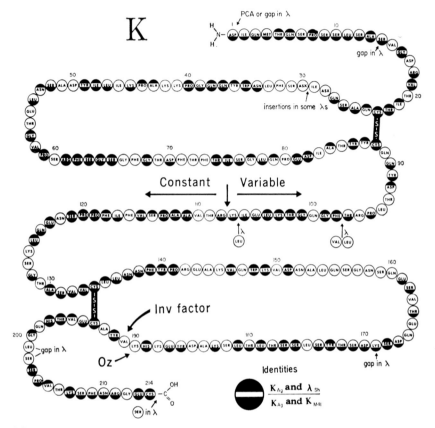

Figure 3. Amino acid sequence of human kappa light chain. Note two loops —one in constant and other in variable portion. (From Putnam, F. W.: Immunoglobulin structure: variability and homology. *Science, 163*:633-644, 1969. By permission of the American Association for the Advancement of Science; and modified from Putnam, F. W., Titani, K., Wikler, M., and Shinoda, T.: Structure and evolution of kappa and lambda light chains. In Cold Spring Harbor Laboratory of Quantitative Biology: *Cold Spring Harbor Symposia on Quantitative Biology.* Volume 32. Antibodies. Cold Spring Harbor, L.I., New York, 1967, pp. 9-29. By permission.)

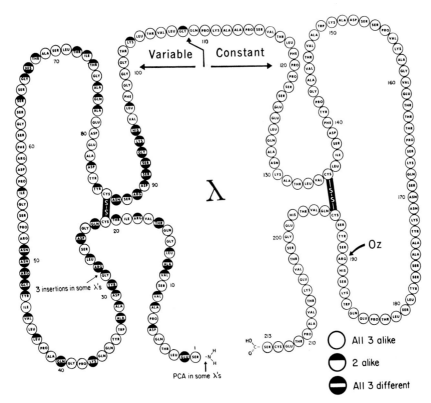

Figure 4. Amino acid sequence of human lambda light chain (note two loops). (From Putnam, F. W.: Immunoglobulin structure: variability and homology. *Science, 163*:633-644, 1969. By permission of the American Association for the Advancement of Science; and from Putnam, F. W., Titani, K., Wikler, M., and Shinoda, T.: Structure and evolution of kappa and lambda light chains. In Cold Spring Harbor Laboratory of Quantitative Biology: *Cold Spring Harbor Symposia on Quantitative Biology*. Volume 32. Antibodies. Cold Spring Harbor, L.I., New York, 1967, pp. 9-29. By permission.)

84 to 91, and 101 to 110 (Capra and Kehoe, 1975) permit the formation of many different antigen-combining sites.

The existence of amino acid differences in the constant portions of the light chains can be related to the presence of certain genetic markers. If the amino acid at position 191 of a κ chain chain is leucine, the protein is designated Inv (1) or Inv (2), whereas if valine is at this position, it is Inv (3). Among λ chains, the comparable marker is Oz (Ein and Fahey, 1967); if lysine is at position 190 the chain is Oz (+), whereas if arginine is present, it is Oz (−). Another genetic marker in λ chains has been designated Kern (+) when glycine is present at position 154 and Kern (−) when serine is there. Further sequence studies of light chains have revealed subgroups of the variable regions; among human kappa chains, three discrete sets of sequences were recognized: subgroups $V_{\kappa I}$, $V_{\kappa II}$, and $V_{\kappa III}$ (Solomon and Mc-Laughlin, 1973). Recently a new kappa variable group has been reported in cold agglutinin disease and designated $V_{\kappa IV}$ (Wang et al., 1973). In the variable portions of human lambda chains, at least five subgroups of sequences have been recognized and similarly designated: $V_{\lambda I}$, $V_{\lambda II}$, $V_{\lambda III}$, $V_{\lambda IV}$, $V_{\lambda V}$ (Solomon and McLaughlin, 1973).

Heavy Chains: Variable and constant regions are found among heavy chains also: V_H and C_H. These have not been studied so extensively as those in light chains, but the variable region of the γ chain is of approximately the same length as the variable region of the light chain—about 110 amino acid residues. The constant regions of the γ chains consist of 310 to 330 amino acids arranged linearly, adjacent regions having homologies with the constant portion of the light chain and also with each other. These portions of the γ heavy chain are called "homology regions" or "domains" and are designated $C_{\gamma 1}$, $C_{\gamma 2}$, and $C_{\gamma 3}$. The first homology region of the constant portion ($C_{\gamma 1}$) corresponds to the constant part of the Fd fragment and runs from about amino acid 110 to approximately 220. The second homology region ($C_{\gamma 2}$) is in the Fc fragment and extends from about 220 up to position 330 to 340, and the third homology region ($C_{\lambda 3}$) extends to the carboxy terminus.

Synthesis: Heavy and light chains are synthesized as one piece, from the amino to the carboxy terminal end, on separate polyribosomes of 300S and 200S, respectively (Buxbaum, 1973). The bulk of the assembly of light and heavy chains occurs after the chains have been released into the cisternae of the endoplasmic reticulum. In many, two heavy chains combine first to form H_2

and then light chains are added singly to produce the complete molecule. Disulfide bonds may be formed first between heavy and light chains, producing a half-molecule consisting of a single heavy and a single light chain (HL); and subsequent polymerization of the two subunits produces the final H_2L_2 structure. In other instances the HL subunit can combine with a free heavy chain to form H_2L and then add a second light chain for completion. Approximately 75% of human IgG myeloma tumors produce an excess of light chains, but not all of the patients have free light chains in the urine. Those tumors producing excess light chains have more monomers intracellularly and more dimers extracellularly, suggesting that the light chains combine after secretion from the plasma cell.

IMMUNOGLOBULIN A (IgA)

Two heavy alpha (α) chains and two light chains (both κ or both λ) form IgA, which was first described by Heremans et al. in 1959 (Tomasi, 1968) (Fig. 5). A symposium on the IgA system has recently been published (Mestecky and Lawton, 1974). There are two subgroups of the α chain, $α_1$ and $α_2$, resulting in IgA1 and IgA2 (Le and He) proteins (Feinstein and Franklin, 1966;

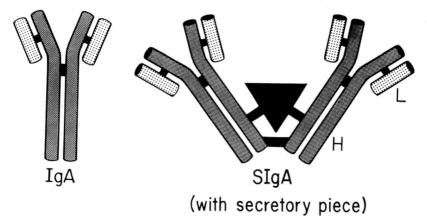

IgA   SIgA
(with secretory piece)

Figure 5. Scheme of IgA and SIgA molecules (L = light chain, H = heavy chain). (Modified from Kyle, R. A., Bieger, R. C., and Gleich, G. J.: Diagnosis of syndromes associated with hyperglobulinemia. *Med Clin North Am,* *54*:917-938, 1970. By permission of W. B. Saunders Company.)

TABLE 13

IgA SUBCLASSES

	Synonym	Frequency	Antigenicity
IgA1	Le	90-94%	"Normal"
IgA2	He	6-10%	Deficient

Kunkel and Prendergast, 1966; Vaerman and Heremans, 1966). These can be distinguished by use of appropriate antisera. Almost 95% of monoclonal IgA proteins are of the IgA1 subclass (Vaerman et al., 1968) (Table 13). In normal individuals almost 90% of plasma cells in the bone marrow stain with IgA1 fluorescent antisera and the remainder with IgA2 antisera (Skvaril and Morell, 1974). IgA2 molecules are unique among the immunoglobulins in that the light chains are bound to the a_2 chains by noncovalent forces instead of disulfide bonds (Grey et al., 1968a) (Table 14). Recently the possibility of a third IgA class was suspected (Penn et al., 1974), but further investigation showed that the myeloma protein was IgA1 with deletion of more than 100 amino acids—probably including the entire CH_3 domain (Despont et al., 1974). IgA protease, a proteolytic enzyme, hydrolyzes IgA1 to Fab and Fc fragments but has no effect on IgA2 (Plaut et al., 1974).

The IgA monomer, whose sedimentation coefficient is 7S, has a propensity to form polymers with sedimentation coefficients of 9 to 13S. These are linked covalently by disulfide bonds and *joining (J) chains*. The J chain is a nonimmunoglobulin with a molecular weight of approximately 15,000 (Koshland, 1975). It consists of 106 amino acids (Mole et al., 1975). It is bound by disulfide bridges to the Fc portion of the heavy chain and thus forms

TABLE 14

GEL ELECTROPHORESIS* OF IgA SUBCLASSES

IgA2 ⟶	Cathodic band (dimer light chain)
IgA1 ⟶	No cathodic band

* In 8 M urea-formate, pH 3.0.

the dimers or polymers of IgA and the pentamer structure of IgM (Halpern and Koshland, 1970). It is never found in IgG or monomers of IgA proteins. Only one J chain is present in each polymer of IgA or pentamer of IgM. Furthermore, the J chain of IgM and IgA is identical (Meinke, 1973). J chain probably does not join the IgM subunits together but may be necessary for the initiation of polymerization (Mestecky et al., 1974). Parkhouse (1974) postulated that the J chain mediated the formation of an oligomeric (probable dimer) form of IgM and then noncovalent forces between the oligomeric and monomeric forms of IgM produced the formation of the 19S molecule. Amino acid sequencing of J chain does not conform to any region of κ or λ chains (Mole and Bennett, 1974); yet, J chain is synthesized by the plasma cell. Kaji and Parkhouse (1975) found J chain in mouse plasma cells synthesizing IgG or only light chains, which do not require J chain; so, it may be synthesized when no apparent function exists. They did not find J chains in plasma cells not producing immunoglobulin.

Study of 13 monoclonal IgA1 myeloma proteins revealed that the major component of 6 was 9S (polymer) rather than 7S. Ultracentrifugation showed that most of the 13 patients had four different components of IgA in their serum, ranging from 7S to 13S. But despite the evidence of four different components, idiotypic antisera proved that all components contained the same monoclonal protein, and J chains were identified in the six cases with the predominant 9S component (Fine et al., 1973b). Two discrete electrophoretic spikes, one of 17S and the other 7S, were found in a case of myeloma. Both spikes consisted of IgA monoclonal protein, monomers in one and polymers in the other (Vaerman et al., 1965). Thus double peaks on the electrophoretic pattern do not always represent biclonal gammopathies.

Production of IgA begins at 4 weeks after birth and approaches the adult level at 1 year (Collins-Williams et al., 1967). No significant changes in concentration occur during adulthood. IgA is catabolized more rapidly than IgG, which accounts in part for its lower serum concentration. Differences in catabolism of the IgA subclasses are a subject of controversy. No difference was found in the catabolic rate of IgA1 and IgA2 in one study (Spiegelberg, 1974), but another disclosed that IgA2 has a slightly higher catabolic rate than IgA1 (Morell et al., 1973). IgA is synthesized in plasma cells in the lamina propria of the mucosa of various organs and may be assembled as a single heavy chain (a) and a single light chain to produce HL, which then combines with another HL to produce $H_2 L_2$ just as in the assembly of IgG (Buxbaum, 1973). The combining of two heavy chains (H_2) and addition of L chain also occurs. Polymers of IgA are usually formed just before, during, or immediately after secretion because the major intracellular IgA component is $a_2 L_2$ (Buxbaum et al., 1974). Synthesis of light chains in excess of a chains occurs just as in IgG myeloma (Buxbaum et al., 1974).

IgA, which contains antibodies to bacteria as well as to viruses, promotes phagocytosis, particularly by monocytes. Aggregated IgA of either major subclass can fix the late components of complement, beginning with C3 (alternate pathway) (Götze and Müller-Eberhard, 1971).

Secretory IgA (SIgA): A special form, termed secretory IgA (SIgA), is found in high concentration in the secretions of many glands lining the respiratory and gastrointestinal tracts, as well as in tears, colostrum, and urine. SIgA has a sedimentation coefficient of 11S and a molecular weight of 390,000. It constitutes 80% of IgA in secretions. Approximately 10% of higher polymers of IgA are dimers and trimers of the SIgA molecule, and about 10% of monomeric IgA is in secretions (Tomasi, 1972). As shown in Figure 5 *(right)*, it is composed of two IgA molecules attached by disulfide bonds and J chains to a glycoprotein (molecular weight, 60,000) called the "secretory piece" (or "S piece"). Secretory piece may be found free in mucous secretions or bound to IgA. The free and bound forms are identical on amino acid sequencing and tryptic digestion maps (Cunningham-Rundles et al., 1974).

The secretory piece protects IgA from digestion by proteolytic enzymes. Recently it has been shown that SIgA is more resistant to papain and pronase than IgA, which in turn is more resistant to digestion than IgG1 (Underdown and Dorrington, 1974).

Also, attachment of secretory piece increases the resistance against digestion by trypsin and pepsin (Lindh, 1975). Electron microscopy has revealed that SIgA contains structures resembling two Y-shaped units linked together (Bloth and Svehag, 1971).

Secretory piece is synthesized in mucosal epithelial cells. SIgA seems to be assembled in the epithelial cell from secretory piece synthesized in the same cell and IgA that enters the epithelial cell after its synthesis in and secretion from a plasma cell (Poger and Lamm, 1974). Although small amounts of IgA may be transported to saliva and to respiratory secretions, at least 95% of salivary IgA and most of the IgA in nasal fluid are synthesized at local sites.

SIgA may be found in serum of patients with intestinal diseases. It exhibits antibacterial and antiviral activity, and recent evidence indicates that SIgA antibodies are preferentially stimulated by upper-respiratory-tract infections. SIgA has a neutralizing effect on viral replication (Tomasi, 1972; DeCoteau, 1974). Also, it may inhibit adherence of streptococci to epithelial cells and could interfere with bacterial infections (Williams and Gibbons, 1972).

IMMUNOGLOBULIN M (IgM)

A third immunoglobulin, IgM, consists of subunits linked by disulfide bonds (Fig. 6) (Metzger, 1970). It constitutes 5 to 10% of the total serum immunoglobulins in the normal human. Approximately three-fourths of this immunoglobulin is intravascular because of its high molecular weight. Its catabolic rate is greater than that of IgG and IgA, and its synthetic rate is less.

The heavy chain of IgM (μ) has a molecular weight of approximately 70,000. Two heavy chains and two light chains compose a subunit, which has a molecular weight of approximately 180,000 to 190,000. Since the molecular weight of IgM is approximately 900,000, it evidently comprises five subunits. J chains identical to those associated with IgA polymers have been isolated from IgM also; these aid in initiating or maintaining the tertiary structure of the molecules. Examination of IgM with the electron microscope has shown figures resembling spiders, each with a central ring where the Fc portions join together and legs

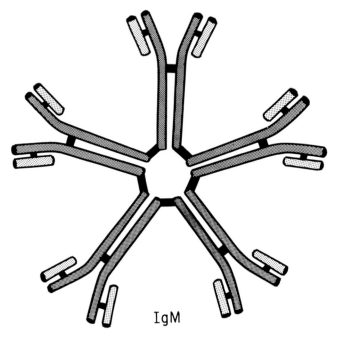

IgM

Figure 6. IgM molecule. (From Kyle, R. A., Bieger, R. C., and Gleich, G. J.: Diagnosis of syndromes associated with hyperglobulinemia. *Med Clin North Am, 54*:917-938, 1970. By permission of W. B. Saunders Company.)

consisting of the Fab fragments (Chesebro et al., 1968). The mu (μ) chain, recently sequenced, consists of one variable (V_H) and four constant ($C_{\mu1,2,3,4}$) domains. V_H and $C_{\mu1}$ are in the Fd piece, $C_{\mu2}$ in the hinge region, and $C_{\mu3}$ and $C_{\mu4}$ in the Fc fragment (Putnam et al., 1973).

IgM has a sedimentation coefficient of 19S, but more rapidly sedimenting molecules of 22S (composed of dimers of the 19S molecule) and 35S occur also. In one instance of Waldenström's macroglobulinemia, monomers (7S), dimers (11S), and pentomers (19S) of IgM were found. The heavy and light chains in each species were identical. Surprisingly, J chain was not identified in the dimer form (Parr et al., 1974). Subclasses of μ chains have been reported from three laboratories (Harboe et al., 1965; Franklin and Frangione, 1968; MacKenzie et al., 1968) (Table

TABLE 15

REACTIVITY OF IgM SUBCLASSES

Harboe Reactivity	*Franklin Reactivity*	*Fudenberg Reactivity*
8 of 21	15 of 41	22 of 40
38%	37%	55%

15), but their subclasses do not correspond and it is doubtful that specific subclasses of IgM exist. In addition, low-molecular-weight (sedimentation coefficient 8S) (McDougal et al., 1975) IgM has been found in patients with various pathologic conditions (Solomon and Kunkel, 1967; Bush et al., 1969), including lupus erythematosus, macroglobulinemia, other lymphoproliferative processes, and cirrhosis. The low-molecular-weight IgM is most likely synthesized as such and is unable to or does not polymerize and is not a breakdown product of 19S IgM.

IgM antibodies are the first produced in a primary immune response. Cold agglutinins, isoagglutinins, rheumatoid factor, and heterophile and Wasserman antibodies, as well as antibodies to various bacteria, are of the IgM class.

Rapid IgM synthesis begins in the first few days of neonatal life, and adult serum levels are attained at 1 year. IgM concentrations have been reported to decrease by the sixth decade (Buckley and Dorsey, 1970). Since the serum IgM levels in females have been reported to be one-third higher than in males, the X chromosome may contain a gene with an effect on IgM concentration (Grundbacher, 1972).

IgM is synthesized in plasma cells, as monomeric molecules. These arise from a combination of a single heavy and a single light chain to form an HL molecule. Two HL molecules combine to form H_2L_2. In the mouse myeloma system, the IgM monomer is seen intracellularly (Buxbaum and Scharff, 1973; Parkhouse, 1973); but three-fourths of samples from humans have had fully assembled 19S IgM inside the cell (Buxbaum et al., 1971).

IMMUNOGLOBULIN D (IgD)

In 1965, Rowe and Fahey found a myeloma protein containing heavy chains unlike those of the other immunoglobulins. This class, named IgD, is present in low concentrations in normal serum, is rapidly catabolized, and has a serum half-life of 2.8 days. Approximately 75% of IgD is intravascular, a distribution that may be due to irregularities in the shape of the molecule. Of patients with IgD myeloma, 80% have λ light chains, in contrast to the 30% of patients with IgG myeloma (Fahey et al., 1968). In addition, the monoclonal IgD protein peak is small and not readily seen on the serum protein electrophoretic pattern. Amino acid sequences of IgD show greater homology to IgE and IgG than to IgM, suggesting that IgD evolved relatively recently and is unlikely to be an ancestral immunoglobulin like IgM (Goyert and Spiegelberg, 1975).

Although antigen-combining activity associated with IgD has been reported, the functions of the molecule that are attributable to the heavy chain have remained obscure (Gleich et al., 1969; Devey et al., 1970). Serum concentrations of IgD may be increased rather than decreased in some patients with immunodeficiency diseases, and this may prove useful in delineating the biologic functions of IgD in the future (Buckley and Fiscus, 1975). It has been reported that IgD is frequently found on the surface of lymphocytes (van Boxel et al., 1972). Antigenic heterogeneity has been reported in IgD heavy chains and may be indicative of subclasses of IgD (Ja and La) (Rivat et al., 1971).

IMMUNOGLOBULIN E (IgE)

A fifth class of immunoglobulins, IgE, has been purified from the serum of allergic patients (Ishizaka et al., 1966), and four cases of IgE myeloma have been reported (Johansson and Bennich, 1967; Ogawa et al., 1969; Fishkin et al., 1972; Stefani et al., 1973). IgE has a molecular weight of 200,000 and a sedimentation coefficient of 8S. The combination of a short biologic half-life of 2.3 days and a very low synthesis rate results in an extremely low serum concentration in normal individuals.

IgE mediates the wheal-and-flare reaction associated with reaginic allergies and binds to basophils. IgE is fixed on normal human target cells, and histamine is released when the cell-fixed IgE reacts with the allergen. An IgE myeloma patient had a negative Prausnitz-Küstner reaction, but it was believed that the IgE-fixing sites on the target cells were saturated with IgE myeloma protein (Ogawa et al., 1971). IgE is often increased in patients with extrinsic asthma, hay fever, and parasitic infections (Johansson, 1967; Yunginger and Gleich, 1973). As expected, the serum IgE level is reduced in patients with B-cell diseases, such as chronic lymphocytic leukemia and multiple myeloma. In contrast, the IgE level was increased in patients with Hodgkin's disease, which is associated with abnormalities of cellular immunity and disorders of T-cell function (Waldmann et al., 1974).

Almost one-fourth of spontaneous ileocecal immunocytomas in inbred LOU/Wsl rats produced a monoclonal rat IgE protein. No IgE-producing tumors had been reported previously in animals (Bazin et al., 1974).

GENETIC BASIS OF IMMUNOLOGIC FUNCTION

Three separate gene regions control the C portions of the immunoglobulin polypeptides—one each for κ and λ and one for the heavy chains. There are also three separate gene pools for the V regions—one for κ, one for λ, and one for all classes of heavy chains. There may be few or many genes in each gene pool, in accord with the germ-line or somatic-mutation hypotheses (Hood and Talmage, 1970). Formation of a single polypeptide chain requires expression of two genes—one for the V region and one for the C region of each chain.

How humans attain antibody diversity is a matter of controversy. The germ-line hypothesis states that all genetic information necessary for the various antibodies is present in each germ-line cell. Information for the synthesis of 1,000 different V_L and 1,000 different V_H chains could produce 1,000,000 different antibodies. Recent studies on the incidence of constant genes in mouse myeloma systems have made this hypothesis unlikely.

According to the other major hypothesis, somatic-mutation, only a few variable (V) genes exist and point mutations account for antibody diversity. These point mutations in the hypervariable region of the V_H and V_L portions then produce an antibody with different specificity. Rapid replication and death of antibody-forming cells could help to account for antibody diversity. The somatic-mutation hypothesis is supported by a large number of stable variants with altered capacity to produce either heavy or light chains in cultured mouse myeloma cells (Baumal et al., 1973)—an observation suggesting that antibody diversity is generated somatically.

Antibody diversity may be enhanced by the existence of multiple-binding or polyfunctional antibody-combining regions. Thus a smaller number of V-region genes need be inherited in order to produce functional antibody diversity (Richards et al., 1975).

CHAPTER III

Relation of Myeloma Proteins and Macroglobulins to Normal Immunoglobulins

ALTHOUGH MYELOMA PROTEINS and macroglobulins have long been considered abnormal, studies during the past several years strongly suggest that they are only normal immunoglobulins in excessive quantities. The striking feature of myeloma proteins and macroglobulins that led investigators to consider them as abnormal is their homogeneity. Whereas normal IgG in human serum is electrophoretically heterogeneous, with mobility ranging from alpha-2 to the slow gamma, IgG myeloma proteins are localized sharply in their electrophoretic mobility.

Kunkel (1965, 1968) showed that each light-chain type and heavy-chain subclass in myeloma proteins has its counterpart among normal immunoglobulins and also among antibodies. After the discovery of the two types of light chains (κ and λ) in myeloma proteins in a ratio of approximately 2:1, these same light-chain types were detected—in essentially the same ratio—among normal immunoglobulins. Similarly, the IgG and IgA subclasses and IgD class were discovered among myeloma proteins and then found as normal serum components. These identifications have gradually weakened the belief that the myeloma proteins and macroglobulins are abnormal and have suggested that they result from overproduction of a normal product by an abnormally functioning cell. Many of the heavy chains found in the heavy-chain diseases show significant deletions of amino acids; thus they are "abnormal" immunoglobulins (Frangione and Franklin, 1973).

Even the antigenic determinants (also termed "individual antigenic specificities" or "idiotypic specificities") (Hopper and Nisonoff, 1971; Natvig and Kunkel, 1973) thought to be associated
uniquely with myeloma proteins have been shown to occur
among antibodies. On the other hand, studies of highly purified
antibodies have revealed a homogeneity approaching that seen in
myeloma proteins. In some instances, after primary immunization with a carbohydrate antigen, group-specific precipitins are
the predominant component of gamma globulin. They are electrophoretically monodispersed, possess individual antigenic specificity, and have a single light-chain type and a single IgG heavy-
chain subclass (Braun et al., 1969; Krause, 1970).

The possibility expressed by Kunkel that myeloma proteins are
individual antibodies and are products of the individual plasma
cells arising from a single clone of malignant cells has been supported by their antigen-combining activity (Eisen et al., 1967;
Potter, 1971). To distinguish between specific antigen-antibody
reactions and nonspecific association of the suspected antigen
and the antibody is difficult. One must first demonstrate that the
antibody activity exists in the isolated monoclonal protein—and
that the antibody is indeed monoclonal (by demonstrating that
the heavy chains are of a single class and that the light chains are
of a single class). Further, one must prove that the antibody activity resides in the Fab fragment of the monoclonal protein and
that no antibody activity or binding is found in its Fc fragment.
In addition, the combining ratio of antigen to antibody should
be similar to conventional antigen-antibody reactions.

In humans, monoclonal antibody activity has been reported in
cold agglutinin disease as well as in a wide variety of bacterial
antigens, including streptolysin O, staphylococcal protein, kleb-
siella polysaccharides, and brucella (Seligmann and Brouet,
1973). The IgA κ monoclonal protein of a patient with myeloma
had antistreptococcal hyaluronidase activity of 5,200,000 U. Its
antibody activity was confined to the Fab portion of the α chain
(Videbaek et al., 1973).

In another case, a monoclonal IgG1 κ protein combined with
transferrin (one molecule with two) and produced a high serum

iron level. All of the transferrin in the patient was bound to the monoclonal protein, which also reacted with transferrin of normal individuals (Wernet et al., 1972). Lindgärde and Zettervall (1974) reported an IgG1 λ monoclonal protein that bound calcium ions at two independent binding sites in the Fab region. Although the light chains were active, isolated heavy chains showed no significant binding activity. The serum concentration of total calcium in this case was persistently high, but the serum level of ionized calcium was normal. Mullinax et al. (1970) reported that a monoclonal IgA protein agglutinated sheep red cells in high titers, and that this agglutination was inhibited by choline chloride, suggesting specific binding of the antibody with choline. Myeloma proteins with phosphoryl choline antibody activity have been found in BALB/c mice (Potter, 1971). Complexes of IgM monoclonal protein and human albumin (Ropars et al., 1972) have been reported, but in the case described, the abnormality was not attributable to an antigen-antibody reaction (Ropars et al., 1973). Recently a monoclonal IgM λ protein has demonstrated antibody-like activity against aggregated albumin (Hauptman and Tomasi, 1974). Binding of the monoclonal IgM protein and albumin was noncovalent and occurred only with the Fab fragment, not with Fc. A human IgG κ monoclonal protein that precipitated horse, rabbit, and pig alpha-2 macroglobulin has been reported. Its binding activity was located in the Fab portion (Seligmann et al., 1973). A patient with an IgM monoclonal protein, high VDRL titer (1:4,096), and negative FTA reacted to cardiolipin and lecithin, suggesting antibody activity (Cooper et al., 1974). Association of a high VDRL titer and negative response to the treponema pallidum immobilization (TPI) test with a monoclonal IgM κ protein has been noted (Drusin et al., 1974), and likewise association of high lactic dehydrogenase isoenzyme activities with monoclonal proteins (Markel and Janich, 1974), and complexes of lysozyme and monoclonal protein (Finkle et al., 1973)—but in the latter instance the protein had both kappa and lambda activity, thus not fulfilling the criteria for a monoclonal protein.

Transient monoclonal proteins have been seen, frequently in

young children with immunodeficiency. These proteins are modest in amount (usually < 1.0 g/dl) and disappear within 2 months. Cytomegalovirus infections may produce transient monoclonal proteins (Danon and Seligmann, 1972; Vodopick et al., 1974). Thus it seems likely that the homogeneity of myeloma proteins and macroglobulins reflects the homogeneity associated with highly purified antibodies, namely that resulting from their production by a single clone of immunoglobulin-synthesizing cells. It is almost certain that more monoclonal human proteins will be found to have antibody activity. Indeed, it has been postulated that all myeloma proteins may have it (Osterland and Espinoza, 1975).

In this view, as illustrated in Figure 7, the heterogeneous normal collection of IgG molecules comprises minute amounts of highly homogeneous proteins from many diverse single clones of plasma cells (and so is polyclonal). If a single clone escapes the normal controls over its multiplication, it reproduces excessively and synthesizes an excess of antibody-like protein of a single heavy-chain class and subclass and single light-chain type (monoclonal). This is neoplastic or potentially so.

Support for the one-cell, one-immunoglobulin concept comes from studies of the cellular localization of these proteins. Experiments performed with antisera to light chains have shown that nearly all individual plasma cells in the red pulp of the spleen in adults contained *either* κ or λ light chains but not both (Pernis and Chiappino, 1964). And most investigators believe that a single antibody-producing cell contains or secretes an immunoglobulin of only one class and subclass (Mäkelä and Cross, 1970). But although most antibody-forming cells release antibody of only one class, a small proportion of them produce two immunoglobulin classes at once (Cunningham, 1973). This is seen in 1.5% of antibody-producing cells and is most likely to occur when a switch from IgM to IgG production occurs (Nossal et al., 1971).

Patterns of Overproduction: Normally, plasma cells produce heavy chains and a slight excess of light chains that spill over into the urine. In IgG myeloma, about three-fourths of patients

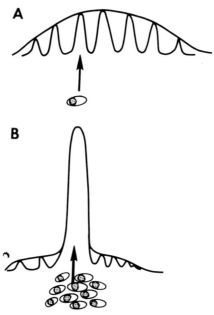

Figure 7. Polyclonal and monoclonal electrophoretic patterns. *A,* Broad outline comprehending small peaks of many different homogeneous proteins (one is represented in normal amount, related by *arrow* to its peak) that have been produced by many different plasma cell clones (polyclonal). *B,* Tall, narrow peak of homogeneous protein (single heavy-chain and single light-chain type) which is excessive output of single clone (monoclonal). (From Kyle, R. A., and Gleich, G. J.: Syndromes associated with hyperglobulinemia. In *Tice's Practice of Medicine.* Vol. 1. Hagerstown, Maryland, Harper & Row, Publishers, 1972, pp. 1-37. By permission.)

have an excess of light chains that may be excreted into the urine as Bence Jones proteinuria or catabolized (Buxbaum, 1973). This small excess of light-chain production could be due to imbalance in translation or transcription within occasional clones or a possible suppression of heavy-chain synthesis in such clones (Bevan et al., 1972). In other instances, no heavy chain is produced by the plasma cell and only excessive quantities of light chains are detected ("light-chain disease") (Williams et al., 1966; Stone and Frenkel, 1975). Finally, a small proportion of myeloma cells do not secrete either heavy or light chains to excess, whether because of a simple failure or some blocking of production ("nonsecretory") (see page 151).

Apart from these patterns, monoclonal proteins with deletions in both the heavy and light chains have been reported (Isobe and Osserman, 1974b). IgG half-molecules consisting of a single heavy chain and a single light chain have been reported. Only one of the five patients had classic multiple myeloma, whereas three had extramedullary plasmacytomas and one plasma cell leukemia (Spiegelberg et al., 1975). In the last-mentioned case a significant deletion of the heavy chain was noted. In amyloidosis, the abnormal tissue deposits seem to be composed of the variable portions of the light chains (see page 233). In cases of so-called heavy-chain diseases, portions of the heavy chains of IgG, IgA, or IgM corresponding to the Fc fragment may be present in serum or urine (see page 223).

CHAPTER IV

Laboratory Methods for Study of Monoclonal Proteins

A NALYSIS OF THE SERUM or urine for monoclonal proteins requires a sensitive, rapid, dependable screening method to detect them and a specific assay to identify them according to their
heavy-chain classes and light-chain types. Electrophoresis on cellulose acetate is commonly used for detection and is superior to
tests on paper (Kohn, 1957); immunoelectrophoresis should be
used to confirm the presence of a monoclonal protein and to distinguish the immunoglobulin class and the light-chain type it represents.

ANALYSIS OF SERUM

Electrophoresis for Detection: When examined by electrophoresis, a monoclonal protein usually appears in the gamma,
beta, or alpha-2 regions—as a narrow peak like a church spire in
the densitometer tracing (Fig. 8) or as a dense, discrete band on
cellulose acetate membrane (Fig. 9). In contrast, a polyclonal increase of immunoglobulins has a broad base but usually is limited to the gamma region (Figs. 10 and 11). Whereas a polyclonal
peak or band consists of increased immunoglobulins of one or
more heavy-chain types with both kappa and lambda light-chain
classes, a monoclonal protein contains a single light-chain type and
a single heavy-chain class and subclass. An occasional serum contains two monoclonal proteins of different immunoglobulin
classes (biclonal) (see page 154).

A tall, narrow, homogeneous peak or discrete band is most suggestive of myeloma, Waldenström's macroglobulinemia, or benign
monoclonal gammopathy; but such monoclonal peaks and bands
may occur also in amyloidosis and in lymphoma. Appreciation of

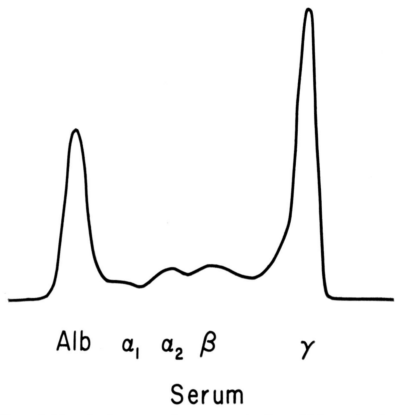

Alb α_1 α_2 β γ

Serum

Figure 8. Monoclonal pattern of serum protein (in multiple myeloma) as traced by densitometer after electrophoresis on paper: tall, narrow-based peak of gamma mobility. (From Kyle, R. A., Bieger, R. C., and Gleich, G. J.: Diagnosis of syndromes associated with hyperglobulinemia. *Med Clin North Am, 54*:917-938, 1970. By permission of W. B. Saunders Company.)

Figure 9. Monoclonal pattern from electrophoresis of serum on cellulose acetate (anode on left): dense band at right.

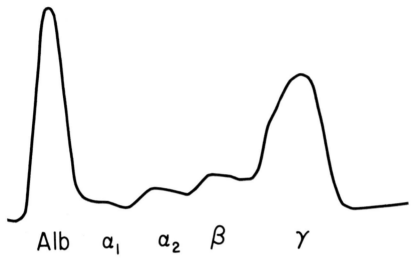

Alb α_1 α_2 β γ

Figure 10. Polyclonal pattern from densitometer tracing after paper electrophoresis: broad-based peak of gamma mobility. (From Kyle, R. A., Bieger, R. C., and Gleich, G. J.: Diagnosis of syndromes associated with hyperglobulinemia. *Med Clin North Am, 54*:917-938, 1970. By permission of W. B. Saunders Company.)

Figure 11. Polyclonal pattern from electrophoresis of serum on cellulose acetate (anode on left): band at right is broad, and advancing and trailing edges both are diffuse.

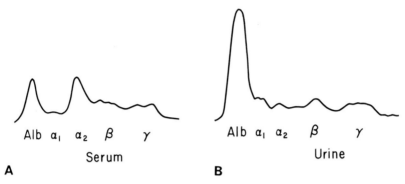

Figure 12. Nephrotic syndrome. *A,* Serum electrophoretic pattern: note decreased albumin and gamma globulin and increased alpha-2 globulin components. *B,* Urinary electrophoretic pattern: most of protein is albumin. (From Kyle, R. A., Bieger, R. C., and Gleich, G. J.: Diagnosis of syndromes associated with hyperglobulinemia. *Med Clin North Am, 54*:917-938, 1970. By permission of W. B. Saunders Company.)

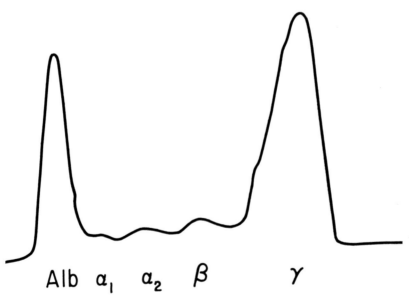

Figure 13. Serum electrophoretic pattern of chronic active hepatitis. (From Kyle, R. A., Bieger, R. C., and Gleich, G. J.: Diagnosis of syndromes associated with hyperglobulinemia. *Med Clin North Am, 54*:917-938, 1970. By permission of W. B. Saunders Company.)

the electrophoretic patterns of certain other conditions is useful. The nephrotic syndrome is distinguished by a distinctive serum pattern featuring low albumin and gamma globulin and an increased amount of alpha-2 globulin. Indeed, the increased alpha-2 globulin often looks like a monoclonal peak or band of rapid mobility and might be mistaken for a myeloma protein. The urinary protein consists mainly of albumin (Fig. 12). Similarly, an increased concentration of transferrin or haptoglobin may be mistaken for a monoclonal peak (Zawadzki and Edwards, 1970b; McPhedran et al., 1972a). Chronic infection, connective-tissue diseases, and chronic liver diseases are characterized by large, broad-based polyclonal patterns on paper (Figs. 10 and 13) or by wide bands with diffuse borders on the cellulose acetate strip (Fig. 11). Occasionally a monoclonal protein also appears as a broad band on cellulose acetate and is mistaken for a polyclonal increase in immunoglobulins. Presumably it is due to the presence of aggregates or polymers, which require immunoelectrophoresis for identification.

Although myeloma, macroglobulinemia, and benign monoclonal gammopathy are associated with monoclonal peaks on filter paper or bands on cellulose acetate, these may be small—particularly in benign monoclonal gammopathy, amyloidosis, and heavy-chain diseases—and thus not readily detected by electrophoresis. It must be emphasized that the patient can have a monoclonal protein when the total protein concentration and the concentration of protein in the globulin compartment are within normal limits (Fig. 14). Even a normal value for quantitative immunoglobulins does not exclude the possibility of a small amount of monoclonal protein; and this is particularly true of IgG.

Cellulose Acetate Versus Filter Paper: The advantages of the cellulose acetate membrane for electrophoresis include lessened absorption of serum on the supporting medium, so there is less "tailing" and a sharper separation of protein bands. On this membrane alpha-1 globulin is well separated from albumin, whereas in filter paper patterns alpha-1 globulin frequently is found in the trailing edge of the albumin peak. In addition, separation oc-

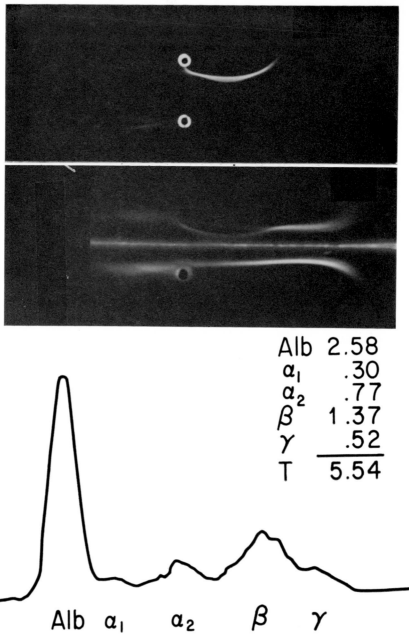

Alb	2.58
α_1	.30
α_2	.77
β	1.37
γ	.52
T	5.54

Alb α_1 α_2 β γ

Figure 14. Myeloma and amyloidosis. *Upper,* Immunoelectrophoretic response to IgD antiserum is sharp arc from patient's serum (upper well) and absence of arc from normal serum (lower well). *Middle,* Immunoelectrophoretic responses to lambda-chain antiserum by same patient's serum (upper well) and by normal serum (lower well), confirming presence of an IgD λ monoclonal protein in patient. *Lower,* Electrophoretic pattern on paper of serum from same patient, showing only modest increase in beta area. (From Kyle, R. A., Bieger, R. C., and Gleich, G. J.: Diagnosis of syndromes associated with hyperglobulinemia. *Med Clin North Am, 54:*917-938, 1970. By permission of W. B. Saunders Company.)

curs in less than half an hour with the microzone apparatus as contrasted to 15 hours with filter paper. With use of cellulose acetate membranes, very small quantities of serum ($< 1 \mu$l) can be used. The stained cellulose acetate strips can be scanned and the components measured in an automated system (Gelman Instrument Company, Ann Arbor, MI). We have compared the results from electrophoretic analysis of 134 sera on filter paper and on cellulose. Significant, detectable differences appeared in more than a third of the cases, proving the superiority of cellulose acetate membranes.

As would be expected, cellulose acetate electrophoresis facilitates the detection of biclonal gammopathies as well as small monoclonal proteins. If the patient's blood does not clot sufficiently, or if plasma rather than serum is sent to the laboratory, fibrinogen remains in the specimen and appears as a discrete band between beta and gamma in the electrophoretic pattern. The presence of fibrinogen may be confirmed by the addition of bovine thrombin or use of immunodiffusion with fibrinogen antisera.

Immunoelectrophoresis for Identification: Immunoelectrophoresis is used to identify the heavy-chain class and light-chain type of the monoclonal protein (Grabar and Williams, 1953). It should be performed in all cases where a sharp peak is found in the cellulose acetate tracing or where myeloma, macroglobulinemia, or a related disorder is suspected; it is particularly helpful in determining whether a solitary plasmacytoma is localized or not.

In this method the serum is placed in a well on a microscope slide covered with 1% agar or agarose and subjected to electrophoresis for a sufficient time (about 1½ hours) to separate the various serum proteins. The slide is then removed from the electrophoretic apparatus. A trough is cut in the agar parallel to the line at migration of components, and the trough is filled with antiserum. Proteins from the electrophoresed sample (antigen) and from the antisera (antibody) are then allowed to diffuse toward each other and to form precipitin lines or arcs at the area of contact between the antigen and the antibody. Most precipitin lines

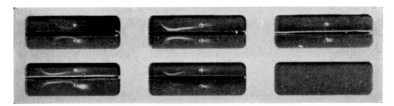

Figure 15. Immunoelectrophoretic patterns in myeloma. Trough of each slide contains monospecific antiserum: upper row—antiserum to IgG in first, to IgA in second, to IgM in third; lower row—antiserum to kappa in first and to lambda in second (no slide in third position). Serum from first patient, placed in upper well of each slide, has produced thickening and bowing of IgG and lambda arcs, indicating presence of IgG λ monoclonal component. Serum from second patient, placed in lower well of each slide, has produced thickening of IgA arc and bowing of kappa arc, indicating IgA κ monoclonal component.

form within 24 hours (Fig. 14); and if one allows the diffusion to continue for more than 24 hours, the arcs become diffuse and interpretation may be very difficult.

Potent antisera to whole human serum produce almost 30 precipitin arcs and create difficulty in interpretation. We therefore use and recommend monospecific antisera to IgG, IgA, IgM, IgD, and IgE and to kappa and lambda light chains. In multiple myeloma, antisera to IgG, IgA, IgD, or IgE produce a deflection of the precipitin arc over a narrow range of mobility (Figs. 15, 16, 17, and 18). In Waldenström's macroglobulinemia, IgM antiserum produces a similarly localized arc (Fig. 19). Additionally, in both situations, one must see a similar deflection from thickening and bowing of the arc by antisera to either kappa or lambda light chains, but not both. This corresponding thickening and bowing of the heavy- and light-chain arcs indicates the presence of a monoclonal protein. As IgG has a wide range of electrophoretic mobility, extending from the slow gamma through the alpha-2 globulin region, the bowing of the IgG precipitin arc may occur anywhere within that range.

The serum protein electrophoretic peak may be relatively broad-based, suggesting a polyclonal increase of immunoglobulins, as in Figure 20 *upper*. Immunoelectrophoresis with mono-

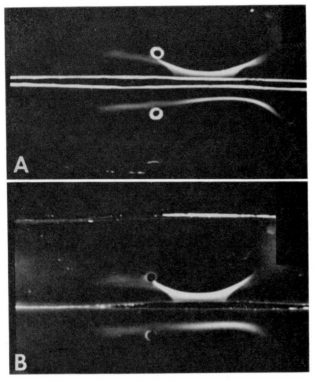

Figure 16. Immunoelectrophoretic patterns in myeloma. *A,* With antiserum to IgG, showing markedly thickened arc from patient's serum in upper well; for comparison, normal arc from normal serum in lower well. *B,* With antiserum to kappa chains, showing thickened arc (top) ; for comparison, normal arc from normal serum (in lower well), indicating monoclonal protein from patient's serum is IgG κ. (From Kyle, R. A., Bieger, R. C., and Gleich, G. J.: Diagnosis of syndromes associated with hyperglobulinemia. *Med Clin North Am, 54*:917-938, 1970. By permission of W. B. Saunders Company.)

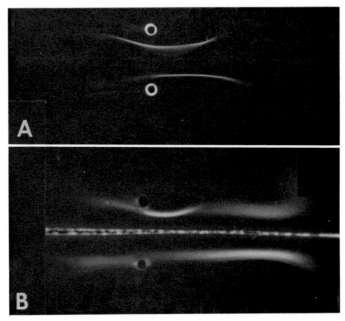

Figure 17. Immunoelectrophoretic patterns in myeloma. *A,* With antiserum
to IgA, showing thickened arc from patient's serum in upper well, compared
with normal arc from normal serum in lower well. *B,* Results from testing
same sera with antiserum to kappa chains. These studies indicate a monoclonal protein of IgA κ type. (From Kyle, R. A., Bieger, R. C., and Gleich,
G. J.: Diagnosis of syndromes associated with hyperglobulinemia. *Med Clin
North Am, 54*:917-938, 1970. By permission of W. B. Saunders Company.)

specific antisera in the illustrated case revealed impressive thickening and bowing of the arc with IgA antisera and a similar
thickening and bowing with kappa antisera, indicating the presence of a monoclonal IgA κ protein (Fig. 20 *middle* and *lower*).
The tendency of IgA monoclonal protein to produce polymers
may be the reason for the broadness of the electrophoretic peak.

Thickening of the IgG arc occurs in many cases with a polyclonal increase of immunoglobulins (Fig. 21). One must find a
localized increase of one—and only one—light-chain arc before
accepting the presence of a monoclonal protein. It must be emphasized again that the densitometer tracing of the monoclonal

band may be very small, or the monoclonal protein may be buried in the normal beta or gamma band and not discovered, until immunoelectrophoresis is done. IgD myeloma classically produces only a small peak or band, as do the monoclonal proteins in the heavy-chain diseases. Therefore immunoelectrophoresis is an essential test when these diseases are suspected. A densitometer tracing of a serum electrophoretic pattern, the band on a cellulose acetate strip, and a localized arc resulting from immunoelectrophoresis of a monoclonal protein are shown in Figure 22.

We find it economical to screen the sera of all our patients with Ouchterlony immunodiffusion, using antisera to IgD and

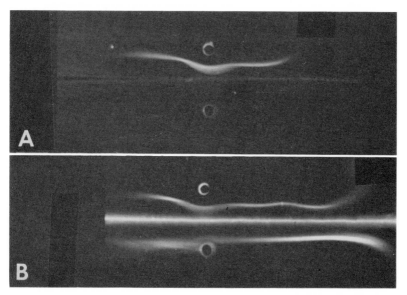

Figure 18. Myeloma and plasma-cell leukemia. *A,* Immunoelectrophoresis with antiserum to IgE: markedly thickened arc from patient's serum in upper well and absence of arc from normal serum in lower well. (IgE serum was a gift of Dr. O. R. McIntyre, Hanover, NH.) *B,* Immunoelectrophoresis with antiserum to lambda chains: same patient's serum in upper well and normal serum in lower well. Results indicate IgE λ monoclonal protein. (From Kyle, R. A., Bieger, R. C., and Gleich, G. J.: Diagnosis of syndromes associated with hyperglobulinemia. *Med Clin North Am, 54*:917-938, 1970. By permission of W. B. Saunders Company.)

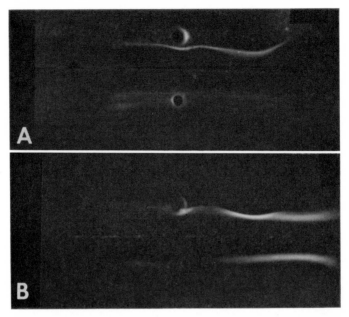

Figure 19. Macroglobulinemia. *A,* Immunoelectrophoresis with antiserum to IgM: thickened arc from patient's serum in upper well and very faint arc from normal serum in lower well. *B,* Immunoelectrophoresis with antiserum to kappa chains: response of patient's serum in upper well confirms presence of IgM κ protein. (From Kyle, R. A., Bieger, R. C., and Gleich, G. J.: Diagnosis of syndromes associated with hyperglobulinemia. *Med Clin North Am, 54:*917-938, 1970. By permission of W. B. Saunders Company.)

IgE against each patient's serum. The central well is filled with a specific IgD or IgE antiserum and each surrounding well is filled with the undiluted serum of the patients. Dense precipitin bands form if the patient has an increased concentration of IgD or IgE protein (Fig. 23). The sera showing a precipitin band are then studied further by immunoelectrophoresis with monospecific antisera to IgD or IgE and to kappa and lambda light chains. The majority of sera produce no reaction on immunodiffusion, and immunoelectrophoresis of them is not necessary. Since four to six sera can be tested with 7 or 8 μl of IgD or IgE antisera by immunodiffusion, whereas 60 μl of antisera are needed to perform immunoelectrophoresis on two sera, prior screen-

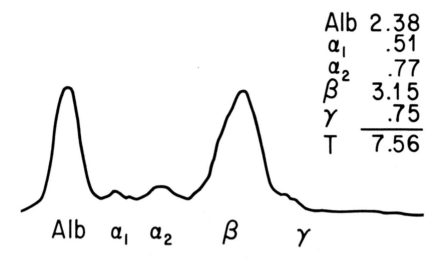

Alb	2.38
α_1	.51
α_2	.77
β	3.15
γ	.75
T	7.56

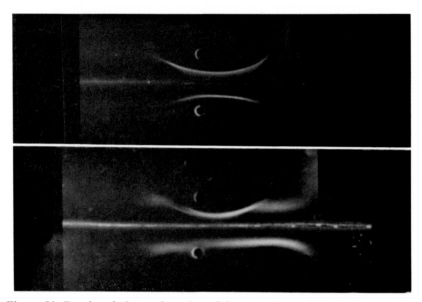

Figure 20. Results of electrophoresis and immunoelectrophoresis of serum of patient with multiple myeloma. *Upper,* Serum electrophoretic pattern on paper with rather broad beta peak appearing polyclonal but consisting of monoclonal IgA κ protein. *Middle,* Result of immunoelectrophoresis of patient's serum (top well) and normal serum (bottom well) with IgA antiserum in center trough; note patient's thickened IgA arc. *Lower,* Result of immunoelectrophoresis, showing reaction to kappa-chain antiserum: prominent arc from patient's serum (upper well) and elongated arc without localized thickening from normal serum (lower well). These results confirm presence of monoclonal IgA κ protein. (From Kyle, R. A., Bieger, R. C., and Gleich, G. J.: Diagnosis of syndromes associated with hyperglobulinemia. *Med Clin North Am, 54*:917-938, 1970. By permission of W. B. Saunders Company.)

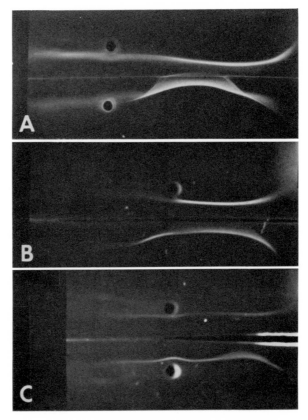

Figure 21. *A,* Immunoelectrophoresis with antiserum to IgG: polyclonal arc (dense but without localized thickening) from serum in top well, thickened precipitin arc from monoclonal IgG protein in lower well. *B,* Immunoelectrophoresis with antiserum to IgA: polyclonal arc from top well and monoclonal arc from lower well. Note asymmetry of the lower arc. *C,* Immunoelectrophoresis with antiserum to IgM (same case as in Figure 19): long, thin arc (polyclonal) from upper well and localized thickened (monoclonal) arc from lower well. Note precipitate around lower well. This precipitate is often seen with euglobulins. (From Kyle, R. A., Bieger, R. C., and Gleich, G. J.: Diagnosis of syndromes associated with hyperglobulinemia. *Med Clin North Am, 54:*917-938, 1970. By permission of W. B. Saunders Company.)

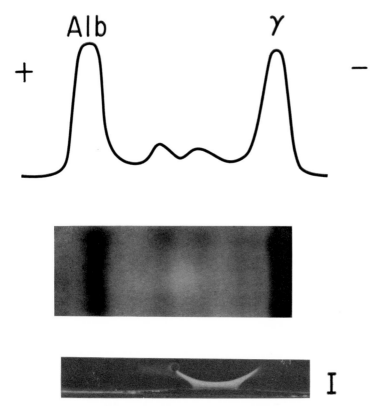

Figure 22. Corresponding determinations of monoclonal serum protein. *Upper,* Densitometer tracing of electrophoretic separation on cellulose acetate membrane. *Middle,* Band separated electrophoretically on cellulose acetate. *Lower,* Localized arc from immunoelectrophoresis.

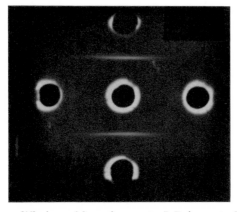

Figure 23. Immunodiffusion with antiserum to IgD in central well and serum of two patients with IgD myeloma in upper and lower wells. Dense precipitin bands indicate presence of IgD protein. Immunoelectrophoresis with IgD, kappa, and lambda antisera must then be done to demonstrate monoclonal IgD protein (see Fig. 14). (From Kyle, R. A., Bieger, R. C., and Gleich, G. J.: Diagnosis of syndromes associated with hyperglobulinemia. *Med Clin North Am,* 54:917-938, 1970. By permission of W. B. Saunders Company.)

ing by immunodiffusion saves a significant amount of antiserum when many specimens are studied.

Further Tests for Special Characteristics: Quantitation of immunoglobulins aids also in the assessment of gammopathies. Usually this is performed by *radial immunodiffusion* (Fahey and McKelvey, 1965; Mancini et al., 1965). With this method, antiserum to the specific immunoglobulin (IgG, IgA, IgM, or IgD) is mixed with agar and layered on a plate or microscopic slide. Known concentrations of the specific immunoglobulin and the unknown serum are placed in wells. The size of the precipitin zones that develop about the wells is proportional to the amount of antigen in the test serum, so the precipitin zone surrounding each well is measured and compared with the known standards. In some cases of macroglobulinemia, the precipitin zone may be very faint and remain unrecognized until the serum is diluted. Low-molecular-weight IgM produces a spuriously elevated IgM value because its rate of diffusion is greater than that of the 19S IgM molecule in the standard. We quantitate the level of immunoglobulins in our laboratory with an automated immunoprecipitin system (Markowitz and Tschida, 1972). In this technique the patient's serum is mixed with a monospecific antiserum; the density of the precipitant, which represents an antigen-antibody reaction, reflects the concentration of immunoglobulin in the specimen. For study of large numbers of sera, this method is more rapid and accurate than and preferable to the immunodiffusion method. Another advantage is accuracy in determining concentrations of 7S (low-molecular-weight) IgM, for which radial immunodiffusion gives spuriously elevated values.

We have seen patients whose sera produced a dense, localized band on cellulose acetate electrophoresis but on immunoelectrophoresis showed only a dense IgM arc without an accompanying similar change in the light-chain arc. The inability to identify a light-chain component suggested the possibility of heavy-chain (μ) disease. However, the IgM was isolated from the sera by *gel filtration* on Sephadex G200 and then the purified monoclonal proteins were readily typed as having a kappa or lambda component, thus excluding the possibility of μ-chain disease. Treatment of the serum with a *reducing* agent, dithiothreitol, for 2 to 5 minutes at room temperature also yielded preparations that could be identified readily as IgM κ or IgM λ monoclonal proteins in most instances. Another way to identify the light-chain type in such situations is to quantitate the light chain by radial immunodiffusion with and without *2-mercaptoethanol (2ME) impregnated agar*. Those sera with an increase in kappa or lambda after incubation with 2ME were considered to have a monoclonal IgM protein of that type (Stein et al., 1973). But this test is not easy to perform as a daily routine; and also, polyclonal increases of IgM can cause confusion.

We believe *serum viscometry* is required in every case with an IgM monoclonal protein or large amounts of IgA or IgG protein, and in any other case with oronasal bleeding, blurred vision, and neurologic symptoms suggestive of a hyperviscosity syndrome (see page 219). The Ostwald-100 viscometer is a satisfactory instrument for this purpose. Distilled water and serum, separately, are made to flow through a capillary tube; and the quotient of the flow durations (serum/water) is the viscosity value. The normal value is 1.8 or less, but symptoms of hyperviscosity are rare unless the value is greater than 4. In fact, some patients with a value of 10 or more do not have symptoms of hyperviscosity. The Wells-Brookfield viscometer (Brookfield Engineering Laboratories, Inc., Stoughton, MA) is preferred, because it is more accurate and requires less serum (about 1.0 ml). In addition, determinations can be made much more rapidly than with the Ostwald viscometer, especially if the viscosity of the serum sample is high. In a series of 100 samples from normal blood bank donors, we found that 95% had a value of 1.8 centipoises or less when determined at a shear rate of 23 sec^{-1} (or 6 rpm). This instrument allows one to determine the viscosity at different shear rates.

The *Sia test* for euglobulins is performed by adding a drop of serum to a tube of distilled water. A positive result is the formation of a precipitate or flocculant as the serum is diluted by the water. This test has been recommended for the diagnosis of macroglobulinemia, but many false positive and false negative reactions are seen. In a study, the Sia test did not distinguish IgM monoclonal proteins from IgG or IgA monoclonal proteins, nor did it separate monoclonal sera as a group from polyclonal sera at the 5% level (Ritzmann et al., 1969). The Sia test is now largely of historic interest and we do not recommend it.

For *measurement of cryoglobulins,* one centrifuges fresh serum in a Wintrobe hematocrit tube at 37°C, incubates the serum at 0°C (in an ice bath in a cold room) for 24 hours, centrifuges the tube and contents at 0°C, and then reads the cryocrit. If the precipitate is due to a cryoglobulin, warming to 37°C will dissolve it (Wintrobe and Buell, 1933; Lerner and Watson, 1947). In some instances the precipitate is very dense after centrifugation and will not dissolve when warmed unless one dilutes the precipitate. Therefore, when we see a precipitate after incubating for 24 hours in the cold, we warm it to 37°C; if it dissolves, we incubate the serum in the cold for another 24 hours and then centrifuge it to obtain the cryocrit. It should be pointed out that cryoglobulins, particularly of the mixed type, may require up to a week to precipitate.

Most often the *detection of pyroglobulins* (see page 218) occurs when serum is inactivated by heating for the VDRL test. At 56°C, these proteins precipitate irreversibly. Since Bence Jones protein precipitates at 40 to 60°C, Bence Jones proteinemia should not be confused with pyroglobulinemia. Bence Jones protein redissolves with boiling and reprecipitates with cooling, in contrast to the irreversible precipitation of pyroglobulins. Also, the two can be distinguished by immunoelectrophoresis with appropriate antisera.

ANALYSIS OF URINE

In studying patients who have gammopathies, analysis of urine is essential. Sulfosalicylic acid (Exton's test) is best for the detection of *protein.* The Albustix® test often does not detect Bence Jones protein and should not be used as a routine screening test for Bence Jones proteinuria. When the reliability of sulfosalicylic acid and Albustix was compared in 18 cases of myeloma with urinary electrophoretic patterns typical of Bence Jones protein, the Albustix test was negative in 11 instances. In the remaining seven the positive Albustix result seemed due to the presence of albumin. All 18 urines were positive with sulfosalicylic acid (Fine and Rees, 1974).

A simple heat test for detection of *Bence Jones protein* consists of mixing 4 ml of centrifuged urine with 1 ml of 2M acetate buffer (pH 4.9) and heating at 56°C in an incubation bath for 15 minutes. Formation of a precipitate that disappears after 3 minutes in a 100°C bath but reappears with cooling indicates the presence of Bence Jones protein (Putnam et al., 1959). When the test is performed in this manner at least 145 mg/dl of protein is necessary to obtain a positive result (Lindström et al., 1968). Occasionally, the result of a heat test is positive even though the patient has no evidence of myeloma or macroglobulinemia and his urine shows no sharp peak in the electrophoretic pattern or evidence of a monoclonal light chain on immunoelectrophoresis. Such false positive results occur in cases of connective-tissue disease, renal sufficiency, or malignancy (Perry and Kyle, 1975). Conversely, in some cases of myeloma, urine containing large amounts of monoclonal light chains has given negative results on the heat test. Study of these proteins revealed the presence of light-chain dimers but no evidence of inhibiting substances. There was no remarkable difference in the isoelectric points of Bence Jones proteins giving negative and positive responses to heat tests. Composition studies revealed similar numbers of amino acid residues and the absence of carbohydrate in both types. It is most likely that a change in the amino acid sequence in the variable region of the light chain accounts for the atypical heat-test result (M. C. Perry, personal communication).

Not all precipitates that form with heating of urine are Bence Jones protein. In one case a precipitate formed after heating of urine for 15 minutes, suggesting the possibility of Bence Jones proteinuria. The urine electrophoretic pattern showed a sharp band of alpha-2 mobility. This paraprotein band was reddish brown when stained with toluidine and was subsequently identified as hemoglobin. Hemoglobin is insoluble at 57°C at a pH of

5.2. Therefore, one must remember that hemoglobinuria can appear as a paraprotein band on electrophoresis and seem to give a positive response to the heat test (Payne, 1972).

In determining the *type of light chain* in the urine, one may use an aliquot from a 24-hour unconcentrated specimen if the concentration of light chains is great enough. Usually the urine must be concentrated 50 to 100 times, for which we prefer ultra-filtration with a Minicon-B15 Concentrator (Amicon Corp., Lexington, MA). If the light-chain amounts are smaller, the urine should be concentrated 200 times and then analyzed by ordinary electrophoresis. Routinely, immunodiffusion is performed with kappa and lambda antisera on unconcentrated urine (Ouchterlony, 1953), and immunoelectrophoresis is done with kappa and lambda antisera on concentrated urine. If electrophoresis reveals a globulin spike, and the response to the heat test for Bence Jones protein gives a negative result, and immunoelectrophoresis does not demonstrate the presence of a monoclonal light chain, one must suspect the possibility of heavy-chain disease and examine the urine for heavy chains.

Although the heat test for Bence Jones protein is useful clinically, one must recognize its shortcomings. *Electrophoresis and immunoelectrophoresis* of an adequately concentrated specimen are the methods of choice for demonstrating a monoclonal light chain in the urine.

CHAPTER V

Multiple Myeloma: Introduction and History

MULTIPLE MYELOMA (also called plasmacytic myeloma, plasma-cell myeloma, myelomatosis, or Kahler's disease) is a malignant disease of plasma cells typically involving the bone marrow but often involving other tissue as well (Waldenström, 1970; Snapper and Kahn, 1971; Azar and Potter, 1973). There is no longer any doubt that the "myeloma cell" is an immature and atypical neoplastic plasma cell. Myeloma may be regarded as a neoplastic proliferation of a single line of plasma cells engaged in the production of a specific protein as if under constant antigenic stimulation. This protein is monoclonal—one class of heavy chains (γ, a, δ, or ϵ) and one type of light chain (κ or λ)—and often is referred to as an "M" or "myeloma" protein. Arbitrarily, we have classified patients having a large amount of monoclonal IgM protein with those having macroglobulinemia.

> Saturday, Nov. 1st, 1845.
> Dear Doctor Jones,—The tube contains urine of very high specific gravity. When boiled it becomes slightly opaque. On the addition of nitric acid, it effervesces, assumes a reddish hue, and becomes quite clear; but as it cools, assumes the consistence and appearance which you see. Heat reliquifies it. What is it? (Bence Jones, 1847b.)

This cryptic note and a urine sample were sent by a leading physician of London, Dr. Thomas Watson, to Henry Bence Jones, a 31-year-old physician at St. Georges Hospital who had already established a reputation as a chemical pathologist. A graduate of Cambridge, Bence Jones had studied medicine at St. Georges Hospital and chemistry at Giessen with Liebig.

57

The patient, Thomas Alexander McBean, was seen in consultation on Oct. 30, 1845, by Dr. William Macintyre, a 53-year-old Harley Street consultant and physician to the Metropolitan Convalescent Institution and to the Western General Dispensary (Clamp, 1967). Mr. McBean, aged 44 and a highly respectable tradesman, had taken a vacation in the country in September of 1844 to regain his strength, which he felt had been impaired by work and a family illness. While vaulting out of an underground cavern he had "instantly felt as if something had snapped or given way within the chest, and for some minutes he lay in intense agony, unable to stir" (Macintyre, 1850). The pain had abated, and after a few days the patient had been relieved by a strengthening plaster applied to the chest by Dr. Macintyre. But 3 or 4 weeks later the pain had recurred, and the patient had been treated by removal of a pound of blood and application of leeches. As might be expected, this had been followed by considerable weakness for 2 or 3 months.

In the spring of 1845 he had had an episode of pleuritic pain in the right side between the ribs and hip. Therapeutic bleeding had produced much greater weakness than before. Wasting, pallor, and slight puffiness of his face and ankles led to consultation with Dr. Watson.

Under a recommended course of steel and quinine therapy, the patient improved rapidly. By the middle of summer he was able to travel to Scotland where ". . . he was capable of taking active exercise on foot during the greater part of the day, bounding over the hills, to use his own expression, as nimbly as any of his companions" (Macintyre, 1850). Diarrhea then developed which proved obstinate and reduced his strength. In September he returned to London in a very debilitated state though free of pain. But in October, sciatic and lumbar pains became severe; and on the 30th he was seen in consultation by Dr. Macintyre.

Because edema had been observed during the patient's illness, Macintyre examined the urine but found no evidence of sugar. When heated, the urine was seen to ". . . abound in animal matter. . . ." With the addition of nitric acid it became clear, but developed a precipitate after an hour. This precipitate ". . . underwent complete solution on the application of heat, but again consolidated on cooling" (Macintyre, 1850). Every movement of the trunk of the patient was attended with excruciating pain. Getting in and out of bed required great care and cautious maneuvering on his part. He developed much flatulence and marked fullness and hardness in the region of the liver, and also had another attack of diarrhea. On Nov. 15, Dr. Bence Jones saw the patient in consultation and recommended alum ". . . with the view of checking the exhausting excretion of animal matter. . . ." He became weaker, continued to have pain, and died, exhausted, on Jan. 1, 1846. The cause of death was listed on the death certificate as "atrophy from albuminuria" (Clamp, 1967). Involvement of the bones was not recognized during the patient's illness.

At postmortem examination great emaciation was noted. The ribs were soft, brittle, and easily broken and could be cut by a knife. Their interior was filled with a soft ". . . gelatiniform substance of a blood-red colour and unctuous feel." The sternum also was involved. The heart and lungs were not remarkable. "The liver was voluminous, but of healthy structure. . . ." The kidneys appeared normal on both gross and microscopic examination. The thoracic and lumbar vertebrae had the same changes as found in the ribs and sternum (Macintyre, 1850).

There is no doubt that John Dalrymple, surgeon to the Royal Ophthalmic Hospital, saw myeloma cells in his examination of two lumbar vertebrae and a rib of Mr. McBean. Nucleated cells formed the bulk of the gelatiniform mass. The greater number were round and about one and a half to two times as large as a red blood cell. Some were oval, and many of these contained two nuclei, each with a distinct nucleolus. Wood engravings made from the drawings by Mr. Dalrymple are consistent with the appearance of myeloma cells (Dalrymple, 1846).

The diarrhea, weakness, emaciation, hepatic enlargement, flatulence, dyspepsia, edema of the ankles and puffiness of the face, and large amounts of Bence Jones proteinuria all suggest the possibility of amyloidosis in addition to myeloma; but the autopsy findings of a normal heart and "voluminous liver of healthy structure" make this unlikely. It should be noted that lardaceous changes (amyloidosis) in the liver were commonly recognized at this time, so it is unlikely that they would have been missed in this case.

As with many so-called first cases, one can find an earlier example. It is most likely that Sarah Newbury, the second patient described by Solly in 1844, had myeloma. She had severe bone pain, skeletal abnormalities, and fractures of her clavicles, both femurs, right humerus, and right radius and ulna. At autopsy the cancellous portion of the bone had been replaced by a red substance that Macintyre said looked like that seen in Mr. McBean. The red matter had replaced all of the femurs except the osseous shell. Solly examined the red matter with Mr. Birkett of Guy's Hospital; and they described the cells as ". . . very clear, their edge being remarkably distinct, and the clear *oval* outline enclosing *one* bright *central* nucleus, *rarely two, never more.*" Dalrymple noted that the microscopic description by Mr. Birkett "accords very nearly" with his description of McBean's marrow.

Having received specimens of urine from both Watson and Macintyre on Nov. 1, Dr. Bence Jones corroborated the finding that addition of nitric acid produced a precipitate which then was redissolved by heat and formed again upon cooling. After an extensive analysis he concluded that the protein was an oxide of albumin, specifically "hydrated deutoxide of albumen" (Bence Jones, 1848). He postulated that chlorine caused this new protein to form from albumin. Bence Jones calculated that there were 66.97 parts of "hydrated deutoxide of albumen" per 1,000 parts of urine and that this was equivalent to the proportion of albumin in healthy blood, so that every ounce of urine secreted was equivalent to the loss of an equal quantity of blood (Bence Jones, 1847a, 1848).

There is some justification for calling myeloma McBean's disease with Macintyre's proteinuria. Although his description of the heat properties of the urine may not have been altogether his own discovery, Bence Jones certainly deserves credit for emphasizing its place in the diagnosis of myeloma, for he said, "I need hardly remark on the importance of seeking for this oxide of albumen in other cases of mollities ossium" (Bence Jones, 1847b).

Henry Bence Jones was an accomplished physician and acquired a large and remunerative practice. Among his patients was the great naturalist Charles Darwin, whom Bence Jones treated with a diet that "half starved him to death." Henry Bence Jones's other discoveries include the first description of xanthine in urine. He died in 1873 at the age of 59 (Rosenbloom, 1919). Macintyre died 7 years after reporting his findings. Thomas Watson went on to become a baronet and physician-in-ordinary to the queen. He was 5 years president of the Royal College of Physicians, and his popular *Principles and Practice of Physic* earned him the title of "the British Cicero."

The term "multiple myeloma" was introduced by Rustizky in 1873 when he found eight separate tumors of bone marrow in an autopsy and designated them as multiple myelomas. (He described a fist-sized tumor in the right frontal area extending into the orbit and producing ophthalmoplegia, an apple-sized tumor in the right fifth rib, a tumor in the left seventh rib producing a fracture, a tumor of the sternum, a tumor of the sixth to eighth thoracic vertebrae producing paraplegia, and three tumors of the right humerus. Although his description of the cells is vague, he did mention cells with eccentric nuclei. He thought these might be fat cells and did not recognize them as plasma cells.) There was little further interest in the disease until 16 years later, when Otto Kahler (1889) described a striking case in Dr. Loos, a 46-year-old obstetrician. He had had recurrent chest pains for 8 years. His course was unusual in its intermittency, which allowed him to practice and travel during the remissions. He developed a marked kyphosis of the upper thoracic spine which became so severe that his chin was pressed against the sternum, producing a decubitus ulcer. Dr. Loos' urine also contained protein that dissolved upon boiling. Kahler concluded that marked "albumosuria" must be a frequent symptom of this bone marrow disease.

The term "plasma cell" was coined by Waldeyer in 1875, but from his description one cannot be certain that he was actually describing such cells. Plasma cells were described accurately by Ramón y Cajal in 1890 while studying syphilitic condylomas; the term "plasma cell" was applied by Unna the following year while describing cells seen in the skin of patients with lupus (Michels, 1931). In 1900, Wright presented a case of multiple myeloma and pointed out that the myeloma tumor consisted of plasma cells. He emphasized that the neoplasm originated, not from red marrow cells collectively, but from only one variety of cells, the plasma cell. In 1928, Perlzweig et al. described a patient with multiple myeloma who had 9 to 11 g of globulin in his serum. He also had Bence Jones proteinuria and probably a small amount of Bence Jones protein in the plasma. They noted that it was almost impossible to obtain serum from the clotted blood because the clot failed to retract even on prolonged centrifugation. Electrophoretic techniques were applied to the study of multiple myeloma proteins by Longsworth et al. in 1939, and 14 years later Grabar and Williams (1953) described immunoelectrophoresis; these procedures have facilitated the diagnosis and contributed greatly to our understanding of the pathophysiology of this disease.

Discrete lytic bone lesions with sharply demarcated borders and no evidence of sclerosis or formation of new bone have been seen in a number of skeletons from 200 to 1300 A.D. and attributed to multiple myeloma (Morse et al., 1974). However, most of these lesions were in young adults or children, which would be strongly against that diagnosis; consequently, it is doubtful that many of these persons actually had myeloma.

CHAPTER VI

Multiple Myeloma: Etiology, Incidence, and Epidemiology

ETIOLOGY

THE CAUSE OF MULTIPLE MYELOMA is unknown. It cannot be related to trauma and there is no compelling evidence that heredity or environmental factors are significant in many instances. Radiation may be a factor in some cases, because the incidence of the disease reportedly is higher among radiologists than in the normal population (Lewis, 1963); also, the incidence among patients exposed to radiation after the atomic blast at Hiroshima appears to be higher than the incidence in an unexposed population, although the number of cases was too small to have unquestioned validity (Anderson and Ishida, 1964). From a follow-up study Nishiyama et al. (1973) reported that the risk of developing multiple myeloma was 4.9 times greater than expected for those survivors in Hiroshima who received 100 rads or more. This increase was not seen in the Nagasaki survivors. However, the numbers again were small and the observations are of questionable significance.

The possibility of a viral cause has been suggested by the presence of virus-like particles in myeloma cells of three patients (Sorenson, 1961, 1965). Alternatively, it has been suggested by some investigators that these "virus-like bodies" are actually deposits of protein in the cell (Fisher and Zawadzki, 1970). Recently a patient having a probably primitive myeloma and a small amount of kappa light chain in the urine was reported to have virus-like particles in the cytoplasm of one-third of the myeloma cells. These virus-like bodies were larger than the usual C-type virus particles and were in the range of poxviruses, suggesting

63

that they may be passenger viruses rather than an etiologic agent (Tavassoli and Baughan, 1973).

Infection of BALB/c mice with Abelson murine leukemia virus after intraperitoneal injection of pristane, a well-defined hydrocarbon, caused development of immunoglobulin-producing plasmacytomas in 28%. Only 4% of animals given pristane alone developed plasmacytomas, and none of those given only the virus developed tumors (Potter et al., 1973). Murine studies have disclosed that intracisternal A particles appear commonly in cases of plasma-cell tumor (Dalton et al., 1961). Two varieties of type C particles have been reported in plasma-cell tumors in mice, but their significance is unknown (Potter, 1973b). Another link with viruses is provided by Aleutian disease of mink. Features of this disease include an extreme, diffuse proliferation of plasma cells, diffuse hyperglobulinemia, and, in some animals, a monoclonal serum protein and Bence Jones proteinuria (Porter et al., 1965). The disease is readily transmissible by cell-free extracts of affected mink tissue; so at least in some cases this virus-induced entity may become a possibly neoplastic overgrowth of the plasma-cell system. A condition very similar to, if not identical to, Aleutian mink disease has been seen in ferrets. Hypergammaglobulinemia and systemic plasma-cell infiltrates were common and some animals had a monoclonal protein (Kenyon et al., 1966).

The presence of a filtrable and viable transmissible agent is suggested by the development of myeloma in adolescent irradiated, thymectomized mice after injection of human myeloma cells (Mitchell et al., 1971, 1974). The myeloma cells found in these animals may develop from replication of the injected myeloma cells or originate from a stem cell in an immunologically deficient host. The incidence of plasma-cell tumors is significantly less in germ-free mice than in mice exposed to normal organisms (McIntire and Princler, 1971). Development of a plasmacytoma of the lung of an immunodeficient child with repeated infections has been reported (Bhan et al., 1974); and possibly the repeated antigenic stimulation of the reticuloendothelial system had some part in this development. But despite all these suggestions of a viral etiology, proof of such a relationship in man is meager.

There is also little significant evidence that chemicals cause myeloma in man, even though occasional reports have linked chemicals and myeloma. Among 35 cases of asbestosis, 2 instances of myeloma were reported (Gerber, 1970); but in 1 of these there was an anaplastic epidermoid cancer of the bronchus with metastases, so a plasma-cell reaction cannot be excluded. Testosterone has been reported to stimulate the growth of established plasma-cell tumors in BALB/c mice (Hollander et al., 1968). Myeloma has developed in a case of Hodgkin's disease with chemotherapy (Cawley et al., 1974).

In BALB/c and NZB mice, plasma-cell neoplasms have been induced with Lucite®, mineral oil, and pristane. These chemical substances produce oil granulomas around which neoplastic plasma cells proliferate. Osteolytic lesions, monoclonal proteins in serum (IgA most common) and urine, and so-called myeloma kidney may occur, as in human myeloma. The major difference between these murine tumors and human myeloma is that in mice the induced tumor arises in relation to lipogranulomas whereas in man multiple myeloma usually arises, de novo, in the bone marrow. Also, the intracisternal type A virus-like particles are seen in practically all plasmacytomas in mice, but virus-like particles are extremely rare in man. Another difference is that amyloid has not been observed in the induced plasmacytomas (Potter, 1973a; Azar, 1974).

Repeated antigenic stimulation of the reticuloendothelial system may induce the development of myeloma. In one study, 2 patients among 78 with plasma-cell dyscrasias had long histories of hyposensitization to allergens; but the investigators did not find any unsuspected monoclonal proteins in another 30 patients who had received allergen injections for at least 5 years (Penny and Hughes, 1970). The authors of another report, which dealt with two patients in whom myeloma developed after hyposensitization for asthma, found no causal relationship between the two events (Imahori and Moore, 1972). Another instance raising the question of antigenic stimulation as a factor in the development of myeloma is the recent report of a patient with multiple myeloma and an IgG κ protein that specifically precipitated equine alpha-2 macroglobulin; the patient had had an injection of horse antitetanus serum in 1930 and another in 1936 (Seligmann et al., 1973). This has led to a "two-hit" hypothesis for myeloma, in which the first hit is stimulation by an antigen of a clone of plasma cells that produce a monoclonal protein (injection of horse serum in the case reported). These clones may involute or subsequently be transformed into myeloma by a "second hit" from an oncogenic virus or other mutagenic stimulant (Salmon and Seligmann, 1974).

Chronic biliary-tract disease has been implicated in the development of plasma-cell dyscrasias, but the incidence of biliary lithiasis reported in such cases (10%) probably does not differ significantly from that in a normal population. Among a control group of 500 patients at the Mayo Clinic who underwent abdominal operations for benign upper gastrointestinal conditions, 47 (9.4%) had cholelithiasis (Diaz-Buxo et al., 1975).

The likelihood of a genetic factor in some cases is supported by the finding of more than one instance of multiple myeloma or monoclonal protein in members of the same family. During a 6-year period we discovered eight families in whom two or more siblings had multiple myeloma. In one family a brother of the two siblings with myeloma had a monoclonal IgG λ protein, the daughter of one of the patients with myeloma had a small monoclonal IgA κ protein, and a nephew of the two patients with myeloma also had multiple myeloma. In another family, one of the siblings originally studied had an apparently benign monoclonal gammopathy but subsequently developed an aggressive myeloma. Immunoelectrophoresis of sera from 72 of the relatives of the 17 patients with myeloma revealed 2 instances of probable benign monoclonal gammopathy. This incidence of monoclonal proteins is not significantly greater than expected, although the occurrence of two cases of benign monoclonal gammopathy and three cases of myeloma within one family certainly is.

We have found 15 well-documented instances of multiple myeloma in two or more first-degree relatives (siblings or parents and children) in the literature. Furthermore, there are several reports of benign monoclonal gammopathy in other relatives of patients with myeloma and macroglobulinemia (Maldonado and Kyle, 1974). Another study found no excess of monoclonal protein in 24 members of two families with familial myeloma and in 124 relatives of 10 patients with myeloma (Odeberg et al., 1974). The occurrence of myeloma in one of a pair of identical twins, both of whom had chromosomal abnormalities, may also be pertinent (Ogawa et al., 1970). It is evident that in some instances genetic factors may have a part in the pathogenesis of multiple myeloma.

Chromosomal abnormalities are found in at least half of the patients with multiple myeloma. Most common is the presence of marker chromosomes, which usually are described as large median or submedian chromosomes resembling those of the A or B group. Also reported are numerical changes (hypodiploidy or hyperdiploidy) and structural abnormalities (including dicentric chromosomes, giant chromosomes, translocations, deletions, breaks, and gaps). These abnormalities have been noted in direct bone-marrow preparations and in peripheral blood cultures. They have also been seen in IgA and IgG myelomas as well as in benign monoclonal gammopathies (Houston et al., 1967; Dartnall et al., 1973). Anday et al. (1974) reported marker chromosomes in 11 of 38 patients with myeloma. They found nine of these after initiation of therapy and noted that an increase of abnormal metaphases and the appearance of marker chromosomes were often associated with relapse. Cytogenic abnormalities are limited to the plasma cells in myeloma (Krogh Jensen et al., 1975).

Among 120 cases of myeloma in Scotland, the share of persons with blood of group A was larger than normal and the share with group O was smaller (Allan, 1970a). The finding that patients with myeloma have a greater incidence of HLA (histocompatibility locus antigen or human leukocyte antigen) of the W18 type than do normal controls also suggests a genetic susceptibility to myeloma (Bertrams et al., 1972).

INCIDENCE AND EPIDEMIOLOGY

Multiple myeloma accounts for about 1% of all malignant disease (Cutler et al., 1975) and approximately 10% of hematologic malignancy. In the United States, the death rate from multiple myeloma has increased from 0.8/100,000 in 1949 to 1.7 in 1963 to 2.0 in 1969, an increase that accords with reports from most countries. In 1969, 4,138 deaths from multiple myeloma were recorded in the United States. Data from the Connecticut Tumor Registry show the age-adjusted rates per 100,000 males rose from 0.4 (1935-1939) to 2.4 (1968) and the corresponding rates for females rose from 0.5 to 1.6/100,000 (Eisenberg, 1966; Christine et al., 1971). In Sweden and in England the incidence rate is approximately 3/100,000; and in northeast Scotland it is 3.4/100,000 (Dawson and Ogston, 1973).

In Olmsted County, Minnesota, the incidence was 2.9/100,000 for the decade 1945 through 1954 and 3.0 for 1955 through 1964. Among patients 30 years of age and older, the rate was 6.3/100,000. No significant difference was found between urban and rural incidence rates (Table 16). The incidence rate increased with age, being highest among males 80 years of age and older (Table 17). It seems probable that the death rate for myeloma has not changed in the last 20 years, and it is likely that the ap-

TABLE 16

MULTIPLE MYELOMA: NUMBER OF CASES AND
INCIDENCE RATE, BY SEX AND RESIDENCE
(OLMSTED COUNTY, MN, 1945-1964)

	Males		Females		Total	
	No.	Rate*	No.	Rate*	No.	Rate*
Rural	10	4.5	3	1.4	13	3.0
Urban	12	3.8	10	2.5	22	3.1
Total	22	4.1	13	2.3	35	3.1

* Per 100,000 residents.

From Kyle, R. A., Nobrega, F. T., and Kurland, L. T.: Multiple myeloma in Olmsted County, Minnesota, 1945-1964. *Blood, 33:*739-745, 1969. By permission of Grune & Stratton.

TABLE 17

MULTIPLE MYELOMA: NUMBER OF CASES AND
INCIDENCE RATE, BY AGE AND SEX
(OLMSTED COUNTY, MN, 1945-1964)

Age, Yr.	Male		Female		Total	
	No.	Rate*	No.	Rate*	No.	Rate*
0-29	...	...	...	...	...	...
30-39	1	1.3	...	...	1	0.7
40-49	1	1.6	1	1.5	2	1.5
50-59	1	2.0	2	3.5	3	2.8
60-69	7	18.6	2	4.6	9	11.1
70-79	7	33.9	6	22.4	13	27.4
80+	5	68.7	2	17.4	7	37.4
Total	22	4.1	13	2.2	35	3.1
Adjusted rate† ..						3.1

* Per 100,000 residents.
† Adjusted to the average 1950 and 1960 US white population.
From Kyle, R. A., Nobrega, F. T., and Kurland, L. T.: Multiple myeloma in Olmsted County, Minnesota, 1945-1964. *Blood, 33:*739-745, 1969. By permission of Grune & Stratton.

parent increase is due to the greater availability and utilization of medical facilities and improved diagnosis (Kyle et al., 1969).

Multiple myeloma occurs in all races and in all geographic locations. Its incidence in Negroes is reportedly twice that in the white race (McPhedran et al., 1972b). In Israel the incidence of myeloma among immigrant Jews from America and Europe is higher than that among Jews from Asia and Africa (4.7 to 3.6/100,000) (Ramot and Salomi, 1961). Myeloma is more common in males; of our series of 869 patients, 61% were men.

Does a patient with multiple myeloma have an increased risk of developing a second malignancy? Berg (1967), in a study of 207 patients with myeloma, found 5 who developed carcinoma, whereas one would expect only 2.49. In a more recent study from the Charity Hospital Tumor Registry, five second neoplasms were reported in white males with myeloma when the expected number was 0.76. Two of these tumors involved the stomach. However, the authors believed that the overall risk of subsequent tumor in patients with multiple myeloma was not increased (Newell et al., 1974). In an autopsy series of 14,944 cases, Cornes et al. (1961) found only 1 carcinoma (of the lung) in 41 instances of myeloma and 1 carcinoma (of the colon) in 2 instances of plasma-cell leukemia.

From a study of occupational factors, Milham (1971) reported that significantly more of the multiple myeloma patients than of matched controls had farming occupations. Priester and Mason (1974) found that in 10 southeastern states the deaths from multiple myeloma, carcinoma of the cervix, and ovarian malignancy were more numerous in counties with high poultry populations; but when age-adjusted mortality rates for myeloma in the entire United States were compared, the significance disappeared. Thus, despite the ubiquity of oncogenic viruses in poultry and poultry products, there is little evidence that these viruses affect the incidence of myeloma in man.

A community cluster of myeloma comprising six cases diagnosed in 1 year (rate, 84/100,000) has been reported (Kyle et al., 1970b) (Table 18). In addition, one case of Waldenström's macroglobulinemia was found in the community during that year. None of the six myeloma patients had a common association except that two of them were a man and his wife. All the rest lived at widely scattered locations within the city; and none had any history of significant exposure to radiation or potential toxic chemicals nor any unusual family history of malignancy. The incidence of leukemia, lymphoma, and congenital malformations

TABLE 18

MULTIPLE MYELOMA IN SIX RESIDENTS OF THIEF RIVER FALLS,
MN, DIAGNOSED 1968

Case	Age, Sex	Race	Onset Symptoms	Diagnosis	Status
1	70, M	White	Apr 1968	Jul 1968	Alive
2	47, F	White	Feb 1968	Aug 1968	Alive
3	59, M	White	Spring 1968	Nov 1968	Dead, Jan 1970
4	58, F	White	Unknown	Dec 1968	Dead, Feb 1971
5	83, F	White	Unknown	Dec 1968	Dead, Dec 1968
6	88, F	White	Unknown	Dec 1968	Dead, Jan 1969

Modified from Kyle, R. A., Herber, L., Evatt, B. L., and Heath, C. W., Jr.: Multiple myeloma: a community cluster. *JAMA, 213:*1339-1341, 1970.

TABLE 19

SERUM-PROTEIN SURVEY IN THIEF RIVER FALLS, MN

Age, Yr.	Male	Female	Total	Incidence of Monoclonal Protein	
				No.	%
50-59	161	246	407	2	0.5
60-69	130	238	368	1	0.3
70-79	113	165	278	5	1.8
80+	55	92	147	7	4.8
Total	459	741	1,200	15	1.25

in this town had not been unduly high during the previous 9 years.

Sera were collected from 1,200 residents of this city who were 50 years of age or older. Monoclonal serum proteins were found in 15 (1.25%) (Table 19), which is not significantly different from the proportion to be expected in a population of this age (Axelsson et al., 1966) (Table 20). The incidence of heavy- and light-chain classes was as expected (Table 21). No clinical, laboratory, or roentgenographic evidence of myeloma or macroglobulinemia was found in any of these 15 patients. The presence of the cluster of myeloma cases in this city might have led one to expect an increased incidence of monoclonal proteins in the same population, but no such increase was found. Assuming that benign monoclonal gammopathy and myeloma have a common etiology, and noting that the prevalence of monoclonal proteins in

TABLE 20

INCIDENCE OF MONOCLONAL PROTEINS IN PERSONS AGED
MORE THAN 50 YEARS

	Present Study, %	Swedish Study, %
Age, yr.		
> 50	1.25	1.6
> 70	2.80	2.5
Sex		
Male	1.70	1.9
Female	0.94	1.3

this group did not differ from that in other populations surveyed, it would be reasonable to conclude that there were no environmental or genetic factors for myeloma or monoclonal proteins in the community (Kyle et al., 1972). The cause and significance of this cluster of myeloma remain unknown.

Although multiple myeloma has been found in four married couples (Table 22), there is no compelling evidence that direct contact influences transmission of the disease. These four couples were recognized during a period of 15 years, during which time at least 20 to 30 instances of myeloma in spouses in the United States could have been expected by chance alone. However, these four certainly are not all of the couples in the country in whom myeloma developed during this period, so the incidence must have been greater (Kyle et al., 1971). We also have seen a woman who died of myeloma and whose husband's second wife also developed myeloma. The fact that the same home was occupied during both marriages raises the question of an environmental effect.

Among a family of four persons, three members each had a different malignant disease during a 3-year period. The mother had multiple myeloma and the father Hodgkin's disease concurrently; and less than 3 years later their only son developed acute granulocytic leukemia. Radiation studies in the home showed more than usual alpha radiation but the excess was of indeterminant significance. No increased incidence of deaths attributed to Hodgkin's disease, acute leukemia, or multiple myeloma was found in the community (Kyle et al., 1976).

TABLE 21

SERUM-PROTEIN SURVEY IN THIEF RIVER FALLS, MN

Age, Yr.	Type of Monoclonal Protein				
	G	A	M	κ	λ
50-59	2				2
60-69	1			1	
70-79	3		2	5	
80-89	5	1	1	5	2
Total	11	1	3	11	4

TABLE 22

MULTIPLE MYELOMA IN FOUR MARRIED COUPLES: CLINICAL DATA

Case	Sex	Birth	Marriage	Diagnosis Myeloma	Follow-up
1	M	Mar 1909		Nov 1968	Dead, Jan 1970
			Apr 1940		
2	F	Jul 1910		Dec 1968	Dead, Feb 1971
3	M	May 1891		Apr 1956	Dead, May 1958
			Jan 1917		
4	F	Jul 1893		Dec 1965	Dead, Jan 1969
5	M	Jun 1906		Dec 1957	Dead, Jun 1958
			1951		
6	F	Mar 1902		Aug 1963	Dead, Aug 1964
7	M	Jun 1895		Apr 1954	Dead, Jun 1960
			May 1913		
8	F	Apr 1898		Jun 1969	Living

From Kyle, R. A., Heath, C. W., Jr., and Carbone, P.: Multiple myeloma in spouses. *Arch Intern Med, 127*:944-946, 1971. By permission of American Medical Association.

Multiple myeloma in pregnancy has been reported, but the off-spring had no persistent electrophoretic abnormalities in the serum on follow-up examination (Kosova and Schwartz, 1966; Rosner et al., 1968; Talerman et al., 1971). Recently a 21-year-old woman with myeloma became pregnant while taking cyclophosphamide orally. Her child was normal except for a 2-g/100 dl discrete monoclonal spike in his serum electrophoretic pattern at birth which disappeared by the time he was 28 months old (Lergier et al., 1974).

A compendium of animal models with myeloma, including cattle, pigs, horses, dogs, and cats, has been published (Cornelius, 1969). It is of historical interest that mollities ossium (myeloma) was noted in "... some hounds there belonging to Lord Middleton, the bones of whose skeletons were softened, the disease attacking one bone after another" (Solly, 1844).

CHAPTER VII

Multiple Myeloma: Basic Series and Clinical Features

Material and Methods of Basic Series: Much of our data on multiple myeloma was obtained from a recent review of 869 cases seen at the Mayo Clinic between Jan. 1, 1960, and Dec. 31, 1971 (Kyle, 1975). The records of all patients with a diagnosis of multiple myeloma, plasmacytic myeloma, plasma-cell myeloma, plasmacytoma, myelomatosis, or Kahler's disease were reviewed and the data were abstracted on sheets suitable for keypunching. The laboratory data for each visit were reviewed, and maximum and minimum values with their dates of occurrence were recorded. Keypunching and abstracting errors were detected by computer. (Examples: a record of a serum protein peak on electrophoresis when there was no record of any serum protein value; a record of the cause of death or a death certificate if the patient was living; and any printout showing an unlikely value such as a leukocyte count of 90,000/mm³.)

The computer was used in tabulating and analyzing the data. Distributions were run for each laboratory test, which made it possible to determine the frequency and distribution of any particular laboratory value. Initial values were those derived from laboratory tests performed within 3 months of the original diagnosis of myeloma; values obtained later, even if that particular test had not been performed before, were excluded from the "initial" category. In the review of data, any value that seemed too extraordinary (e.g., more than 5% immature leukocytes, or more than 10% plasma cells in peripheral blood) was reassessed. Character counts of each abstract card provided the number of entries for each value.

Follow-up letters were written to every patient not seen or heard from during the previous year, and to his physician. If those failed, letters were written to other contacts such as hospitals or other medical institutions where the patient had been. Death certificates were requested from the department of vital statistics of the state of residence of the patient. Even when the date of death was not known, the death certificate was often obtainable when we suggested the 2-year or 3-year interval in which it seemed likely that the patient had died. Retail credit searches produced follow-up information in some instances.

The diagnosis of multiple myeloma was based on the following findings: (1) increased number of abnormal, atypical, or immature plasma cells in the bone marrow or histologic proof of plasmacytoma; (2) the presence of a monoclonal protein in the serum or urine; or (3) bone lesions consistent with those of myeloma. Patients with plasma-cell reactions to connective-tissue diseases, liver disease, metastatic carcinoma, or chronic infections were excluded. Also excluded were patients with benign monoclonal gammopathy (monoclonal serum protein concentration < 2 g/dl), normal serum albumin, fewer than 5% plasma cells in the bone marrow, absence of myeloma bone lesions, Bence Jones proteinuria, anemia, and absence of change or development of

TABLE 23

MULTIPLE MYELOMA: SEX DISTRIBUTION AND AGE AT DIAGNOSIS
(869 MAYO CLINIC CASES)

Age, Yr.	Sex Distribution, %	
	Males (N = 529) (61%)	Females (N = 340) (39%)
< 40	2	2
40-49	8	11
50-59	25	29
60-69	40	37
70-79	22	18
80-89	3	3
(Mean age, yr)	(62)	(61)

Modified from Kyle, R. A.: Multiple myeloma: review of 869 cases. *Mayo Clin Proc, 50:29-40,* 1975.

these abnormalities during at least 3 years of observation. Patients presenting with solitary plasmacytoma, extramedullary plasmacytoma, or plasma-cell leukemia were also excluded from this review.

Clinical Findings. *Sex; Age at Onset:* Among our cases, 61% of the patients were males.

The onset of myeloma usually occurs between the ages of 40 and 70, with its peak incidence in the seventh decade of life. It is uncommon before the age of 40 (2% of our patients were less than 40 years old) and rare before the age of 30 (Table 23).

Myeloma in children has been reported (Slavens, 1934; Porter, 1963; Maeda et al., 1973), but serum and urinary proteins typical of the disease were not always found. When the tissue of the Slavens case was reexamined some years later, it was concluded that the histopathology was that of malignant lymphoma. Such cases may not represent the same disease as myeloma seen in adults. It must be emphasized that a diagnosis of myeloma before the age of 30 is to be accepted only after critical evaluation of all data.

History: Multiple myeloma is predominantly a disease of the bone marrow, with secondary osteolysis. Bone pain, typically in the back or chest and less often the extremities, is present at the time of diagnosis in almost 70% of cases (Table 24). The pain

TABLE 24

MULTIPLE MYELOMA: FREQUENCY OF VARIOUS FEATURES IN HISTORY
(869 MAYO CLINIC CASES)

Feature	Frequency, %
Bone pain, as initial finding	68
Infection, bacterial	12
Herpes zoster	2
Fever (from myeloma)	1
Bleeding, gross	7
Other malignancy	
Patient	7
Family	6

From Kyle, R. A.: Multiple myeloma: review of 869 cases. *Mayo Clin Proc,* *50:*29-40, 1975 usually is induced by movement and does not occur at night except with change of position. This is in contrast to the pain of metastatic carcinoma, which frequently is worse at night. The pain of myeloma often is sudden in onset, frequently becomes intense, and may be protracted or transient, moving from one location to another or involving more than one region at a time without reason apparent to the patient. Bone tenderness and deformity are common. Persistent localized pain of sudden onset usually indicates a pathologic fracture, which often occurs with only minimal trauma. The patient's height may be reduced by several inches because of vertebral collapse and kyphosis.

Weakness and fatigue are common symptoms and often associated with anemia. Weight loss and night sweats are not prominent until the disease is advanced. Fever from the disease itself occurs much less frequently than in lymphoma or acute leukemia: only 1% of our patients had fever attributed to their myeloma. Most myeloma patients with fever have an infection. Gross bleeding occurred in 7% of our patients, most often as epistaxis —but gastrointestinal bleeding also was noted.

A history of an additional malignancy was reported by 7% of our patients. A history of malignancy in first-degree relatives was recorded in 6% of our cases.

In some cases major symptoms resulted from acute infection, renal insufficiency, hypercalcemia, or amyloidosis. Hypercalcemia may be manifested by nausea, vomiting, apathy, weakness, polydipsia, polyuria, and constipation. Congestive heart failure, the nephrotic syndrome, joint pains, the carpal tunnel syndrome, or steatorrhea may reflect associated amyloidosis, which occurs in ap-

TABLE 25

MULTIPLE MYELOMA: SIZE OF LIVER AND SPLEEN
(869 MAYO CLINIC CASES)

	Liver	Spleen
Not palpable	687	826
Palpable	182 (21%)	43 (5%)
< 5 cm	142	38
≥ 5 cm	40	5

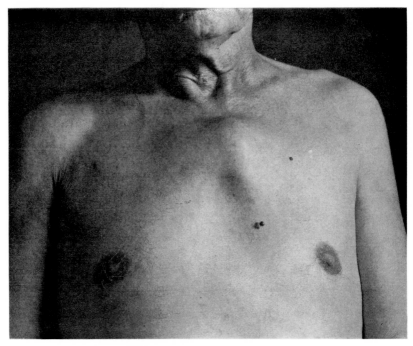

Figure 24. Multiple myeloma: prominence of sternum.

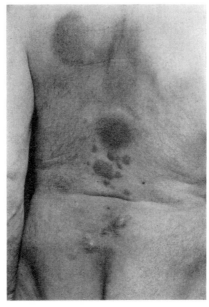

Figure 25. Multiple myeloma: subcutaneous extramedullary plasmacytomas.

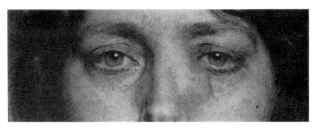

Figure 26. Multiple myeloma: extramedullary plasmacytoma adjacent to nose.

proximately 10% of patients with myeloma. Cryoglobulinemia may cause symptoms on exposure to cold. Rarely, extramedullary tumors in the upper respiratory tract, conjunctiva, or other parts of the body produce local symptoms.

Physical Findings: Pallor is the most common physical finding. Bone deformity, pathologic fracture, bone tenderness, and tumor formation also are seen. The liver was palpable in 21% of our patients, but in only 5% was it 5 cm or more below the costal margin. The spleen was palpable in 5%, but extended more than 5 cm below the costal margin in only 0.6% (Table 25). Lymphadenopathy likewise was relatively uncommon, being detected in only 4% of patients. In a number of these, the "lymphadenopathy" consisted of submandibular swelling from macroglossia due to amyloidosis. Involvement of the sternum may present as a painless, progressive swelling with subsequent deformity or fracture (Fig. 24). Purpura may be prominent, particularly if amyloidosis is present. Extramedullary plasmacytomas are uncommon but may present as large, exceedingly vascular subcutaneous masses having a purplish hue (Fig. 25). Findings due to local lesions depend, of course, on their location; for example, extradural cord compression results in paraplegia. Extramedullary plasmacytomas have been found in almost all tissues (Fig. 26). Amyloidosis may produce such diverse abnormalities as defects of cardiac conduction, congestive heart failure, macroglossia, joint pains, or the carpal tunnel syndrome.

CHAPTER VIII

Multiple Myeloma: Laboratory Findings

HEMATOLOGIC DATA

A NORMOCYTIC, NORMOCHROMIC ANEMIA occurs eventually in nearly every case of multiple myeloma. Such anemia was present at the time of diagnosis in 62% of our patients. It may be severe: 8% of our patients presented with hemoglobin values less than 8 g/dl (Table 26). The anemia of multiple myeloma is due mainly to inadequacy of red-cell production, which results from displacement by excessive numbers of abnormal plasma cells or some other factors inhibiting erythropoiesis; but a mild shortening of red-cell survival as well as iron deficiency and extravascular blood loss may also have an influence (Cline and Berlin, 1962). Increased plasma volume, which probably arises from the osmotic effect of the large amount of monoclonal protein, commonly produces hypervolemia in myeloma and decreases the hemoglobin and hematocrit concentrations (Bjørneboe and Jensen, 1969; Kopp et al., 1969). Thus, significant anemia may be

TABLE 26

MULTIPLE MYELOMA: INITIAL HEMOGLOBIN VALUE
(741 MAYO CLINIC CASES)

Hb, g/dl	Cases, %
≤ 8.0	8
8.1- 9.0	9
9.1-10.0	15
10.1-11.0	15
11.1-12.0	15
> 12.0	38
(Mean: 11.1)	

suggested by the hemoglobin or hematocrit value when the red-cell mass is only slightly diminished.

Overt hemolytic anemia has been reported in myeloma, but the incidence is low (Bohrod and Bottcher, 1963; Pirofsky, 1969; Pengelly et al., 1973). Ten of our patients had a positive Coombs test, but an overt hemolytic process was documented in only one of them. More commonly, shortened red-cell survival with a negative Coombs test contributes to anemia.

Deficiency of folic acid may contribute to the anemia of some patients with multiple myeloma. Hoffbrand et al. (1967) reported that 6 of 32 patients had intermediate megaloblastic changes. Folic acid deficiency was the predominant cause, and in two patients was severe enough to contribute to the anemia. They postulated that the folic acid deficiency was due to excess utilization of the vitamin by the tumor.

Low serum concentration of vitamin B_{12} without evidence of megaloblastic anemia has been reported in multiple myeloma (Hippe et al., 1974). In 23 patients with multiple myeloma the vitamin B_{12} serum level was statistically less than in 23 normal control patients. The mean value for hemoglobin, mean corpuscular volume, and mean erythrocyte folate level were similar to those of a group of patients with normal serum B_{12} levels. Schilling test responses were normal, and no megaloblastic changes were seen in the bone marrow. The authors concluded that there is a significant decrease of vitamin B_{12} serum level in myeloma, but considered it a result of dilution of circulating vitamin B_{12} rather than a reflection of vitamin B_{12} deficiency.

Typically, the erythrocyte sedimentation rate (ESR) is increased: 76% of our patients had a value greater than 50 mm in 1 hour (Westergren) (Table 27). But 10% of our patients had ESRs less than 20 mm in 1 hour, and it must be emphasized that a normal sedimentation rate does not exclude the diagnosis of myeloma. Rouleau formation of grade 3 or 4 was present in 61% of 772 patients and of grade 1 or 2 in 27%; only 12% showed no increase in rouleau formation. The common blue-gray staining of the background of the peripheral blood smear is attributed to the increased protein content of the serum.

TABLE 27

MULTIPLE MYELOMA: MAXIMUM ERYTHROCYTE SEDIMENTATION
RATES* (841 MAYO CLINIC CASES)

Rate, mm in 1 Hour	Cases, %
< 10	6
10-20	4
21-50	14
51-100	38
> 100	38
(Mean: 82.5)	

* Westergren.
Modified from Kyle, R. A.: Multiple myeloma: review of 869 cases. *Mayo Clin Proc, 50*:29-40, 1975.

The initial leukocyte count in myeloma is usually normal, but it was less than 4,000/mm³ in 16% of our patients and greater than 10,000 in 9% (Table 28). During the course of the disease, immature leukocytes were recorded in the differential count in 50% of cases, but their proportion exceeded 5% in only 6% of cases. A leukemoid reaction consisting of more than 15% immature leukocytes in the peripheral blood occurred in 10 patients but we were unable to make a diagnosis of leukemia in all of them. Of course leukemia might have developed if the patients had survived longer, but the leukemoid reaction may not be related to an evolving acute leukemia. Though usually sparse, atypical plasma cells or myeloma cells identical to those in the marrow were found in the peripheral blood of 16% of our cases on routine examination of the blood smear. The proportion of

TABLE 28

MULTIPLE MYELOMA: INITIAL LEUKOCYTE COUNT
(737 MAYO CLINIC CASES)

Count/mm³	Cases, %
< 4,000	16
4,000-10,000	75
> 10,000	9
(Mean: 6,450)	

plasma cells exceeded 5% in only 16 of the patients in this series. Rarely, patients develop clear-cut plasma-cell leukemia, with leukocyte counts greater than 50,000/mm³ and large numbers of myeloma cells in the peripheral blood (see Plasma-Cell Leukemia, p. 148).

The platelet count is usually normal or slightly decreased (Table 29). Thrombocytopenia occurs in far-advanced disease with extensive marrow replacement or after radiation therapy or chemotherapy. Thrombocytosis has been reported (Waldenström, 1970; Zimelman, 1973) and was present in 12% of our patients.

In the absence of a fracture with callus formation, serum alkaline phosphatase values usually are normal, but elevated values have been reported (Adams et al., 1949; Dillman and Silverstein, 1965). Careful evaluation may show another cause for elevation of the alkaline phosphatase value, such as liver disease, Paget's disease, or healing bone fractures (Ginsberg, 1967). The serum alkaline phosphatase concentration was elevated (greater than 60 IU) in 25% of 336 of our patients. Most of these elevations were modest (mean total value 55 IU), but 8 of the 336 patients had concentrations exceeding 200 IU. Three of these patients had amyloidosis, one had chronic ulcerative colitis with hepatomegaly, one had Paget's disease, and one had hepatosplenomegaly of indeterminate etiology. No cause other than myeloma was found for the increase in alkaline phosphatase in the other two instances. Thus, myeloma per se appears to be an uncommon cause of significant serum alkaline phosphatase elevation.

The serum acid phosphatase value also may be elevated in my-

TABLE 29

MULTIPLE MYELOMA: INITIAL PLATELET COUNT
(543 MAYO CLINIC CASES)

Count/mm³	Cases, %
< 100,000	12
100,000-300,000	76
301,000-500,000	11
> 500,000	1
(Mean: 195,000)	

TABLE 30

MULTIPLE MYELOMA: MISCELLANEOUS LABORATORY FINDINGS
(MAYO CLINIC)

Test	No. Pts.	% Positive
Rheumatoid factor	74	8
Coombs' test	58	17
LE clot	110	1
Serum viscosity (> 1.7)	80	89
Cryoglobulin	325	5
Pyroglobulin	500	1

Modified from Kyle, R. A.: Multiple myeloma: review of 869 cases. *Mayo Clin Proc, 50*:29-40, 1975.

eloma, even in the absence of prostatic carcinoma—and in this situation the possibility of multiple myeloma may be overlooked in differential diagnosis (Frenkel and Tourtellotte, 1962). The serum acid phosphatase concentration was elevated (> 10 IU) in 14 of the 94 of our cases in which it was measured. All of the 14 patients were men. Tartrate inhibition was less than 20% in three cases and carcinoma of the prostate was excluded at autopsy in six others. In one case the acid phosphatase value was normal on repeat determination, and Paget's disease was associated in another. Digital examination revealed a firm prostate in one patient, but further studies were not done and carcinoma cannot be excluded. In the remaining two cases, no further information was available. It does appear that serum acid phosphatase may be increased in multiple myeloma.

Values for serum creatinine, serum calcium, uric acid, liver function, and urinary findings are presented in Chapter IX, and results of miscellaneous laboratory studies in Table 30.

ELECTROPHORETIC AND IMMUNOELECTROPHORETIC DATA

Electrophoresis and immunoelectrophoresis are important aids in the diagnosis of multiple myeloma. These examinations of the serum and concentrated urine should be made in all cases of myeloma, whether known or suspected. They are particularly helpful in determining the response to treatment for solitary or extramedullary plasmacytomas as well as multiple myeloma.

TABLE 31

MULTIPLE MYELOMA: RESULTS OF ELECTROPHORESIS OF SERUM
(MAYO CLINIC)

	Cases	
	No.	(%)
Mobility of peak		
Gamma	457	(53)
Beta	182	(21)
Alpha-2	9	(1)
"Polyclonal" peak	8	(1)
Hypogammaglobulinemia	78	(9)
"Normal"	124	(15)
Total	858	(100)

Modified from Kyle, R. A.: Multiple myeloma: review of 869 cases. *Mayo Clin Proc, 50:*29-40, 1975.

They are beneficial in determining recurrence of large plasmacytomas and detecting the development of widespread disease.

Serum Findings. *Electrophoretic:* A tall, sharp peak on the densitometer tracing (Fig. 8) or a dense localized band on the cellulose acetate strip (Fig. 9) was seen in the gamma range in 53% of our cases, in the beta area in 21%, and in the alpha-2 range in 1% (Table 31); and a polyclonal-appearing peak was found in an additional 1%. Such a broader peak is most likely to be made of IgA monoclonal proteins, which have a tendency to form polymers. Among the 554 patients with a serum globulin spike, the globulin concentration exceeded 2 g/dl initially in 83% (Table 32).

Hypogammaglobulinemia was present in 78 (9%) of the series (Table 31) and was usually associated with a large monoclonal globulin peak in the urine (Bence Jones proteinuria) (Fig. 27). Urine electrophoresis performed in 66 of these 78 cases produced a globulin spike in 56 (85%). Of the remaining 10 patients, 5 had amyloidosis in addition to myeloma (4 of them excreting 4 g or more of albumin daily) and 3 had a small amount of monoclonal protein in the serum or urine. The remaining two patients had a normal-appearing urinary electrophoretic pattern, but immunoelectrophoresis was not done. The presence of hypogammaglobulinemia in myeloma needs emphasis

TABLE 32

MULTIPLE MYELOMA: FREQUENCY OF INITIAL GLOBULIN PEAK
ON SERUM ELECTROPHORESIS (554 MAYO CLINIC CASES)

Globulin, g/dl	Cases, %
1.0-2.0	17
2.1-3.0	26
3.1-4.0	21
4.1-5.0	16
5.1-6.0	11
6.1-8.0	8
> 8.0	1
(Mean: 3.6)	

Modified from Kyle, R. A.: Multiple myeloma: review of 869 cases. *Mayo Clin Proc, 50:*29-40, 1975.

because myeloma should be considered in all cases of adults who develop hypogammaglobulinemia and proteinuria.

In 124 (15%) cases the serum electrophoretic pattern appeared normal or contained only a very small spike or band (Table 31). Urine electrophoresis, performed in 102 of these 124, revealed a globulin spike in 83 (81%) of them. Among the remaining 19 were 7 with a monoclonal protein that was not visible on electrophoresis of either the serum or the urine. (In only three cases did immunoelectrophoresis fail to show a monoclonal protein in

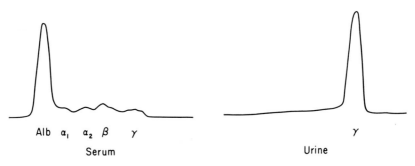

Figure 27. Multiple myeloma and hypogammaglobulinemia: electrophoretic patterns of serum and urine. Narrow peak in urine was positive for Bence Jones protein. (From Kyle, R. A., Bieger, R. C., and Gleich, G. J.: Diagnosis of syndromes associated with hyperglobulinemia. *Med Clin North Am, 54:* 917-938, 1970. By permission of W. B. Saunders Company.)

TABLE 33

MULTIPLE MYELOMA: RESULTS OF IMMUNOELECTROPHORESIS
OF SERUM (MAYO CLINIC)

	Cases	
	No.	(%)
Immunoglobulin		
IgG	316	(59)
IgA	126	(23)
IgD	6	(1)
Negative (heavy chain)	89	(17)
Total	537	(100)
Light chain		
Kappa	320*	(60)
Lambda	158*	(30)
Negative	55	(10)
Total	533	(100)

* Includes Bence Jones proteinemia.
Modified from Kyle, R. A.: Multiple myeloma: review of 869 cases. *Mayo Clin Proc, 50:*29-40, 1975.

both the serum and urine, which therefore were instances of "nonsecretory" myeloma.)

Looking at it from another aspect, 23 of the patients with hypogammaglobulinemia or an apparently normal serum electrophoretic pattern had a small monoclonal heavy chain revealed in the serum by immunoelectrophoresis. This illustrates the need for immunoelectrophoresis to identify the abnormal protein when serum protein electrophoresis fails to display a distinctive peak. One patient with a minor serum electrophoretic spike had more than 30% abnormal plasma cells in his marrow and extensive amyloidosis. Thus, electrophoretic abnormalities may be minimal when overt multiple myeloma is first seen. The cellulose acetate membrane displays small amounts of monoclonal protein better than filter paper (Kohn, 1957). Even so, in our experience it is unusual to see a band on the cellulose acetate tracing in the presence of Bence Jones proteinemia. Presumably these monoclonal light chains are buried in the beta or gamma regions. Others also have emphasized the use of immunoelectrophoresis to detect a monoclonal protein when the cellulose acetate tracing appears normal (Ironside, 1970).

Immunoelectrophoretic: In 537 cases, immunoelectrophoresis of serum was performed (Table 33). There was no monoclonal heavy chain in 89 (17%) of them, but 38 of this group (8% of the total) had a monoclonal light chain (Bence Jones proteinemia). Thus a monoclonal serum protein was detected in 91% of our myeloma patients. It is noteworthy that the light chains were of the lambda type in 22 (58%) of the 38 cases mentioned, which is appreciably greater than the usual frequency of about 35%. Of patients with a monoclonal heavy chain in the serum, 71% had IgG, 28% had IgA, and 1% had IgD. The ratio of kappa to lambda light chains was 2:1. In 10% of cases the type of the monoclonal light chain was not distinguished. In many of these instances, immunoelectrophoresis was done when our antisera were less satisfactory than now. The light-chain class of some IgA monoclonal proteins—particularly the lambda class—may be difficult to establish. Immunoelectrophoresis was done in four instances when light-chain antisera were not available.

Urinary Findings: Electrophoresis of urine (concentrated 50 to 100 times) was done in 551 cases (Table 34). There was a globulin peak in 75%, a peak with the mobility of albumin in 10%, and neither in 15%. The incidence of globulin peaks in the urine was higher than expected, but probably would have been lower if urine electrophoresis had been performed in all 869 cases, for electrophoresis probably was requested less frequently

TABLE 34

MULTIPLE MYELOMA: RESULTS OF ELECTROPHORESIS OF URINE (MAYO CLINIC)

	Cases	
	No.	(%)
Mobility of peak		
Gamma	188	(34)
Beta	215	(39)
Alpha-2	11	(2)
Protein mainly albumin	54	(10)
"Normal"	83	(15)
Total	551	(100)

Modified from Kyle, R. A.: Multiple myeloma: review of 869 cases. *Mayo Clin Proc, 50:*29-40, 1975.

TABLE 35

MULTIPLE MYELOMA: SIZE OF INITIAL GLOBULIN AND
ALBUMIN PEAKS ON URINE ELECTROPHORESIS
(MAYO CLINIC)

Excretion, g/24 h	Cases, % Globulin (N = 171)	Albumin (N = 41)
< 1.0	16	54
1.0- 3.0	45	24
3.1- 5.0	13	7
5.1-10.0	17	13
> 10.0	9	2
(Mean, g/24 h)	(3.9)	(2.2)

Modified from Kyle, R. A.: Multiple myeloma: review of 869 cases. *Mayo Clin Proc, 50*:29-40, 1975.

in cases where routine urinalysis revealed little or no proteinuria. The sizes of the urinary globulin and albumin peaks at the time of diagnosis in a smaller number of cases are indicated in Table 35.

Immunoelectrophoresis of concentrated urine showed a monoclonal light chain in 80% of 198 cases (Table 36). Among cases wherein the class of monoclonal light chain was identified, it was kappa in 58% and lambda in 42%. There was no monoclonal protein in the urine in 20% of patients.

Three of our patients had "nonsecretory" myeloma (no detectable monoclonal protein in either serum or urine), which is

TABLE 36

MULTIPLE MYELOMA: RESULTS OF IMMUNOELECTROPHORESIS
OF URINE (MAYO CLINIC)

Light Chain	Cases No.	(%)
Kappa	93	(47)
Lambda	66	(33)
Negative	39	(20)
Total	198	(100)

Modified from Kyle, R. A.: Multiple myeloma: review of 869 cases. *Mayo Clin Proc, 50*:29-40, 1975.

TABLE 37

MULTIPLE MYELOMA: QUANTITATION OF SERUM
IMMUNOGLOBULINS (340 MAYO CLINIC CASES)

Immunoglobulins, mg/ml	Cases, %
IgG	
< 6.4	29
6.4-14.3	15
> 14.3	56
(Mean: 28.2)	
IgA	
< 0.3	51
0.3-3.0	30
> 3.0	19
(Mean: 4.6)	
IgM	
< 0.2	73
0.2-2.0	26
> 2.0	1
(Mean: 0.3)	

Modified from Kyle, R. A.: Multiple myeloma: review of 869 cases. *Mayo Clin Proc, 50*:29-40, 1975.

similar to the finding of 3 such cases among the 262 reported by Osserman and Takatsuki (1963).

Quantitations of serum immunoglobulins in 340 of our cases are summarized in Table 37. The IgG value was elevated in 56% and the IgA value in 19%.

CHAPTER IX

Multiple Myeloma: Involvement of Organs and Systems

ORGANS

Renal: Proteinuria is very common in multiple myeloma and was present in 88% of our patients. Its severity was graded 3 or 4 in 38% and 1 or 2 in 25% each. Bence Jones proteinuria was detected in 49% of the 631 cases in which the heat test was performed. (Among cases excluded from review were 27 in which the heat test gave equivocal results.)

Renal insufficiency is common in myeloma (Martinez-Maldonado et al., 1971), and an elevated serum creatinine concentration was an initial finding in 54% of 238 males and 56% of 151 females in our series. Almost one-third of these patients had an initial serum creatinine value greater than 2 mg/dl (Table 38). The possibility of myeloma must be considered in the case of any older patient with renal failure of obscure cause. This point is em-

TABLE 38

MULTIPLE MYELOMA: INITIAL SERUM CREATININE
CONCENTRATIONS, BY SEX
(MAYO CLINIC)

Creatinine, mg/dl	% of 238 Males	% of 151 Females
Normal		
Males, < 1.3	46	
Females, < 1.0		44
Elevated		
—2.0	22	30
2.1- 5.0	19	19
5.1-10.0	8	4
> 10.0	5	3
(Mean, mg/dl)	(2.8)	(2.1)

phasized by the report of Hanicki et al. (1972) that 10 of 622 patients admitted to their nephrology service with a diagnosis of chronic glomerulonephritis or pyelonephritis had multiple myeloma.

Causes of Renal Insufficiency: One of the most important causes of renal insufficiency is hypercalcemia. This condition was noted in 30% of our patients initially (Table 39). In contrast, hypocalcemia was present in only 1%. Hypercalcemia must be suspected in the presence of anorexia, nausea, vomiting, polyuria, increased constipation, weakness, confusion, stupor, or coma. If recognized early and if therapy is promptly instituted, the results are good; frequently, renal function is improved (see page 189).

Another common cause of renal insufficiency is the so-called myeloma kidney, in which the distal and occasionally proximal convoluted tubules and collecting tubules become obstructed by large laminated casts (Fig. 28). These casts are eosinophilic and usually homogeneous, but some have a granular appearance (Zlotnick and Rosenmann, 1975). Electron microscopy of tubular casts in one case showed amyloid fibrils (Abrahams et al., 1966). But similar fibrils were seen in the tubular cells; and although Congo red and thioflavin T staining was negative, one cannot exclude amyloidosis in this case.

Contrary to the widespread belief that these casts are composed of precipitated Bence Jones protein, they actually contain albu-

TABLE 39

MULTIPLE MYELOMA: INITIAL SERUM CALCIUM CONCENTRATIONS
(611 MAYO CLINIC CASES)

Serum Calcium, mg/dl*	Cases, %
< 8.0	1
8.0-10.1	69
10.2-15.0	28
> 15.0	2
(Mean: 10.1)	

* Upper limit of normal = 10.1.
Modified from Kyle, R. A.: Multiple myeloma: review of 869 cases. *Mayo Clin Proc, 50:*29-40, 1975.

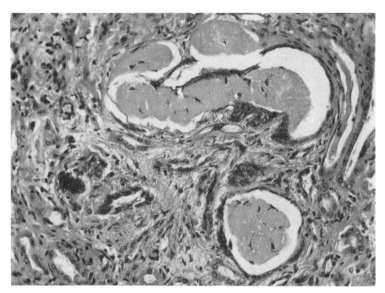

Figure 28. Multiple myeloma: large laminated cast in renal tubule. (Hematoxylin and eosin; ×225.)

min, IgG, and light chains of both kappa and lambda types rather than only one of them (Levi et al., 1968). Multinucleated syncytial epithelial cells (giant cells) often are seen at the periphery of the casts.

Dilatation and atrophy of the tubules occur. Hyaline droplets have been found within tubular epithelial cells (Bell, 1933). These droplets may consist of Bence Jones protein, which damages the tubular cells and leads to atrophy and degeneration. In the experience of some, atrophy of renal tubular epithelial cells has correlated better than the presence of casts with renal failure (Levi et al., 1968). Interstitial fibrosis and nephrocalcinosis may occur. Glomeruli usually are not affected initially in myeloma unless amyloidosis occurs. However, eventually the entire nephron becomes distorted and ceases to function, thus affecting all modalities of renal function. Yet renal tubular casts may form without accompanying renal insufficiency, whereas extensive tubular atrophy can occur in the absence of casts.

In a review of kidney tissue obtained at autopsy or biopsy in

146 cases of myeloma, Schubert et al. (1972) found typical evidence of myeloma kidney in 29% and signs of low-grade myeloma kidney in an additional 14%. There was evidence of severe pyelonephritis in 8% of their cases, while 28% had no abnormalities. The blood pressure usually is normal, even in the presence of marked renal insufficiency.

Glomerular nodules indistinguishable from those seen in diabetic glomerular sclerosis were seen by Schubert and Adam (1974) in three patients with multiple myeloma who did not have diabetes mellitus. Amyloid could not be demonstrated by either light or electron microscopy. The authors believed that the nodules consisted of protein deposits. There was a unique collagen material in the marginal part of the nodules and in the periglomerular interstitium.

Hyperuricemia, present in 39% of 305 males and 61% of 184 females in our series, may contribute to renal insufficiency (Table 40). The incidences are higher than one would expect, probably because of biased patient selection: the serum uric acid was determined initially in only a little more than half of our cases, and it is likely that more of those with hyperuricemia were measured than of those with normal values.

Acute and chronic pyelonephritis are uncommon in our experience but may contribute to renal insufficiency. Infiltration of the

TABLE 40

MULTIPLE MYELOMA: SERUM URIC ACID CONCENTRATIONS, BY SEX
(MAYO CLINIC)

Uric Acid, mg/dl	% of 305 Males*	Uric Acid, mg/dl	% of 184 Females*
≤ 4.2	6	≤ 2.2	2
4.3- 8.0	55	2.3- 6.0	37
8.1-10.0	16	6.1-10.0	49
10.1-15.0	19	10.1-15.0	10
> 15.0	4	> 15.0	2
(Mean, 8.3)		(Mean, 7.0)	

* Upper limits of normal: 8.0 for males, 6.0 for females.
Modified from Kyle, R. A.: Multiple myeloma: review of 869 cases. *Mayo Clin Proc, 50:*29-40, 1975.

kidney by plasma cells is usually not of clinical significance, though it may aggravate renal insufficiency. Excessive blood viscosity, by reducing renal blood flow, may also contribute to renal failure.

Amyloid deposition also may produce the nephrotic syndrome or renal insufficiency, or both. Histologic documentation of amyloidosis was found in 61 (7%) of our patients with myeloma. This rather low incidence may be explained by the fact that biopsy for amyloid was not generally done unless the patient had suggestive symptoms or findings. Also, there were a number of patients in whom amyloid was suspected on the basis of such conditions as congestive heart failure or carpal tunnel syndrome, but histologic proof was not sought because it would not have altered the course of their therapy. Schubert et al. (1972) reported amyloid in 7.5% of their series of 146 myeloma patients whose renal tissue was studied. Deposition of amyloid may produce the nephrotic syndrome or renal insufficiency. Rarely, the nephrotic syndrome occurs in myeloma without amyloidosis. In one instance it was attributed to extensive changes in the glomerular mesangial foam cells and alterations in the basement membrane that were thought to be related to IgA monoclonal protein and low-density lipoprotein complexes (Rosen et al., 1967b). Severe renal insufficiency has occurred in a myeloma patient whose urinary protein consisted mainly of the Fc fragment of IgG and only small amounts of light chain. Large mesangial nodules resembling those in diabetic nodular glomerular sclerosis developed in their patient (Sølling and Askjaer, 1973).

Intravenous urography has been followed by acute renal failure (Bartels et al., 1954; Brown and Battle, 1964), but it appears that the risk is slight if dehydration from water deprivation and laxatives is minimized and if abdominal compression and hypotension are avoided during the procedure (Morgan and Hammack, 1966; Myers and Witten, 1971). Occasionally, acute renal failure may occur in the absence of prior urography and may respond to dialysis (Bryan and Healy, 1968; Duarte-Amaya and Mansour, 1972). Hypercalcemia may be a significant factor in the precipitation of acute renal failure (DeFronzo et al., 1975).

Adult Fanconi's Syndrome: Multiple myeloma may be associated with adult Fanconi's syndrome (Engle and Wallis, 1957; Horn et al., 1969; Finkel et al., 1973). Among the three of our patients with acquired Fanconi's syndrome, myeloma developed in one after 8 years and amyloid in another after 17 years, and inclusions were found in the renal tubular cells and bone marrow of the third. In 11 of the 17 reported cases of Fanconi's syndrome with Bence Jones proteinuria, features typical or suggestive of the syndrome preceded the development of myeloma or amyloidosis. In three instances the two diagnoses were made simultaneously. Typing in seven cases showed the Bence Jones protein was of the kappa class. Osteomalacia is the most common skeletal abnormality, but osteoporosis or lytic lesions also occur. All except one reported case have had plasmacytosis or frank myeloma in the marrow. Crystalline cytoplasmic inclusions were found in the lymphoplasmacytic elements of the marrow in six cases and similar inclusions were found in the renal tubular cells in eight. It is likely that acquired Fanconi's syndrome with Bence Jones proteinuria derives from a plasma-cell disorder characterized by a slowly evolving myeloma with or without deposition of amyloid. One may postulate an association of intracellular defect in the synthesis of light chains and crystallization of protein in the endoplasmic reticulum of the plasma cells. This protein, presumably light chains, is reabsorbed by the renal tubules, leading to dysfunction and Fanconi's syndrome (Maldonado et al., 1975b).

Implications of Bence Jones Protein: What Bence Jones protein has to do with renal failure is not yet clear. Some investigators believe that Bence Jones protein may be the primary factor in the development of renal insufficiency and that individual Bence Jones proteins may differ in their nephrotoxicity (DeFronzo et al., 1974). Others have suggested that the degree of renal impairment is related to the amount of aggregation of each individual Bence Jones protein. Fine et al. (1973a) reported Bence Jones protein with a molecular weight of 92,000 in patients with renal failure but only 44,000 in those without renal insufficiency.

Animal studies have shown that the onset of azotemia correlated with the deposition of casts containing Bence Jones protein in the distal tubule of the kidney. It was thought that the intrarenal deposition of Bence Jones protein resulted from its relative insolubility at an acid pH and the increase of protein load presented to the kidney with an increase in tumor mass (Shuster et al., 1970). It has been shown that kappa light chains may crystallize within the proximal renal tubules, producing an adult Fanconi-like syndrome (Clyne et al., 1974). Preuss et al. (1974) reported that ammoniagenesis and gluconeogenesis by rat kidney slices were significantly less with incubation in urine proteins from patients with myeloma than with incubation in urine proteins from patients with the nephrotic syndrome. This suggests that proteins found in urine of patients with myeloma do have a part in disturbance of tubular function. One cannot altogether exclude the possibility that proteins other than light chains were responsible for the changes noted.

Although overproduction of lysozyme (muramidase) has been postulated as a cause of renal tubular dysfunction in myeloma (Muggia et al., 1969), it also has been suggested that the influence of lysozyme is not significant (Rudders and Bloch, 1971). In animal plasma-cell tumor, serum concentrations of Bence Jones protein and creatinine, tumor weight, and degree of cast formation were found to be interrelated (Bryan and McIntire, 1974). Cast formation in this study was lowest in a group treated with diuretics. These studies suggest that sustained diuresis may be helpful in treatment for myeloma.

Clearance of free light chains from plasma was inversely proportional to creatinine clearance in myeloma patients, indicating that improved renal function might lessen light-chain excretion, perhaps by increasing the fraction that is catabolized by the kidney (Fermin et al., 1974). Thus, decrease in the amount of urinary light chains might not reflect successful chemotherapy but rather improved renal function. Conversely, decreased renal function might result in increased light chain excretion without an actual increase in the myeloma tumor mass. Ward and Preston (1974) reported fibrin deposition on the endothelium of the glomerular capillaries in 15 of 35 patients with myeloma. Fibrin thrombi were seen occluding intertubular capillaries in three and extrarenal large vessels in three others. Proliferation of the mesangial complex was seen in 16. There was no obvious correlation between the presence of intraglomerular fibrin and Bence Jones proteinuria. The authors believed that the deposition of fibrin from intravascular coagulation might be a factor in the genesis of the renal lesions in myeloma.

Acute Renal Insufficiency: Acute renal insufficiency may be the presenting symptom of myeloma. We have seen several patients who were in apparent good health until acute renal insufficiency developed, and after that the diagnosis of myeloma did not become apparent until Bence Jones protein was recognized or some other feature suggesting myeloma was found.

Other authors have reported the development of acute renal failure as the first manifestation of multiple myeloma in patients not previously subjected to intravenous pyelography or dehydration. Occasionally, normal renal function has been documented shortly before the onset of acute renal failure (Kjeldsberg and Holman, 1971; Booth et al., 1974). Ladefoged et al. (1970) described seven patients in whom acute renal insufficiency was the first symptom of myeloma. Six of these patients had Bence Jones proteinuria. Three patients were treated with melphalan and prednisone, and their renal condition improved. Melphalan alone in the fourth case and symptomatic therapy in the remaining three produced no improvement of renal function. DeFronzo et al. (1975) have emphasized the role of hypercalcemia in acute renal insufficiency.

We have seen two patients who excreted more than 1 g of Bence Jones protein daily for more than 7 years without any further evidence of multiple myeloma or other malignant disease. Neither patient has developed renal insufficiency yet, so evidently Bence Jones proteinuria is not always significantly nephrotoxic (Kyle et al., 1973b).

Other investigators have identified myeloma cells in urine (Rees and Waugh, 1965; Kunwar and Kumar, 1966). Recently, plasma cells were seen in the urinary sediment of 11 of 18 patients with myeloma (Pringle et al., 1974). In eight of these, fluorescent staining indicated only a single light-chain type. No correlation was found among the presence of plasma cells in the urine, the patient's light-chain type, and the presence of renal insufficiency. The presence of myeloma cells in the urine indicates extramedullary disease, and it is possible that myeloma cells in the kidney may contribute to renal insufficiency.

Salt-wasting has been reported in cases of myeloma (Kahn and Levitt, 1970). Hyponatremia has been noted in 8 of 33 patients with myeloma. The authors postulated that the myeloma protein had a positive charge and behaved as a cation, thus displacing normal cations such as sodium. The serum sodium level returned to normal in two patients in whom the paraprotein was reduced by therapy (Frick et al., 1967).

Neurologic: Involvement of the nervous system is not uncommon in myeloma (Silverstein and Doniger, 1963). Radiculopathy is the single most frequent neurologic complication and usually is lumbosacral. Root pain results from compression of the nerve by the vertebral lesion or by the collapsed bone itself. Compression of the spinal cord or cauda equina, usually produced by myeloma arising in the marrow cavity of the vertebra with extension to the extradural space, has been reported in 5 to 10% of patients with myeloma (Svein et al., 1953). The incidence of spinal-cord compression has declined in the past decade, from 10% before 1960 to 3.8% between 1960 and 1970 (Callis and Sheets, 1974). The thoracic cord is most commonly involved, and paraplegia is not uncommon. Peripheral neuropathy may occur, disturbing both motor and sensory modalities (Victor et al., 1958). It is usually symmetric and involves the lower extremities more than the upper. Frequently it is associated with osteosclerosis (see page 110). Peripheral neuropathy is more common than expected; in one series of 23 patients with myeloma, 3 patients had clinical neuropathy and 6 more had electrophysiologic evidence of peripheral neuropathy (Walsh, 1971). Because peripheral neuropathy may precede the diagnosis of myeloma and dominate the clinical pattern, one needs to exclude multiple or solitary myeloma in all cases of peripheral neuropathy without known cause (Davis and Drachman, 1972).

Intracranial plasmacytomas are usually extensions of myelomatous lesions of the skull. Infrequently plasmacytoma of the dura mater, independent of skull lesions, has been reported. Disseminated myeloma is rare in these cases. One of our patients presented with lethargy, stupor, and papilledema from increased intracranial pressure and died from compression of the brainstem. Autopsy disclosed myelomatous involvement of the dura mater and leptomeninges which was unrelated to bony lesions (Figs. 29 and 30). Review of 110 additional autopsies that had included examination of the central nervous system of patients with myeloma did not reveal any other case of intracranial involvement independent of bone lesions (Maldonado et al., 1970). A plasma-

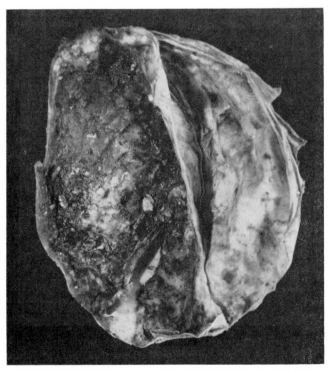

Figure 29. Thick layer of myelomatous infiltration on inner aspect of cerebral dura on left side over convexity of brain. (From Maldonado, J. E., Kyle, R. A., Ludwig, J., and Okazaki, H.: Meningeal myeloma. *Arch Intern Med, 126:*660-663, 1970. By permission of American Medical Association.)

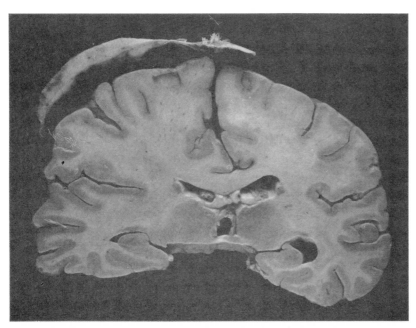

Figure 30. Cross section of cerebral hemispheres at posterior thalamic level with piece of dura over left convexity. Compression of left cerebral hemisphere with edema of underlying white matter, compression of left lateral ventricle, shift of midline structures to right, subfalcial cingulate gyral herniation, and transtentorial herniation of left uncus. (From Maldonado, J. E., Kyle, R. A., Ludwig, J., and Okazaki, H.: Meningeal myeloma. *Arch Intern Med, 126:*660-663, 1970. By permission of American Medical Association.)

cytoma involving the meninges but not accompanied by lytic lesions in the skull or other evidence of disseminated myeloma has been reported by Kennerdell et al. (1974). Initially, the symptoms resembled those of optic neuritis. An abnormal gammaglobulin band formed by electrophoresis of the cerebrospinal fluid disappeared after subtotal resection of the tumor and irradiation of the remainder. Plasmacytomas may involve the brain: Lesions in the hypothalamus (French, 1947), temporal cortex (Kramer, 1963), corpus callosum (Case Records of the Massachusetts General Hospital, 1973), and posterior fossa (Someren et al., 1971) have been described. Orbital involvement has been reported in 30 cases, the majority of which presented as proptosis (Rodman and Font, 1972). Orbital involvement may produce characteristic angiographic changes (Rosenbaum et al., 1970). The optic nerve also may be involved (Gudas, 1971). Destruction of the sella has been reported, with involvement of the third, fourth, and sixth cranial nerves.

Patients with IgG or IgA monoclonal proteins in the serum usually have monoclonal proteins in the cerebrospinal fluid, but this does not seem to increase the total CSF protein concentration (Weiss et al., 1965). There is no correlation between the concentration of monoclonal protein or total protein in the serum or CSF and the presence of clinical polyneuropathy or severity of EEG abnormality (Frantzen et al., 1969). Myeloma cells were reported in the cerebrospinal fluid of two patients with myeloma (Afifi, 1974).

Amyloid deposits in cases of myeloma may compress the median nerve, producing the carpal tunnel syndrome, or may involve the autonomic nervous system, contributing to orthostatic hypotension (see page 252). Rarely, amyloid deposits may be found in the nerves of patients with myeloma and peripheral neuropathy (Davies-Jones and Esiri, 1971; Dayan et al., 1971). Neurologic symptoms may occur with hypercalcemia or uremia. Multiple myeloma may be associated with progressive multifocal leukoencephalopathy (DelDuca and Morningstar, 1967; Gordon et al., 1971).

Gastrointestinal: Multiple myeloma may involve the stomach and present as a prominence of the rugal folds. But in a review of 900 cases of myeloma, the gastrointestinal tract was affected in only 16 (Feingold et al., 1969). Habeshaw et al. (1975) reported a patient with multiple myeloma who was producing an IgG κ protein and who subsequently was found to have a plasmacytoma of the stomach producing an IgA λ protein.

Evidence of hepatic involvement in our series included palpability of the liver in 21%. Decreased serum albumin concentration, increased sulfobromophthalein (Bromsulphalein, BSP) retention, and elevated serum alkaline phosphatase levels were common (Table 41).

Thomas et al. (1973), at autopsy in 64 cases of myeloma,

TABLE 41

MULTIPLE MYELOMA: LIVER FINDINGS—PHYSICAL AND FUNCTIONAL
(MAYO CLINIC)

	Cases	
Finding	*No.*	*(%)*
Liver palpable	869	(21)
Serum alkaline phosphatase increased*	336	(25)
BSP elevated (> 5% in 1 hour)	202	(39)
Serum albumin (initial) ≤ 3.0 g/dl†	727	(52)

* Upper limit of normal, 60 U/liter; mean value in these cases, 55.
† Mean value in these cases, 3.0.
Modified from Kyle, R. A.: Multiple myeloma: review of 869 cases. *Mayo Clin Proc, 50:*29-40, 1975.

found hepatomegaly in 58% and jaundice and ascites in 14% each. BSP retention was the most sensitive index of hepatic dysfunction, having been abnormal in almost 90% of those tested. Serum albumin, prothrombin, and serum glutamic-oxaloacetic transaminase each had had abnormal values in more than one-half of cases. Seven of the nine patients with jaundice had died within 3 weeks of the onset of icterus. At autopsy, plasma-cell infiltration of the liver was seen in 40%, appearing as tumor nodules or diffuse sinusoidal infiltration.

It is apparent that hepatic involvement is more common late in the disease than one would suppose.

One might expect a predominance of IgA myeloma protein with extramedullary involvement, but only 21 of the above series of 64 patients had immunoelectrophoresis and there was no predominance of IgA myeloma protein.

Hemorrhagic ascites was reported in one case with an IgG κ myeloma. The patient had many plasma cells in the ascitic fluid as well as multiple peritoneal plasmacytomas (Poth and George, 1971). Involvement of the gallbladder and bile ducts in myeloma has been described (Abt and Deppisch, 1969), and plasma-cell infiltration may produce jaundice by involvement of the ampulla of Vater and head of the pancreas (Derechin et al., 1970). In two cases myeloma produced obstruction of the large bowel (Elias et al., 1969).

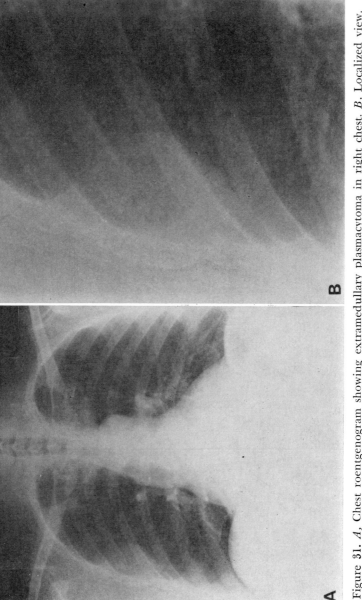

Figure 31. *A*, Chest roentgenogram showing extramedullary plasmacytoma in right chest. *B*, Localized view.

Respiratory: Intrathoracic plasmacytomas, reported in more than 50 cases, may present as a mass in the mediastinum or lung (Herskovic et al., 1965). At the time of diagnosis, myeloma is most often found in multiple areas of the body. The site of origin in most instances is the ribs, but plasmacytomas can arise from the vertebrae or subcutaneous tissues as well as the mediastinum or lung. Roentgenographically, plasmacytomas often appear as soft-tissue masses with destruction of the involved rib. Occasionally, destruction of the rib may not be recognized initially and the roentgenogram suggests only a primary tumor of the lung (Figs. 31 and 32).

Pleural effusion of significant degree, producing dyspnea, may appear in patients with myeloma (Safa and Van Ordstrand, 1973; Badrinas et al., 1974; Ghosh and Sayeed, 1974). Frequently myeloma cells can be seen in the pleural fluid if it is examined carefully. Electrophoresis and immunoelectrophoresis of the pleural fluid usually reveal the same monoclonal protein found in the serum. Biopsy of the pleura also is helpful in making the diagnosis. Myeloma may produce a pulmonary infiltration, but this is not distinguishable roentgenographically from infiltration

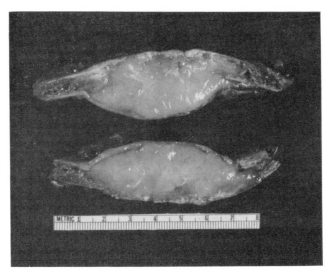

Figure 32 (same case as in Figure 31). Gross specimen of tumor. Note tumor has arisen in rib. Microscopic examination showed plasmacytoma.

caused by infections (Gabriel, 1965; Sparagana, 1970). Metastatic calcification involving the alveolar septa and alveolitis producing severe dyspnea have been noted in a patient with multiple myeloma and hypercalcemia treated with sodium sulfate and sodium phosphate (Fayemi and Wisniewski, 1973).

Cardiac: Myeloma involving the pericardium may produce cardiac tamponade (Derechin et al., 1970; Goldberg and Mori, 1970). We have also seen pericardial perfusion and acute tamponade from pericardial involvement in a patient with an IgA myeloma. Garrett et al. (1972) noted gross invasion of the myocardium, pericardium, and great vessels which produced pleural effusion, pericardial effusion, and cardiac tamponade. Plasma cells were identified in the pericardial fluid. Plasmacytomas up to 5 cm in diameter in the cardiac atria have been reported in multiple myeloma (Ghosh and Sayeed, 1974). Atrial fibrillation resistant to digoxin may result from extramedullary plasmacytoma involving the sinoatrial node (Atkinson et al., 1974).

Skeletal: Conventional roentgenograms evidenced skeletal abnormalities in 79% of our patients (Table 42). This proportion undoubtedly would have been higher if roentgenography had been done more extensively throughout each patient's illness. More than half of our patients had a combination of osteoporosis, lytic lesions, or fractures. Punched-out lytic lesions without associated osteoblastic changes are characteristic of myeloma

TABLE 42

MULTIPLE MYELOMA: SUMMARY OF ROENTGENOGRAPHIC FINDINGS
(MAYO CLINIC)

Finding	Cases No.	(%)
Lytic only	108	(13)
Osteoporosis only	50	(6)
Fractures only	22	(3)
Osteoporosis, lytic, or fractures	473	(57)
Negative	171	(21)
Total	824	(100)

Modified from Kyle, R. A.: Multiple myeloma: review of 869 cases. *Mayo Clin Proc, 50:*29-40, 1975.

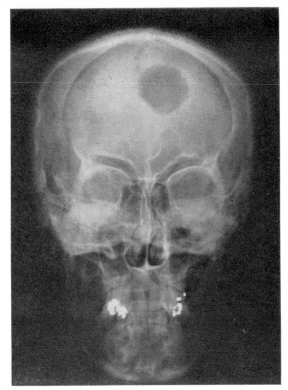

Figure 33. Skull roentgenogram of patient with multiple myeloma, showing large defect in frontal bone.

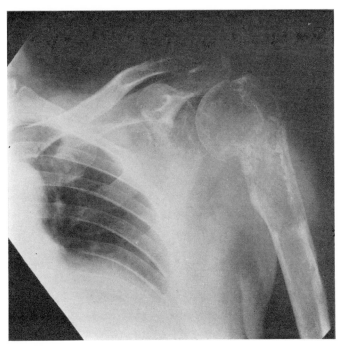

Figure 34. Roentgenogram of left shoulder, showing destruction of bone in multiple myeloma.

(Fig. 33). They may be sharply circumscribed or, when seen against a background of diffuse bone demineralization, poorly defined. To decide whether ill-defined rarefaction is abnormal may be difficult, particularly in distinguishing venous lakes from lytic lesions of the skull; moreover, multiple lytic lesions are not pathognomonic of myeloma and cannot be distinguished roentgenographically from those caused by metastatic carcinoma.

The vertebrae, skull, thoracic cage, pelvis, and proximal humeri and femurs are the usual sites of involvement (Fig. 34). Lesions in the distal portions of the extremities generally are rare,

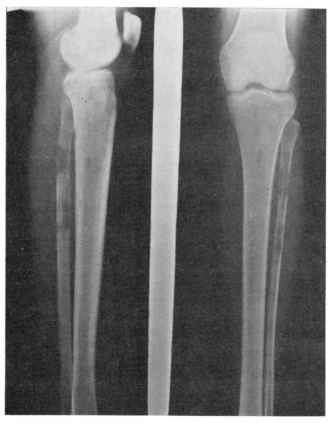

Figure 35. Leg of patient with multiple myeloma. Note involvement and fracture of fibula.

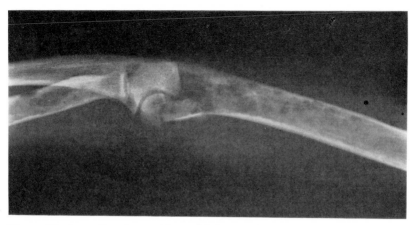

Figure 36. Arm of patient with multiple myeloma, showing involvement of distal humerus and of proximal radius and ulna.

but more would be found if more roentgenograms were taken (Figs. 35 and 36). Involvement of the mandible is not infrequent, and several of our patients have suffered a pathologic fracture while eating. Pathologic fractures, especially vertebral, are common and should always suggest the possibility of myeloma. In contrast to the frequency with which they are the site of metastatic carcinoma, the vertebral pedicles are rarely involved by myeloma. Lesions frequently extend into the soft tissues, particularly from the ribs and vertebral column, and this feature should suggest myeloma.

Distannous ethane-1-hydroxy-1,1-diphosphonate labeled with Technetium-99m (^{99m}Tc-SN-EHDP) bone scans are generally inferior to conventional roentgenograms for detecting lesions in myeloma (Wahner et al., unpublished data), but yet more effective in regard to rib and sternal lesions. In addition, roentgenographic metastatic surveys do not usually include the distal extremities, but the scans do. The facial bones, neck, skull, and anterior pelvis are difficult to evaluate with the scan because of increased uptake in the facial bones, thyroid, and urinary bladder. If one must choose between the two methods, roentgenograms are superior; yet, bone scans are of value in selected cases.

We have seen positive bone scans and negative roentgenograms of myeloma patients having severe pain from localized myeloma. However, metastatic carcinoma from the prostate to bone is much more likely to be detected by ^{99m}Tc-SN-EHDP scans than by roentgenograms (Wahner et al., unpublished data). The reason for the difference is that many of the lesions in myeloma are lytic and have minimal bone reactions, which are much less evident than metastatic carcinoma.

Osteosclerosis, resembling that associated with metastases, is rarely seen in multiple myeloma. When it does occur, osteosclerosis may be diffuse, involving almost every bone, or it may have the form of solitary or multiple focal lesions (Odelberg-Johnson, 1959; Langley et al., 1966; Evison and Evans, 1967; Brown and Paterson, 1973; Meszaros, 1974). Rarely a sclerotic margin of bone may surround a destructive myelomatous lesion in the absence of chemotherapy or radiotherapy (Getaz et al., 1974). Sclerotic bone lesions are often associated with a chronic, symmetric, sensorimotor polyneuropathy (Morley and Schwieger, 1967). Among 36 reported cases of osteosclerosis in myeloma, 13 had chronic polyneuropathy (Mangalik and Veliath, 1971). Characteristic lytic lesions are uncommon in patients with osteosclerosis, and CSF protein usually is increased. These patients have an atypical myeloma. In addition, sclerotic bone lesions may be produced by Paget's disease or metastatic carcinoma; so these disorders must be excluded.

Miscellaneous: Involvement of the eye in myeloma may consist of an intraorbital plasmacytoma producing exophthalmos (Henderson, 1973) (see page 146). In one case of multiple myeloma, plasmacytoma of the conjunctiva and orbit developed (Benjamin et al., 1975). Protein-filled cysts of the ciliary epithelium (pars plana) are common (Sanders et al., 1967) but usually asymptomatic and not readily visible clinically. In one case they may have contributed to unilateral angle-closure glaucoma (Baker and Spencer, 1974).

Myeloma may involve the skin and produce large, reddish purple, subcutaneous nodules. Many of these resemble reticulum-cell sarcoma histologically, but it is likely that they are merely extramedullary plasmacytomas less well differentiated than the usual myeloma (River and Schorr, 1966). Occasionally, morphologic features may suggest both reticulum-cell sarcoma and myeloma (Okano et al., 1966). Thickening of the skin of the neck, arms, trunk, and face, resembling scleroderma or amyloid infiltration, was seen in a patient with myeloma. Extensive biopsies of multiple organs disclosed no evidence of scleroderma, amyloidosis, or plasma-cell infiltration. Treatment with melphalan and prednisone produced marked improvement in the skin lesions and disappearance of Bence Jones proteinuria. The skin lesions worsened when therapy was withdrawn temporarily (Jablońska and Stachow, 1972).

Breast masses have been reported as the initial finding in myeloma (Rosenberg et al., 1963). Hypopituitarism has been caused by a myelomatous sellar lesion that destroyed the pituitary gland (Miturzyńska, 1962; Wolfe, 1970).

In addition to these extraosseous sites of myeloma, lesions may occur in the lungs, spleen, liver, lymph nodes, adrenal glands, and retroperitoneal regions (Hayes et al., 1952; Durant et al., 1966; Edwards and Zawadzki, 1967; Pasmantier and Azar, 1969; Oberkircher et al., 1972). Patients with extramedullary involvement are reported to have a preponderance of IgA myeloma proteins (Edwards and Zawadzki, 1967); but IgG and IgD myeloma also may have extramedullary involvement.

SYSTEMS

Immunologic: Bacterial infections were recorded in 12% of our patients; six patients had more than five acute bacterial infections each. Undoubtedly the infection rate would have been higher if it had been possible to follow the patients closely throughout the duration of their illness. Fahey and colleagues (1963) reported that the incidence of infection was more than six times as great in patients with myeloma as in hospitalized patients with other diseases. *Diplococcus pneumoniae* and *Staphylococcus aureus* were the most frequent pathogens in pulmonary infections, and *Escherichia coli* was the organism most frequently encountered in urinary-tract infections. The incidence of infections among patients with myeloma did not depend on the type or quantity of the myeloma protein. Although in most patients with myeloma proteins the concentrations of the other immunoglobulins were less than normal, there was no correlation between the frequency of infection and the IgG or IgM values. However, the IgA values were generally higher in those patients without recurrent infection. Antibody response to typhoid, diphtheria, and mumps antigen was less in the myeloma patients than in normal controls. There was an inverse correlation between the frequency of bacterial infections and the capacity to respond to antigens.

The predominance of gram-negative organisms in myeloma has been emphasized by Meyers et al. (1972), who reported that 29 infections were found in 55 patients with myeloma and that gram-negative organisms accounted for 72% of the 39 isolates from these patients. This is contrary to the predominance of gram-positive organisms seen in the past. Unusual bacterial infections, including clostridial pyoarthritis of the shoulder (Schlenker et al., 1972) and pneumococcal infection in the knee joint (Smith and Phelps, 1972), have been reported.

The immune deficit in myeloma is clearly related to abnormalities of B lymphocyte production (Harris and Copeland, 1974). Significant impairment of the synthesis of antibodies to *Streptococcus pyogenes, D. pneumoniae,* and *S. aureus* in myeloma has been reported (Dammacco and Clausen, 1966). Prolongation of the induction time of humoral-antibody production (IgM), more rapid switching from IgM to IgG production, and poor maintenance of antibody concentrations thereafter were noted in myeloma patients immunized with keyhole-limpet hematocyanin (Harris et al., 1971). These patients also had smaller delayed skin reactions than did controls tested with the same antigen, and this finding suggests some impairment of cellular immunity. Failure to develop sensitivity to 2,4-dinitro-1-fluorobenzene (DNFB) has been noted in myeloma (Cone and Uhr, 1964). Depression of reticuloendothelial function, as measured by aggregated albumin, may contribute to infections in myeloma

(Groch et al., 1965). And decrease of neutrophil migration, as measured by the skin-window technique (Rebuck and Crowley, 1955), and reduced phagocytosis of yeast particles may contribute also (Penny et al., 1971).

The impairment of antibody response, deficiency of the normal immunoglobulins, reduction of delayed hypersensitivity, and in some instances, depression of reticuloendothelial function and impairment of activity of the neutrophils may all contribute to susceptibility to infections in myeloma patients; and the propensity to infection is further increased by chemotherapeutic depression of the immune response and production of neutropenia.

Of the viral diseases, herpes zoster reportedly occurs in 2 to 3% of patients with myeloma (Williams et al., 1959; Shanbrom et al., 1960; Saidi et al., 1973). In contrast, it has been reported recently that malignant plasma cells produce increased amounts of interferon; and the authors speculated that this could have a protective effect against viral infections in myeloma (Epstein and Salmon, 1974). Finally, cerebral toxoplasmosis (Theologides et al., 1966) and infections due to *Pneumocystis carinii* (Callerame and Nadel, 1966; Gordon et al., 1971) have been found in myeloma. Undoubtedly these opportunistic infections occur more often than is reported, and they must be considered in every case of myeloma with fever of undetermined cause.

Studies of lymphocyte transformation by phytohemagglutinin (PHA) have given conflicting results. Catovsky et al. (1972b) reported a normal lymphocyte response on the basis of the percentage of blast cells found and the incorporation of tritiated thymidine; but they recognized binucleated blast cells, which probably represented an abnormal response (Catovsky et al., 1972a). On the other hand, a diminished response to PHA was reported from two other studies (Salmon and Fudenberg, 1969; Campbell et al., 1975). Mellstedt and Holm (1973) found that the stimulative effect of pokeweed mitogen on DNA synthesis was decreased significantly by treatment with melphalan and prednisone, whereas the effect of stimulation by concanavalin A and phytohemagglutinin was not. This suggests that melphalan and prednisone impair the function of B-lymphocytes that respond to pokeweed antigens. Normal T-cell and macrophage function in myeloma has been reported (Twomey and Douglass, 1974).

Coagulation: Bleeding diathesis may be a prominent feature in multiple myeloma. Perkins et al. (1970) reported that 15% of their patients with myeloma had bleeding; it was more common with IgA than with IgG types. The most frequently abnormal features were the bleeding time and platelet adhesiveness, indicating abnormality of platelet function.

The increased bleeding tendency in multiple myeloma may be related to a number of causes. Qualitative platelet abnormalities may occur, including abnormal platelet adhesiveness, decreased availability of platelet factor 3, impaired aggregation of platelets, and interference with platelet function by the monoclonal protein. The presence of inhibitors to Factor VIII, as well as nonspecific inhibitors of the thromboplastin generation test, may contribute. Factor X deficiency (which is usually associated with primary amyloidosis) and depression of Factors II, V, VII, and X and of fibrinogen have all been reported. Thrombocytopenia from plasma-cell replacement of the bone marrow or from chemotherapy may produce bleeding (Lackner, 1973). Antithrombin and antithromboplastin activity has been reported in a patient with an IgG λ myeloma and excessive bleeding (Harbaugh et al., 1975).

Abnormal clot retraction resulting in a gelatinous bulky clot from which one could obtain almost no serum was noted in the first myeloma patient recognized to have hyperglobulinemia (Perlzweig et al., 1928). Study of seven such patients revealed that they had lambda-type myeloma proteins, and it was believed that the Fab fragments of the myeloma proteins bound to fibrin during clotting and prevented clot retraction (Coleman et al., 1972).

In addition, increased bleeding is a common manifestation of the hyperviscosity syndrome (see page 219). Other potential causes of bleeding in myeloma are renal insufficiency and azotemia, liver disease, intravascular coagulation, and amyloid deposition (Lackner, 1973).

A tendency to thrombosis manifested by a shortened coagulation time, increased fibrinogen concentration, and decreased antiplasmin concentration has been detected (Sanchez-Avalos et al., 1969), and the observation is supported by recognition of an increased concentration of Factor VIII (Weiss and Kochwa, 1968). In one series of 376 patients with myeloma, 14 had major thrombotic phenomena and 6 of them died of pulmonary embolism (Catovsky et al., 1970). However, there was no control series; and because patients with myeloma are in the older age groups and may be debilitated and bedridden, all of which circumstances contribute to thrombosis, the significance of these findings is open to question.

CHAPTER X

Multiple Myeloma: Diagnosis

B ONE PAIN, ANEMIA, and excessive erythrocyte sedimentation or increased rouleaux constitute a triad that strongly suggests multiple myeloma. A number of other findings are suggestive by themselves: multiple osteolytic lesions, pathologic fractures, bone tumors, osteoporosis, hypercalcemia, uremia, cryoglobulinemia, pyroglobulinemia, hyperglobulinemia, Bence Jones proteinuria, and protein electrophoretic abnormalities. Blood typing or counting of erythrocytes may prove difficult; indeed, the inability to type or crossmatch blood for transfusion may be an initial clue to the diagnosis of myeloma. The diagnosis depends upon demonstration of increased numbers of atypical, immature plasma cells.

BONE-MARROW PLASMA CELLS

From the time of Thomas Alexander McBean's illness and Bence Jones's investigations until the turn of the century, the essential question was: What kind of disease is multiple myeloma? By 1900, when Wright's observations implicated a proliferation of plasma cells, the following histopathologic diagnoses had been made of myelomatous lesions: lymphosarcoma, myelogenous pseudoleukemia, lymphadenoma, hyperplasia of marrow, vascular endothelioma, sarcoma, small round cells, and lymphoid cells (Bayrd, 1948).

Plasma-cell myeloma then became the principal form identified; but even so, promyelocytic, myelocytic, myeloblastic, erythrocytic, lymphocytic, hemocytoblastic, and megakaryocytoblastic myelomas were reported into the 1940s. The understanding that gradually supplanted these concepts developed from Arinkin's introduction of bone-marrow aspiration and the increasing familiarity with results from its use in the 1930s. Whereas 33 cases of myeloma ascribed to origins other than the plasma cell had

116

been reported prior to the advent of bone-marrow cytology, only 10 of 150 cases diagnosed from marrow aspirates in the next 15 years were so regarded (Bayrd, 1948).

No longer are we concerned with other cell types that might produce myeloma, for no other does. Thus the designation of "plasma-cell" myeloma may be redundant. We now grapple with the problems of distinguishing "benign" monoclonal gammopathy from slowly progressive or rapidly progressive myeloma, distinguishing plasma-cell reactions from non-neoplastic conditions and neoplasia, and distinguishing lymphoidal disease from plasma-cell proliferation.

Cellular and Extracellular Features: In myeloma, plasma cells may show striking variations on light microscopy. These include differences in cytoplasm, staining characteristics, size, inclusions, vacuolization, polyploidy, and the nucleus and nucleoli. A typical bone-marrow aspirate is shown in Figure 37.

Among the most striking features may be the "flaming" plasma cells (characterized by diffuse eosinophilic coloring of the cytoplasm which resembles a sunset glow, strongest at the margins,

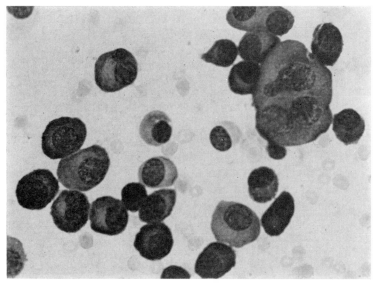

Figure 37. Typical multiple myeloma with extensive replacement of marrow. Nucleoli are common and polyploidy is present. (Wright's stain; ×470.)

Fig. 38 *A*) and thesaurocytes (large flaming cells, each with a nucleus that is pushed to the side and appears pyknotic, Fig. 38 *B*). These phenomena have been reported in IgA myeloma (Paraskevas et al., 1961; Drivsholm and Clausen, 1964), but they are not specific for the IgA type; indeed, some flaming may be seen in non-neoplastic plasma cells. More often, of course, the cytoplasm is some shade of blue, usually more intense than the normal plasma cell but not uniformly so. The cytoplasm is commonly fragmented, ragged, and extended. Free cytoplasmic pieces may be numerous. The cytoplasm may range in amount from enormous, distended by lacunae and larger than megakaryocytes, to a scant fringe. An occasional myeloma cell may have the appearance of a Gaucher cell. Present in some cases are Russell bodies, acidophilic, hyaline, cytoplasmic structures that usually are PAS-positive. Ordinarily they appear as red granules; but they may take the form of rods, amorphous red globs, angular clear crystals, and spicules resembling Auer rods. It is likely that the Rus-

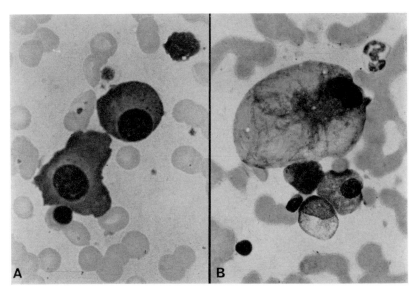

Figure 38. "Flaming" plasma cells. *A,* Typical examples, with staining more intense at periphery and streaming of cytoplasm in one cell. (Wright's stain; ×1,300.) *B,* Thesaurocyte adjacent to two conventional myeloma cells. (Wright's stain; ×800.)

sell bodies are made up of stored protein (Fisher and Zawadzki, 1970). They may be seen in normal plasma cells as well as myeloma cells. Needle-like crystals may be seen in the extra-cisternal portions of the cytoplasm (Stavem et al., 1975).

Nuclei usually are exceeded twofold to threefold in volume by cytoplasm and tend to be eccentric where cytoplasm is ample. The pattern of chromatin may be dense and either lymphoidal or reticular; but there is likely to be some degree of blocking or clumping (abortive and dispersed in dysplastic cases) with some definition of parachromatin. Polyploidy is not uncommon; and whereas diploidy is perhaps as frequent in reactive marrows as in malignant, very few reactive cells have more than four nuclei. Nucleoli are common and in some cases conspicuous, multiple, and large. Frequently a relatively clear area (hof) is seen in the cytoplasm adjacent to the nucleus. The area is occupied by the Golgi region.

Myeloma cells have been found in direct contact with cytoplasmic processes of dendritic macrophages. In these areas of contact there was a characteristic thickening of the inner leaflet of the cytoplasmic membrane of the plasma cell (Blom, 1973). Whether such contact areas between plasma cells and macrophages have a relation to abnormal plasma-cell proliferation is not known at present.

Intranuclear inclusion bodies distinct from Russell bodies (which are of cytoplasmic origin) were described by Brittin et al. (1963); but another report suggested that these intranuclear inclusions consist of entrapped portions of cytoplasm (Fisher and Zawadzki, 1970). Recently Stavem et al. (1974) reported the presence of one or more bluish hyalin nuclear inclusions in one-third of the bone-marrow plasma cells of a patient who had an IgG λ myeloma. The intranuclear inclusions were nearly always surrounded by a narrow brown rim that was much darker than the rest of the nucleus. Immunofluorescent microscopy disclosed that many intranuclear inclusions stained with IgG antisera, but they seemed to have an unstained dark core. Electron microscopy revealed dense inclusion bodies surrounded by a single triple-layered membrane. The inclusions had no features suggesting a viral origin. The absence of cytoplasmic structures in the inclusions, the lack of inclusion material in nuclear indentations, and the presence of a single membrane surrounding the inclusions are all strong evidence that they were true intranuclear inclusions and not of cytoplasmic origin. The central core, which did not react with specific immunoglobulin antisera, requires further investigation.

Intranuclear inclusions that were not electron-dense have been found in the plasma cells of a patient with multiple myeloma producing only Bence Jones lambda protein (Cohen and Lefer, 1975). More than half of the plasma cells had one to four pale blue nuclear inclusion bodies. They stained light blue with bromphenol blue and demonstrated positive immunofluorescence with lambda-chain antiserum. Electron microscopy showed a single limiting membrane surrounding each inclusion, the contents of which consisted of an amorphous granular proteinaceous material. No electron-dense inclusions were seen. The authors believed that the low-electron-density intranuclear inclusions were from dilute concentrations of protein, whereas electron-dense inclusions might have had a more concentrated proteinaceous material. They postulated that the inclusions rose within the nucleus as a result of intranuclear protein synthesis but could not exclude the possibility that inclusions arose from intranuclear invagination of perinuclear cisternal material. The intranuclear invagination could result in an inclusion bound by an inner nuclear membrane and containing proteinaceous material of the same nature as in the cytoplasm. The possibility of intranuclear protein synthesis was supported by the absence of intracytoplasmic inclusions and the lack of dilatation of the perinuclear cisternae.

Electron microscopy of the plasma cell reveals a prominent, well-developed endoplasmic reticulum (ergastoplasm) and a prominent, well-organized Golgi region (Maldonado et al., 1966a, Figs. 39 and 40). In the typical cell the endoplasmic reticulum is abundant and lamellar in configuration; but variations in shape and amount lead to differing degrees of endoplasmic dilatation and dense-body formation, as shown by Maldonado and associates. A highly anaplastic myeloma cell is shown in Figure 41. The

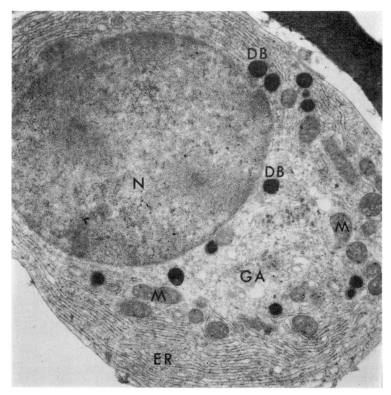

Figure 39. Mature myeloma cell. Nucleus *(N)* is ovoid and peripherally located. Cytoplasm is abundant and rich in endoplasmic reticulum *(ER)*, which is of lamellar type. Golgi area *(GA)* is prominent. There are some dense osmiophilic bodies *(DB)* and numerous mitochondria *(M)*. (Epon; ×10,000.) (From Maldonado, J. E., Brown, A. L., Jr., Bayrd, E. D., and Pease, G. L.: Ultrastructure of the myeloma cell. *Cancer, 19:*1613-1627, 1966. By permission of the American Cancer Society, Inc.)

rough endoplasmic reticulum is the primary site of protein synthesis and may be dilated from protein storage. Protein may also be stored in the Golgi region prior to secretion.

Diagnostic Interpretation: Smetana et al. (1973) emphasized asynchrony of nuclear and cytoplasmic maturation in myeloma cells. This feature, detectable by electron microscopy, may be useful in distinguishing myeloma from reactive plasmacytosis and benign monoclonal gammopathy (Graham and Bernier,

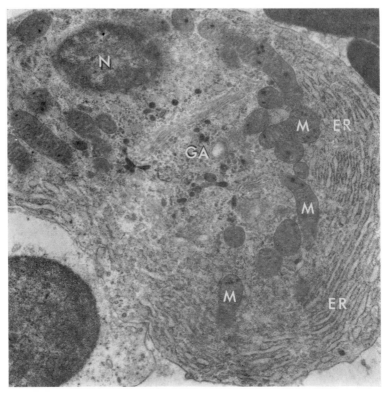

Figure 40. Myeloma cells showing prominent Golgi area *(GA)* with numerous profiles and granules of different size, shape, and density. Large mitochondria *(M)* have prominent granulation, with bizarre morphology in some. N = nucleus, ER = endoplasmic reticulum. (Epon; ×15,350.) (From Maldonado, J. E., Brown, A. L., Jr., Bayrd, E. D., and Pease, G. L.: Ultrastructure of the myeloma cell. *Cancer, 19*:1613-1627, 1966. By permission of the American Cancer Society, Inc.)

1975). Larger nuclei and nucleoli are seen in plasma cells in myeloma than in benign monoclonal gammopathy (Turesson, 1975).

Myeloma cells may have a very lymphoid appearance on light microscopy, which may cause myeloma to be confused with lymphosarcoma or macroglobulinemia (Maldonado et al., 1966b, Fig. 42). Electron microscopy has been useful in demonstrating a spectrum from lymphocytes to plasma cells (Figs. 43, 44, and 45).

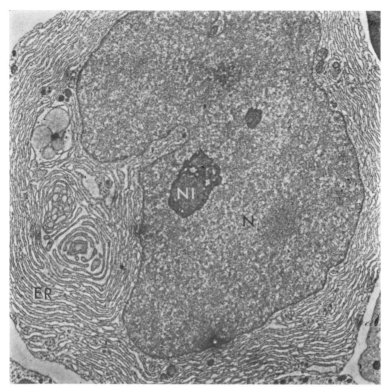

Figure 41. Highly anaplastic myeloma cell. Nucleus *(N)* and large nucleolus *(N1)* have abnormal shape, but endoplasmic reticulum *(ER)* is abundant. (Methacrylate; ×2,500.) (From Maldonado, J. E., Brown, A. L., Jr., Bayrd, E. D., and Pease, G. L.: Ultrastructure of the myeloma cell. *Cancer, 19*:1613-1627, 1966. By permission of the American Cancer Society, Inc.)

However, the distinction between lymphocytes, stimulated lymphocytes, and plasma cells is often arbitrary and one of degree.

Of course familiarity with normal plasma-cell morphology is essential to interpretation, for qualitative differences may be as significant as quantitative, or more so. To be emphasized is the fact that normally reactive plasma cells exhibit some pleomorphism and immaturity along with classically normal forms, and in addition may contain Russell bodies, have vacuoles, manifest diploidy, and lack clearly defined parachromatin. The hof, or paranuclear clear area, is usually seen and has some value in dif-

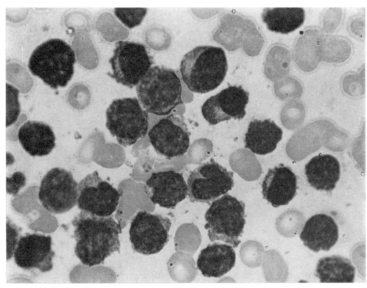

Figure 42. Bone marrow smear of lymphoid myeloma. Predominant cell element (94.5% in unconcentrated preparations) is lymphoid-appearing cell with scanty cytoplasm. (Wright's stain; ×1,200.) (From Maldonado, J. E., Kyle, R. A., Brown, A. L., Jr., and Bayrd, E. D.: "Intermediate" cell types and mixed cell proliferation in multiple myeloma: electron microscopic observations. *Blood, 27*:212-226, 1966. By permission of Grune & Stratton, Inc.)

ferentiating plasma cells from lymphocytes, but does not differentiate neoplastic from benign plasma cells. We believe that the normal upper limit of plasma cells in the bone marrow is 3%.

Neoplastic myeloma cells may differ clearly from reactive plasma cells, singly or in the aggregate. Recurring homogeneity ("clonal maturation") suggests myeloma even when an individual cell may not (Fig. 46). Such a pattern may be noted in marrow sufficiently replaced that a single field is diagnostic or so scantily involved that extensive and careful review is necessary. Although many myelomas are characterized by a uniform plasma-cell pattern, some are not; and indeed, many of the most malignant myelomas show striking pleomorphism.

In some cases the degree of atypia is neither diagnostic in individual cells nor convincingly so overall, and one is unable to dis-

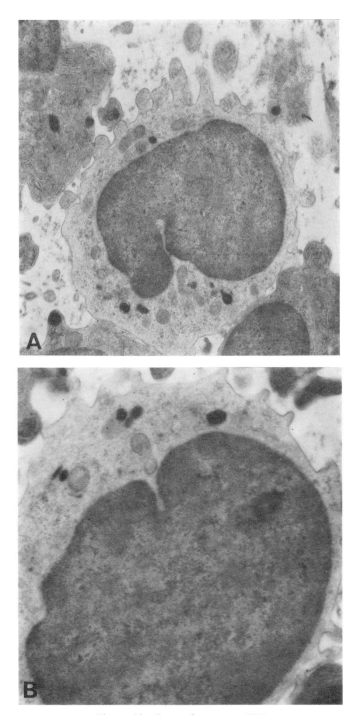

Figure 43. (Legend on page 127.)

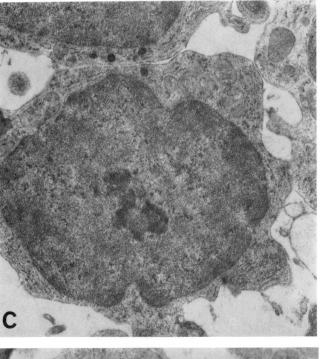

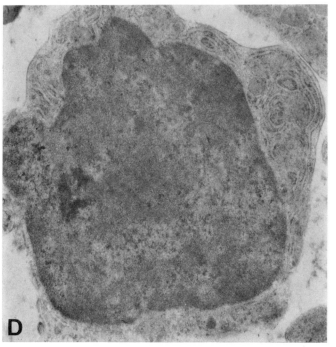

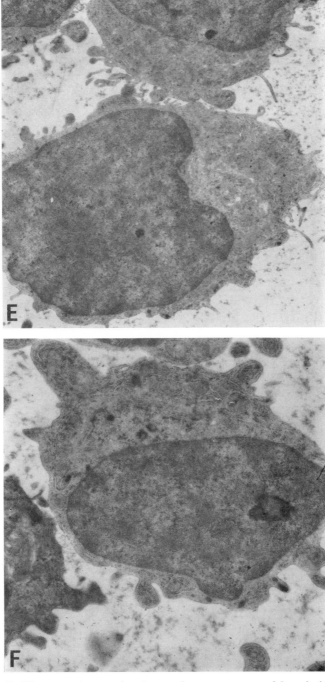

Figure 43. Electron microscopic pictures from same case of lymphoid myeloma as in Figure 42. Cell characteristics range from normal lymphocytic (*A, B*) through intermediate (*C, D*) to plasmacytic (*E, F*) features (Epon; *A* ×4,900, *B* ×7,450, *C* ×7,750, *D* ×7,450, *E* ×4,900, *F* ×4,900.) (From Maldonado, J. E., Kyle, R. A., Brown, A. L., Jr., and Bayrd, E. D.: "Intermediate" cell types and mixed cell proliferation in multiple myeloma: electron microscopic observations. *Blood, 27*:212-226, 1966. By permission of Grune & Stratton, Inc.)

tinguish the reactive plasma cell from the well-differentiated myeloma cell. Then it is helpful to look specifically for the fully normal plasma cell, as depicted in Figure 47, because coexistence of neoplastic plasma cells and plasma cells capable of such complete differentiation is rare and the presence of the latter militates against a diagnosis of myeloma.

Marrow plasmacytosis is not peculiar to multiple myeloma; it can be found in patients with carcinoma, connective-tissue diseases, liver diseases, hypersensitivity states, and viral and bacterial infections. Rarely, patients with plasma-cell reactions to these disorders have more than 20% plasma cells in their marrow (Fadem, 1952); and in many of these instances one sees mature plasma cells in a perivascular distribution, whereas in myeloma the plasma cells often are immature and may be diffuse or nodular in distribution (Liu and Dahlke, 1967; Canale and Collins,

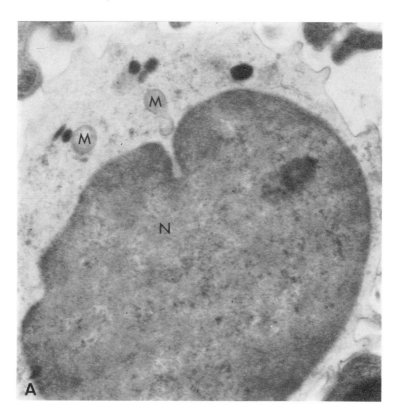

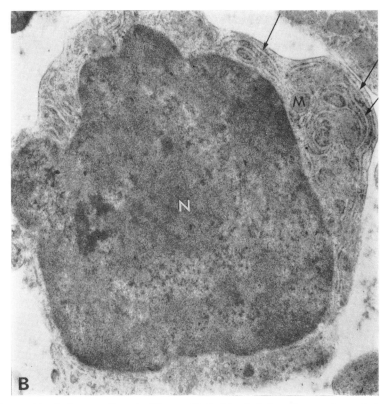

Figure 44. *A,* Same cell as in Figure 43 *B.* Typical lymphocyte has minimal endoplasmic reticulum in its cytoplasm. Nucleus *(N)* occupies large area of cell section: M = mitochondria. *B,* Same cell as in Figure 43 *D.* Like cell in *A,* this cell has relatively large nucleus *(N).* Scanty cytoplasm, however, shows well-developed endoplasmic reticulum *(arrows);* M = mitochondria. (From Maldonado, J. E., Kyle, R. A., Brown, A. L., Jr., and Bayrd, E. D.: "Intermediate" cell types and mixed cell proliferation in multiple myeloma: electron microscopic observations. *Blood, 27*:212-226, 1966. By permission of Grune & Stratton, Inc.)

1974). Therefore the diagnosis of multiple myeloma depends on the qualitative characteristics as well as the number and distribution of plasma cells.

Although plasma cells generally are 10% or more of all nucleated marrow cells in myeloma, they may amount to less than 5% or almost 100% of the marrow cells. They may present diffusely,

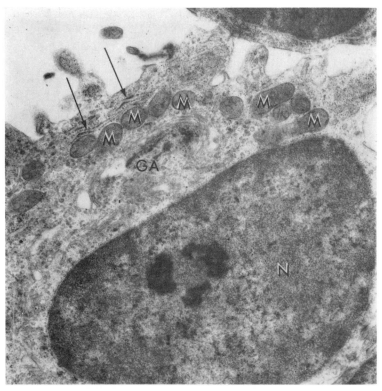

Figure 45. (Same case as in Figures 42, 43, and 44.) Cell corresponding to that depicted in smaller magnification in Figures 43 *E* and *F*. Plasmacytic features are some endoplasmic reticulum *(arrows)*, large numbers of mitochondriae *(M)*, and very prominent Golgi area *(GA)*. Nucleus *(N)* has ovoid configuration and rather peripheral location. (Epon; ×15,500.) (From Maldonado, J. E., Kyle, R. A., Brown, A. L., Jr., and Bayrd, E. D.: "Intermediate" cell types and mixed cell proliferation in multiple myeloma: electron microscopic observations. *Blood, 27*:212-226, 1966. By permission of Grune & Stratton, Inc.)

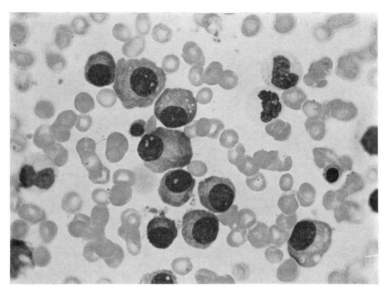

Figure 46. Multiple myeloma. Close similarity of size, shape, and differentiation suggests proliferation of uniform character. Intranuclear inclusions are present.

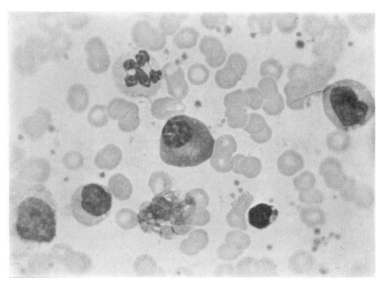

Figure 47. Normal plasma cell demonstrating classic features including chromatin blocking of nucleus, absence of nucleolus, well-defined parachromatin, hof, dark-staining characteristics of cytoplasm, eccentricity of nucleus, and normal nuclear-cytoplasmic ratio. (Wright's stain; ×800.)

in small clumps, in syncytia, or in large sheets. Marrow involvement is often focal rather than diffuse; consequently, separate specimens often vary strikingly. One may consist of nothing but myeloma cells, while one from another site may be normal or almost normal. Thus a negative bone-marrow aspirate does not exclude the diagnosis of myeloma. Repeated marrow examinations may be necessary, and needle aspirations of tender areas are often productive. Fractures of the sternum have occurred after sternal punctures in patients with myeloma; and aspiration from the posterior iliac crest is preferred as safer, easier for the patient to tolerate, and equally productive. If the aspirate is inadequate, a bone-marrow biopsy should be done. We prefer the Jamshidi needle (Jamshidi and Swaim, 1971).

To sum up, bone-marrow diagnosis depends on the number of plasma cells present, their location, and the observer's skill in distinguishing reactive and neoplastic forms.

Qualitative appraisal of individual cells requires an appreciation of the normal and abnormal; of the ranges and frequencies of secretory, tinctorial, and morphologic responses; and of patterns of repetition and distribution that have been depicted and described many times over but must still be seen and studied often enough to develop one's discriminative sense. Diagnosis also includes the differentiation of metastatic carcinoma, some forms of leukemia, left-shifted dyserythropoietic normoblasts, osteoblasts, osteoclasts, other gammopathies, and lymphoma.

Although problems of differential diagnosis reach their ultimate in distinguishing low-grade early multiple myeloma, benign monoclonal gammopathy, and primary amyloidosis from reactive processes, the decision usually is not critical, for among conditions such as these, even the cases that may ultimately prove to be multiple myeloma will be of such low grade that years may go by before treatment is needed.

Our Experience: The bone-marrow aspirate was diagnostic of multiple myeloma in 92% of cases in our series. In 1%, plasma cells appeared lymphoid and initially suggested the possibility of lymphosarcoma or macroglobulinemia (Fig. 42). In 6%, either the increase in the number of plasma cells was insufficient for the diagnosis of myeloma or a nondiagnostic aspirate was obtained. In several of these patients, examination of the bone-marrow biopsy indicated myeloma. A bone-marrow aspirate was not obtained in 1%. Where the diagnosis of myeloma was not made from bone-marrow aspirate, it was made by autopsy, open biopsy of a skeletal lesion, or identification of an extramedullary plasmacytoma. Plasma cells were counted or estimated initially in 326 cases. Among these, 84% had 10% or more plasma cells with a mean plasma-cell value of 36%. The proportion of plasma cells in bone-marrow aspirate may range from less than 5% to almost 100%.

PROTEINS

Although the presence of a large quantity of monoclonal protein favors the diagnosis of myeloma, it is not pathognomonic. Cryoglobulins and pyroglobulins are infrequent overall, but when present in large amounts suggest myeloma or macroglobulinemia. Bence Jones proteinuria also is observed rarely in patients without multiple myeloma. Polyclonal hyperglobulinemia accompanies a number of seemingly unrelated disorders such as liver disease, connective-tissue diseases, chronic infections, sarcoidosis, and kala-azar. A sharp homogeneous peak obtained by electrophoresis of the serum or urine is suggestive of myeloma; but benign monoclonal gammopathy (see page 284), macroglobulinemia (see page 197), amyloidosis (see page 229), and lymphoma may produce similar electrophoretic patterns. Again, the diagnosis depends on demonstration of increased numbers of abnormal atypical plasma cells.

Bence Jones proteinuria is detectable by the heat test in about one-half of cases of myeloma, but electrophoresis of urine reveals an abnormal protein with the mobility of globulin in approximately three-fourths of cases. In approximately 1% of proved cases of myeloma there is no detectable monoclonal protein in either the serum or urine; but in some of these cases monoclonal proteins have been identified within the plasma cell. This entity has been designated "nonsecretory" myeloma (see page 151).

Approximately 70% of monoclonal serum proteins in myeloma

are of the IgG type, 1% are IgD, and the remainder are IgA (Hobbs, 1969a; Fine, 1970). Approximately two-thirds of the IgG and IgA monoclonal proteins are of the kappa class and the remaining one-third are lambda. In contrast, the light-chain class is lambda in 80% of IgD myelomas.

Infrequently, electrophoresis of serum from a patient with myeloma reveals two separate monoclonal protein peaks. Most often these are formed by IgG and IgA heavy chains, but combinations of IgG and IgM have been reported also (Rosen et al., 1967a). One needs to exclude a biclonal peak of IgA with IgA polymers; and in some instances Bence Jones proteinemia may be manifested as a second peak in the serum electrophoretic pattern (Zinneman and Seal, 1969).

CONCLUSION

Although the protein abnormalities mentioned above are strongly suggestive of myeloma, the diagnosis ultimately depends on the demonstration of increased numbers of abnormal plasma cells. For purposes of most protocols one may utilize the diagnostic criteria prepared by a Committee of the Chronic Leukemia-Myeloma Task Force of the National Cancer Institute (1973). Patients with a monoclonal protein in the serum or urine may be regarded as having myeloma if one or more of the following are found: more than 5% plasma cells in the bone marrow (rheumatoid arthritis, chronic infection, collagen disease, carcinoma, lymphoma, or leukemia should be excluded unless other features make the diagnosis of myeloma clear); biopsy tissue showing replacement and distortion of normal tissue by plasma cells; more than 500 plasma cells per cubic millimeter of blood; or osteolytic lesions unexplained by other causes.

In the absence of a serum or urinary "myeloma protein," the diagnosis of myeloma may be made if there are either palpable tumors or radiologic evidence of osteolytic lesions, plus one or both of the following: more than 20% plasma cells in bone marrow from two sites, in the absence of another disease capable of causing plasmacytosis; or tissue biopsy specimens demonstrating replacement and distortion of normal tissue by plasma cells. But, since approximately 99% of patients with myeloma have a monoclonal protein in the serum or urine, the latter set of criteria rarely is necessary.

CHAPTER XI

Multiple Myeloma: Association With Other Diseases

Rheumatoid Arthritis: Association of rheumatoid arthritis has been reported with each of the following disorders: benign monoclonal gammopathy, multiple myeloma, Waldenström's macroglobulinemia, and heavy-chain disease (Goldenberg et al., 1969; Zawadzki and Benedek, 1969). The onset of rheumatoid arthritis antedated detection of the protein abnormality by an average of 15 years. Often the rheumatoid factor decreased during progression of myeloma (Wegelius et al., 1970). It is postulated that stimulation of the reticuloendothelial and lymphoid systems in rheumatoid arthritis causes a single clone of immunocytes to become neoplastic. In our experience, the incidence of multiple myeloma among 279 consecutive patients with rheumatoid arthritis did not appear significantly greater than that in a control group. Moreover, joint pains are not uncommon in myeloma; and we have seen several instances of "rheumatoid arthritis" with myeloma in which deposits of amyloid were found in the joints (see page 259). Under such circumstances the diagnosis of rheumatoid arthritis must be made with caution.

Serum Lipids and Xanthomatosis: The serum cholesterol concentration is lower than normal in many cases of multiple myeloma. It was 150 mg/dl or less in 26% of 300 of our patients (Table 43). The mean was 203 mg/dl in our series and 131 mg/dl in another (Lewis and Page, 1954). Such values may correlate with larger globulin concentrations. The serum triglyceride concentration was decreased in 13% of 131 of our patients.

However, the serum concentration of cholesterol was elevated in only 6% of our patients, and greater than 500 mg/dl in only 1%

(Table 43). The association of myeloma and hyperlipidemia has been reported in 19 cases and usually in conjunction with xanthomas (Özer et al., 1970). Several of these cases are difficult to evaluate because some patients had diabetes mellitus, which may produce hyperlipidemia, and others had a family history of hyperlipidemia. The association of familial xanthelasma, hyperlipidemia, and myeloma has been recorded also (Sawkar, 1971). Recently, an IgA monoclonal protein of a myeloma patient bound—through choline side chains—free lipids, lipoproteins, and sheep red cells. The investigators believed that the lipid-binding site and antigen-binding sites were separate (Mullinax et al., 1970).

Plane xanthomatosis, a rare entity characterized by diffuse, tannish, or yellowish areas of varied shape and size, located on the head, eyelids, neck, upper trunk, and extremities, has been reported in 15 cases of multiple myeloma (Moschella, 1970). Seven of the patients had a mixed type of hyperlipidemia (hypercholesterolemia and hypertriglyceridemia), five had normal lipids, two had hypercholesterolemia, and one had hypertriglyceridemia. Plane xanthomatosis usually antedates the discovery of myeloma, but occasionally it occurs during the course of myeloma (Marien and Smeenk, 1973). We have seen three patients with myeloma and plane xanthomatosis in our practice. The significance of this relationship is not known. Xanthoma disseminatum, a rare

TABLE 43

MULTIPLE MYELOMA: CONCENTRATIONS OF SERUM LIPIDS
(MAYO CLINIC)

Concentration, mg/dl	Cholesterol, % 300 Cases	Triglycerides, % 131 Cases
< 50	0	13
50-150	26	71
151-300	68	14
301-500	5	0
> 500	1	2
(Mean, mg/dl)	(203)	(105)

Modified from Kyle, R. A.: Multiple myeloma: review of 869 cases. *Mayo Clin Proc, 50:*29-40, 1975.

mucocutaneous, granulomatous, histiocytic, proliferative disorder with normal serum lipid levels, has been reported in myeloma (Maize et al., 1974). However, the relationship between myeloma and xanthoma disseminatum, if any, is obscure.

Neoplasms: Myeloma and carcinoma of the colon have been associated (Shanbrom, 1963). Isobe and Osserman (1971) found 2 cases of carcinoma of the rectosigmoid among 303 cases of myeloma; other neoplasms were found in 15.5% of the series.

Multiple myeloma has developed during the course of chronic lymphocytic leukemia (Vander and Johnson, 1960; Shuster et al., 1971). Chronic lymphocytic leukemia and multiple myeloma have been discovered simultaneously in two cases, and nodular lymphocytic lymphoma and myeloma in one case (Narasimhan et al., 1975). It is impossible to tell whether myeloma and the lymphoproliferative disorders are separate entities occurring by coincidence in the same patient or whether they are different manifestations of a single B-lymphocyte disease.

One most unusual patient developed chronic lymphocytic leukemia and was treated with intermittent courses of chlorambucil. Three years later a malignant melanoma was excised. The following year, multiple osteolytic lesions, a monoclonal IgG serum protein, and increase of plasma cells in the bone marrow developed. Two years later the bone marrow contained 75% plasma cells and the monoclonal protein had increased to 6.19 g/dl. Chlorambucil treatment was discontinued and melphalan and prednisone were given. The patient also received radiation for large osteolytic lesions in the femurs and the right humerus. Acute myeloblastic leukemia developed 8 years after the onset of chronic lymphocytic leukemia (Clinicopathologic Conference, 1975). Lohrmann et al. (1972) described a patient in whom carcinoma of the rectum, chronic lymphocytic leukemia, and light-chain myeloma were found simultaneously. It is of interest that the patient's sister had an IgG plasmacytoma. The association of myeloma, carcinoma of the colon, and hypernephroma has been reported also (Cohen et al., 1970). The association of Kaposi's sarcoma and myeloma or plasma-cell leukemia has been noted (Mazzaferri and Penn, 1968; Law, 1974).

Myeloproliferative Diseases: Myeloma has been observed in association with polycythemia vera and myelofibrosis with myeloid metaplasia (Brody et al., 1964b; Heinle et al., 1966). In another case, a well-documented myeloma was associated with probable myeloid metaplasia (Corwin, 1972). One patient who had had polycythemia vera for 9 years was found to have two paraproteins in the serum (IgG κ and IgA λ) and two proteins that resembled Bence Jones protein in the urine in the last year of her life. Two clones of plasma cells were found in the marrow by immunofluorescence and each produced one type of heavy chain. These two types of plasma cells were morphologically indistinguishable from each other (Dittmar et al., 1968).

Miscellaneous Diseases: Associations of multiple myeloma and other diseases have been reported, but one must use adequate controls in order to be sure whether it is an actual increase or merely coincidence. The association of myeloma, red-cell aplasia, and thymoma has been noted (Gilbert et al., 1968; Lindström et al., 1968). Multiple myeloma with pernicious anemia has been reported in a number of instances (Larson, 1962; Fraser, 1969; Gomez and Harley, 1970; Twomey et al., 1971). Myeloma in association with preexisting Paget's disease of bone has been reported in 11 cases, but whether this is attributable to an etiologic relation or mere coincidence is not known (Grader and Moynihan, 1961; Scurr, 1972).

Myeloma has developed in the sinus tract of chronic osteomyelitis and may be related to chronic irritation by the infection. One patient who had had drainage from his lower thigh due to chronic osteomyelitis for 40 years developed a myeloma tumor 15 by 20 cm in the area of the previous incisions (Fig. 48). Bone-marrow aspiration, serum electrophoresis, Bence Jones protein tests, and skeletal roentgenograms showed no evidence of disseminated myeloma; but while receiving radiation to the right hip he developed large subcutaneous masses of tumor in the right flank and the left trochanter (Baitz and Kyle, 1964).

Refractory sideroblastic anemia has been reported in myeloma (Catovsky et al., 1971). Sideroblastic anemia, prior to the development of acute leukemia, has also been seen in patients with

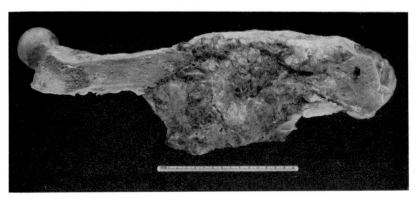

Figure 48. Gross specimen showing myelomatous involvement of femur and massive extraosseous extension. (From Baitz, T., and Kyle, R. A.: Solitary myeloma in chronic osteomyelitis: report of case. *Arch Intern Med, 113*:872-876, 1964. By permission of American Medical Association.)

multiple myeloma treated with alkylating agents (Khaleeli et al., 1973) (see page 179). The Sturge-Weber syndrome with myeloma has been reported, but the association may have been fortuitous (Kiely and Perry, 1969). Multiple myeloma has been associated with lichen myxedematosus (papular mucinosis) (Perry et al., 1960) (see page 293). Other disorders reported as associated with multiple myeloma are hyperaminoaciduria and deposition of crystalline material in the cornea and lens (Handley and Arney, 1967), hypercupremia (Goodman et al., 1967), hypoglycemia (Heffernan, 1972), Gaucher's disease (Pinkhas et al., 1965), sarcoidosis (Selroos et al., 1974), and pancreatitis secondary to hypercalcemia (Meltzer et al., 1962).

CHAPTER XII

Multiple Myeloma: Variant Forms

SOLITARY PLASMACYTOMA (SOLITARY MYELOMA) OF BONE

THERE CAN BE NO DOUBT that some plasmacytomas develop singly and remain solitary; but in many instances widespread
multiple myeloma develops years after the initial lesion. In fact,
many regard solitary plasmacytoma as only the first manifestation of multiple myeloma (Kyle, 1967). The diagnosis of the
plasmacytoma rests upon histologic evidence of a tumor consisting of plasma cells identical to those seen in myeloma. Vertebral
bodies are the bones most commonly involved; but the pelvis,
femur, or humerus may be the initial site. The roentgenographic
picture may closely resemble that of giant cell tumor of bone or
a large osteolytic lesion. In addition to histologic confirmation of
the identity of the lesion, complete skeletal roentgenograms must
show no other lesions of myeloma; the bone-marrow aspirate
must contain no evidence of multiple myeloma; and electrophoresis and immunoelectrophoresis of the serum and concentrated urine should show no monoclonal protein spike for the
plasmacytoma to be regarded as solitary.

A few exceptions to the last-mentioned criterion occur, however. An example is a patient who had a plasmacytoma of the
jaw and a small serum spike of gamma mobility. This peak
disappeared several months after removal of the tumor and did
not recur subsequently (Lane, 1952). In another patient with
a plasmacytoma of the third lumbar vertebra and a narrow gamma globulin spike of 2.2 g/dl serum, the protein peak disappeared after a tumoricidal dose of radiation and 12 years later
there was no evidence of recurrence (Kaplan and Bennett, 1968).
A patient presented with a hard mass, 5 by 5 cm, in the clavicle
and a monoclonal IgG λ protein of 1.2 g/dl, but no other evidence
of myeloma. The plasmacytoma was excised and the monoclonal

protein in the serum gradually diminished to an undetectable level over a period of 9 months. During the 2 years of follow-up, no further evidence of myeloma developed (Carter and Rushman, 1974).

Two of 12 patients with a presumed solitary myeloma of bone had a serum electrophoretic spike. In one case the spike disappeared after radiation therapy and there was no further myeloma in a 12-year follow-up; in the other instance the spike persisted after radiation therapy, but it was 9 years before disseminated myeloma became clinically apparent (Meyer and Schulz, 1974). Bence Jones proteinuria with solitary plasmacytoma has been reported (Benedict, 1970), but its occurrence strongly suggests multiple myeloma.

Meyer and Schulz (1974) reported that 9 of their 12 patients with solitary myeloma showed dissemination 2 to 10 years after diagnosis (average 5 years). The mean age of their patients was 47 at the time of diagnosis, which is significantly less than the mean age of 61 in our series of multiple myeloma.

The most uncertain criterion for the diagnosis of solitary plasmacytoma of bone is the length of observation necessary before one can be sure that the disease is not generalized. Dissemination or recurrence of plasmacytoma has developed 9 to 12 years after discovery of the initial lesion (Yentis, 1956; Kaye et al., 1961); in one case it was as late as 21 years after discovery (Cohen et al., 1964). The potential for multiple myeloma to develop in a patient who has had a solitary plasmacytoma exists for many years; indeed, one never can be absolutely certain that multiple myeloma will not occur at some later date. Yet the existence of solitary plasmacytoma is supported by cases without evidence of multiple myeloma for as long as 16, 22, 24, and 35 years after histologic diagnosis of solitary plasmacytoma (Christopherson and Miller, 1950; Wright, 1961; McLauchlan, 1973). There may be validity in the adage that a true solitary plasmacytoma is one whose growth is slow enough for the patient to die of some other disease.

Solitary myeloma may be associated with peripheral neuropathy. In one instance the patient developed severe peripheral neuropathy, and subsequent studies revealed a sacral plasmacytoma displacing the rectum anteriorly. The lesion was removed surgically and the site irradiated. The peripheral neuropathy began improving 1 week postoperatively, and during the 6-year follow-up there was no recurrence of either plasmacytoma or peripheral neuropathy (Davidson, 1972). Another patient presented with peripheral neuropathy and a routine chest film showed a lytic, partly sclerotic lesion in the left humeral head which proved to be a plasmacytoma. This was curetted and the site irradiated. The peripheral neuropathy disappeared, and at 10 months no evidence of myeloma or neuropathy was observed (Philips et al., 1972).

Severe paresis of the lower extremities was the presenting symptom of a patient who had osteosclerosis of the ninth thoracic vertebra and a complete block demonstrated by myelography. Laminectomy showed an extradural plasmacytoma. The autopsy revealed myeloma and marked osteosclerosis of the body and neural arch of the ninth thoracic vertebra and no evidence of myeloma elsewhere. The gamma globulin concentration had been increased, but immunoelectrophoresis had not been done (Roberts et al., 1974).

Of the 15 patients with an apparently solitary plasmacytoma of the sternum described by Moazzenzadeh et al. (1973), 6 had died of disseminated disease and the majority of those living also had developed systemic myeloma at the time of their report.

Two unusual patients who had a solitary plasmacytoma of the skull without evidence of disseminated myeloma were described by Kutcher et al. (1974). The first presented with a soft mass the size of an orange on the left side of the head, and roentgenography demonstrated a large lytic defect in the parietal bone. At surgery, a large plasmacytoma involving the bony tables and dural surface was identified. The other patient presented with weakness and numbness of his left arm and leg. The skull films showed a lytic defect of the parietal bone, and surgery revealed a plasmacytoma destroying both bony tables and extending beyond the meninges to infiltrate the sensory motor region of the brain. Radiation was given to both patients, and after 2 years of follow-up no evidence of multiple myeloma was present in either. During preoperative study, carotid angiography showed hypertrophy or prominence of an extracranial artery as well as displacement of intracranial vessels by dural extension in both patients. Pathologic vessels were not frequent, and the tumor blush was less intense and of shorter duration than with meningioma or vascular metastasis and occupied only a small portion of the involved area. Thus carotid angiography may be helpful in the diagnosis of plasmacytoma.

An unusual patient with recurrent plasmacytomas survived for 30 years or more (Pankovich and Griem, 1972). This patient presented in 1941 with a plasma-cell tumor of the right ischium, which was irradiated. Over the ensuing years the ischial lesion extended and new lesions were seen in the right ilium. In 1952, further extension of the lesion was seen in the ilium and ischium and radiation was given. A lytic rib lesion was found in 1956 and left untreated. In 1961 there was an extensive lytic lesion of the right humerus that produced a pathologic fracture, for which the treatment was fixation with an intramedullary rod and irradiation. Although no new lesions were detected during the next 10 years, the lesions in the ilium and sacrum remained "active." An elevation of globulins was first noted in 1950, and in 1958 a monoclonal IgG protein was demonstrated. Repeated bone-marrow biopsies showed no evidence of myeloma and Bence Jones proteinuria did not develop. This patient's disease started as solitary myeloma and developed as multiple solitary recurrences.

Treatment for solitary plasmacytoma consists of supervoltage irradiation in the range of 4,000 to 5,000 R. Local recurrence has been noted often when the initial radiation dose has been 3,000 R or less (Meyer and Schulz, 1974). There is no evidence that surgical removal of the plasmacytoma is superior to adequate irradiation, and amputation is not indicated for solitary plasmacytoma. Electrophoresis and immunoelectrophoresis are helpful in following the course of plasmacytomas after irradiation (Maruyama and Thomson, 1970).

EXTRAMEDULLARY PLASMACYTOMA

Extramedullary plasmacytomas are plasma-cell tumors that arise outside the bone marrow. These tumors may behave benignly, may be extensions of or metastases from multiple myeloma already existing (Hayes et al., 1952; Durant et al., 1966; Edwards and Zawadzki, 1967), or may disseminate later to produce widespread disease. They may be single or multiple and may be invasive or not. The upper respiratory tract, including the nasal cavity and sinuses, nasopharynx, and larynx, is the location of approximately 80% (Dolin and Dewar, 1956). The next most common site is the conjunctiva, where the tumors generally have a benign course (Hellwig, 1943). Plasmacytoma, believed to arise from the middle ear, has been reported (Noorani, 1975).

Epistaxis, rhinorrhea, and nasal obstruction are the most frequent symptoms. Extramedullary plasmacytomas may spread locally or develop into widespread multiple myeloma. Among a series of 19 patients with solitary extramedullary plasmacytoma of the upper air passages or oral cavities, multiple myeloma eventually developed in 6. Of 11 patients in this study who were followed for 10 years or more, 7 remained alive and free of recurrence (Webb et al., 1962).

Radiation for localized disease is beneficial. Of 16 patients given radiation as primary therapy, 8 were alive without disease when last seen. The median survival at last follow-up in these 16 cases was 6.8 years (Kotner and Wang, 1972). Castro et al. (1973b) reported that, of 24 patients with plasmacytoma of the paranasal sinuses and nasal cavity, 52.9% survived 5 years. Electron microscopy may be needed for proper identification of poorly differentiated plasmacytomas (Booth et al., 1973).

Extramedullary plasmacytomas may involve any portion of the gastrointestinal tract. A plasmacytoma of the lower esophagus was found to be the cause of dysphagia in one patient; and at autopsy 14 months later, no evidence of myeloma could be found in any organ (Morris and Pead, 1972).

Remigio and Klaum (1971) reported that of 13 patients with extramedullary plasmacytoma of the stomach, only 3 were alive at 5 years. Six of the others had died of recurrence, spread, or complication of their plasmacytoma; and four had died in the immediate postoperative period. Ten were treated with partial or total gastric resection. A plasmacytoma of the stomach was found in a 76-year-old man with anorexia, weakness, and weight loss. Autopsy disclosed a large plasmacytoma in the upper abdomen—involving the stomach, spleen, tail of the pancreas, and splenic flexure of the colon—and numerous peritoneal and hepatic nodules (Godard et al., 1973). Extramedullary plasmacytomas may involve the small bowel (Douglass et al., 1971; McCaffrey et al., 1972). Primary plasmacytoma of the colon was discovered in one patient upon proctoscopy for the investigation of pain (Nielsen et al., 1972). In another instance a patient admitted to the hospital with abdominal pain was found to have a large cecal mass that had perforated and produced peritonitis. Postmortem examination revealed a plasmacytoma in the cecum and myeloma in the marrow (Naqvi et al., 1970). Solitary plasmacytoma of the liver producing obstructive jaundice has been reported (Bark and Feinberg, 1967).

Plasmacytomas of both eyelids of a 30-year-old woman, interfering with vision, have been described. At surgery a plasmacytoma was found to involve the lacrimal gland on the left and another plasmacytoma was removed from the right orbit. No evidence of generalized disease was noted, but there was no followup (Darbari et al., 1972). Gupta et al. (1974) described an 18-year-old youth presenting with plasmacytoma of the cervical nodes, pleural effusion, and subcutaneous nodules. He was found to have a monoclonal protein in the serum and responded to radiotherapy.

Extramedullary plasmacytoma localized to the kidney has been reported (Farrow et al., 1968). A plasmacytoma of the kidney with metastasis to regional lymph nodes and to the liver was found in a patient who 8 years before had undergone partial right temporal lobectomy for a plasmacytoma (Catalona and Biles, 1974). Primary plasmacytoma of the skin has been reported in eight cases (LaPerriere et al., 1973), but care must be taken to exclude an inflammatory plasma-cell reaction. Extramedullary plasmacytomas of the skin may be the initial presentation of multiple myeloma (Stankler and Davidson, 1974).

Plasmacytoma presenting as vaginal bleeding from a large mass filling the upper vagina was reported. The patient had been treated with prednisone for 15 years and azathioprine (Imuran®) for 3 years for systemic lupus erythematosus. She had had a solitary plasmacytoma in the left groin 4 years earlier and a plasmacytoma of the right jaw 3 years after that (Neuberg, 1974). A patient who presented with a plasmacytoma of the chest subsequently developed gross hematuria and was found to have a large plasmacytoma of the prostate (Estrada and Scardino, 1971). Another patient presented with a large painful mass in the left thigh which had been gradually increasing in size for 4 years. Roentgenograms showed a large soft tissue mass; and although there was thinning of the outer cortex and some periosteal bone proliferation, it was felt that these changes were secondary to the enlarging mass rather than to intrinsic involvement of the bone itself. Biopsy showed sheets of moderately differentiated plasma cells as well as amyloid deposits. No evidence of multiple myeloma could be found. The tumor responded poorly to radiation therapy and to subsequent chemotherapy (Upstate Medical Center, 1974). Extramedullary plasmacytomas of the testes have been reported; and in one series of seven such cases, extra testicular myeloma developed in six (Levin and Mostofi, 1970). A patient treated for Hodgkin's disease subsequently developed extramedullary plasmacytomas in the testes that later spread to the skin and to the bone. The tumors produced monoclonal lambda light chains (Oldham and Polmar, 1973).

Rarely, extramedullary plasmacytomas have arisen in the salivary glands (Pascoe and Dorfman, 1969) or lymph nodes (Suissa et al., 1966). Slow response to radiation therapy was noted in a patient with a large plasmacytoma involving both vocal cords. Biopsy of the tissue 3 months after radiation still showed tumor cells, but subsequent biopsies were negative and no evidence of disease was found at 3-year follow-up (Griffiths and Brown, 1974). A single patient with a solitary plasmacytoma of the spleen and a polyclonal increase of IgG has been reported by two investigators (Stavem et al., 1970; Bjørn-Hansen, 1973). Angiograms of the spleen were consistent with a malignant tumor. This patient underwent splenectomy and was asymptomatic 3 years later.

PLASMA-CELL LEUKEMIA

Increased numbers of plasma cells in the peripheral blood characterize plasma-cell leukemia, which should be considered as a facet of multiple myeloma and not a separate entity (Bichel et al., 1952; Pruzanski et al., 1969; Kyle et al., 1974a). We have seen 17 patients with plasma-cell leukemia (defined as a neoplastic disorder with more than 20% plasma cells in the peripheral blood and an absolute plasma-cell content of at least 2,000/cu mm) during a period when 675 patients with multiple myeloma were seen, making the relative incidence 1.6%. Twelve patients were already leukemic when myeloma was diagnosed; in 5 the myeloma was diagnosed first. The patients who presented with plasma-cell leukemia without previously recognized myeloma were younger and had greater frequency and severity of hepatomegaly and splenomegaly, higher leukocyte and plasma-cell counts, lower incidence of monoclonal proteins in the serum and urine, less bone pain, and fewer skeletal lesions than did the patients whose myeloma developed before their plasma-cell leukemia (Table 44). Among the entire group with plasma-cell leukemia—as might be expected—there was a distinctly higher incidence of hepatosplenomegaly, renal insufficiency, leukocytosis, peripheral plasmacytosis, and low hemoglobin values than among a group of multiple-myeloma patients who did not develop plasma-cell leukemia (Table 44).

The possibility of plasma-cell leukemia should always be considered in apparently lymphocytic leukemia if the circulating cells are unusually basophilic, with nuclei eccentric or blocked. The blast cells of plasma-cell leukemia may be highly undifferentiated and not readily recognized as plasma cells; electron microscopy may be necessary for establishing the plasmacytic origin of the circulating leukemia cells (Thijs et al., 1970). In some cases the most primitive cells may be difficult to classify as plasmablasts because of the absence of ergastoplasm (Jean

TABLE 44

MULTIPLE MYELOMA: COMPARISON WITH PLASMA-CELL LEUKEMIA
(MAYO CLINIC CASES)

	Plasma-Cell Leukemia: With Previous Myeloma		Myeloma Without Plasma-Cell Leukemia
	No	*Yes*	
Cases	12	5	869
Symptoms to diagnosis, mean mo.	3.5	16.6	...
Diagnosis to death, mean mo.	9.2*	5.0	...
Age at diagnosis, mean yr.	51	65	62
Bone pain, % cases	50	100	68
Hepatomegaly, % cases	75	0	21
Splenomegaly, % cases	50	20	5
Hemoglobin $\leq$ 10 g/dl			
% cases	75	80	32
Mean, g/dl	7.2	7.7	11.1
Leukocytes > 10,000/mm^3			
% cases	92	100	9
Mean/mm^3	38,200	18,200	6,450
Plasma cells in differential count			
% cases	100	100	16
Mean/mm^3	25,671	7,469	...
Platelets < 100,000/mm^3			
% cases	70	100	13
Mean/mm^3	107,000	28,000	195
Calcium, mean mg/dl	11.3	10.3	10.1
Creatinine > 1.2 mg/dl			
% cases	100	80	48
Mean, mg/dl	6.3	5.2	2.5
Sedimentation (Westergren), mean mm in 1 h	86	138	83
Bone lesions, % cases	50	100	79
Serum spike			
% cases	50	80	76
Mean, g/dl	3.2	5.5	3.6
Urine globulin spike			
% cases	85	100	75
Mean, g/24 h	2.5	3.0	3.9

* Patient surviving 149 months not included.

Modified from Kyle, R. A., Maldonado, J. E., and Bayrd, E. D.: Plasma cell leukemia: report on 17 cases. *Arch Intern Med*, *133*:813-818, 1974. By permission of American Medical Association.

et al., 1971). The presence of less immature plasma cells may aid in the identification of plasma-cell leukemia. Many of our patients were thought to have a lymphoproliferative disorder until Bence Jones proteinuria, monoclonal serum protein, or the distinguishing characteristics of the circulating cells were recognized.

The incidence of plasma-cell leukemia appears to be high in both IgD and IgE myeloma.

Acute renal failure may occur in plasma-cell leukemia and may respond to dialysis and chemotherapy (Richards and Hines, 1973). Rarely, hyperviscosity may complicate the course of plasma-cell leukemia (Sawkar, 1972). A patient with Kaposi's sarcoma developed plasma-cell leukemia, but the relationship between these two entities is uncertain (Law, 1974). One unusual patient was regarded as having chronic lymphocytic leukemia for $8\frac{1}{2}$ years and was treated with chlorambucil. She then developed an acute leukemic process and a small amount of IgM (0.7 g/dl) monoclonal protein. Nearly all metaphases contained a large marker chromosome with a subterminal centromere like the chromosomal findings in macroglobulinemia. The cells in the peripheral blood had the appearance of plasma cells (Fitzgerald et al., 1973). Plasma-cell leukemia has been reported with both a γ heavy-chain fragment (γ heavy-chain disease) and an IgM κ monoclonal protein (Keller et al., 1970). A most unusual case of plasma-cell leukemia was reported with a γ chain as well as both kappa and lambda chains in the urine. The authors postulated a defective association of light and heavy chains (Polliack et al., 1974). However, the reaction of the urinary protein with both kappa and lambda antisera makes it doubtful that a monoclonal light chain was present. Extramedullary tumors also may occur in plasma-cell leukemia, as illustrated by development of a large plasmacytoma of the left testis and a 4-cm subcutaneous nodule in the back of one patient (Andaloro and Babott, 1974).

Treatment for plasma-cell leukemia is generally unsatisfactory, with only limited responses to melphalan or cyclophosphamide. Recently a patient obtained a partial remission with a combination of cyclophosphamide, vincristine, cytosine arabinoside, and prednisone. Melphalan and prednisone were given intermittently for maintenance of the remission, but the patient died of the disease 13 months later (Shaw et al., 1974). Occasionally a good result occurs. We have seen a patient with plasma-cell leukemia who presented with 8,600 leukocytes per cubic millimeter, 41% plasma cells in the peripheral blood, hemoglobin 9.3 g/dl, a monoclonal IgG λ protein 6 g/dl, and 100% plasma cells in the bone marrow. With intermittent courses of melphalan and prednisone, her differential count returned completely to normal and the monoclonal spike in her serum disappeared. Administration of melphalan and prednisone was continued, but 18 months later she returned with severe anemia (hemoglobin 6.5 g/dl), a gamma spike of 4.1 g, leukocytes 3,800, and 43.5% plasma cells in peripheral blood. Though cyclophosphamide was given intravenously, the monoclonal protein increased, hypercalcemia and renal insufficiency developed, and a pathologic fracture of the humerus occurred.

NONSECRETORY MYELOMA

Occasionally in well-documented cases of myeloma no detectable monoclonal protein can be identified in either the serum or the urine; and as an entity, this condition has been designated "nonsecretory" myeloma (Hurez et al., 1970; Azar et al., 1972). Yet in some cases, monoclonal proteins have been identified within the plasma cell itself. The presence of a single type of light chain in the plasma cells confirms the impression that the protein is synthesized but fails to be secreted (Arend and Adamson, 1974). In other cases no evidence of a monoclonal protein can be seen within the plasma cell, suggesting the absence of synthesis of a monoclonal protein (Gach et al., 1971; Indiveri et al., 1974). Stein and Kaiserling (1974) described a patient who secreted a monoclonal IgG protein but also had an excess of 7S IgM that was not secreted from the cell. It was assumed that the IgM was on the cell surface and that the plasma cell had just switched from IgM to IgG synthesis.

In one case of multiple myeloma, no monoclonal protein could be detected in either the serum or the urine. Immunofluorescence revealed kappa chains in the majority of the marrow plasma cells. Melphalan and prednisone produced a remission. Three years later, at relapse, no monoclonal protein was detected in the serum or urine but immunofluorescence revealed IgG and kappa in the plasma cells (Stites and Whitehouse, 1975). Presumably this patient had begun to produce IgG κ monoclonal protein during the relapse.

Patients with nonsecretory myeloma may have a better prognosis than those with ordinary myeloma. Five patients without a monoclonal protein in either the serum or the urine responded well to chemotherapy and had a longer survival than expected (Kim et al., 1972). Approximately 1% of patients with multiple myeloma do not have a demonstrable monoclonal protein in the serum or the urine (Osserman and Takatsuki, 1963).

IgD MYELOMA

IgD myeloma differs enough in a number of respects from IgG and IgA myeloma to warrant discussion as a separate entity. Since the discovery of IgD immunoglobulin in 1965 (Rowe and Fahey), more than 130 cases of IgD myeloma have been reported (Jancelewicz et al., 1975). Initially the small size of the monoclonal IgD peak, frequency of Bence Jones proteinuria, and renal insufficiency were emphasized (Hobbs et al., 1966). In a review of IgD myeloma Fahey et al. (1968) noted the exceptionally high frequency (80%) of lambda light chains and estimated the incidence of IgD myeloma at about 1% among patients with multiple myeloma. Hobbs and Corbett (1969) in a report of 30 cases emphasized the higher incidence of extraosseous plasmacytomas, osteolytic lesions, and renal failure in IgD myeloma. Fine et al. (1974), in reviewing 60 cases of monoclonal IgD sera, emphasized that the monoclonal protein was not detectable by electrophoresis in 20% of them. They reported that 85% of the IgD monoclonal proteins had Ja antigenic determinants and 15% belonged to the La group. As others have noted, they found a high percentage of lambda (87%) and frequent Bence Jones proteinuria (90+%).

In a comprehensive review of 133 cases of IgD myeloma, including 9 personal cases, Jancelewicz et al. (1975) reported that 76% of the patients were males and the median age was 56 years. This is a somewhat greater incidence among men and perhaps a slightly earlier onset than is usual with multiple myeloma. Hepatosplenomegaly or lymphadenopathy was found in 55% of patients. Extraosseous infiltrates were common, yet symptoms with IgD were similar to those with myeloma of other kinds. Anemia was common, and azotemia was found in two-thirds of the patients.

The concentration of serum monoclonal protein was less than that seen in IgG and IgA myeloma: indeed, 12.5% of Jancelewicz and associates' series had no visible monoclonal component on serum electrophoresis. Bence Jones proteinuria was found in 92% of cases. Plasma-cell leukemia was present in 5%, which is three times the incidence with IgA or IgG myeloma. Amyloidosis was noted in 44% of patients, which is also distinctly more than in myeloma with other classes of heavy chains. The increased incidence (about 80%) of lambda light chains in IgD myeloma may account for some of this, because the incidence of lambda light chains is higher than that of kappa in patients with amyloidosis.

One of our patients with IgD myeloma had most unusual skin lesions. She presented with hypercalcemia and lytic bone lesions. Melphalan and prednisone produced improvement; but 4 months later non-thrombocythemic purpura developed, and it progressed to large infarctions of the skin with epidermal necrosis secondary to obstructive vascular lesions. The necrotic lesions increased in size, covering most of the body; and the patient died.

We have seen 8 of approximately 30 patients with IgD myeloma who also had systemic amyloidosis.

Survival with IgD myeloma is shorter than with other classes. Among 54 patients about whom information was available, the median survival was 9 months, with 60% dying in less than 12 months and only 17% surviving more than 24 months. However, one of our patients with IgD myeloma has done much better. He presented with back pain in January 1965 and was found to have an extradural plasmacytoma at laminectomy 2 months later. No evidence of multiple myeloma was found, and radiation was given. But 6 months later, when the patient returned with chest and back pain, there were lytic lesions in his skull, pelvis, and ribs as well as pathologic fractures of the ribs. Bence Jones proteinuria, lambda type, was present (6.1 g in 24 h). The bone marrow contained 25% plasma cells, and subsequent immunoelectrophoresis of serum revealed an IgD λ monoclonal protein. The patient was treated with continuous low dosages of melphalan, prednisone, and testosterone as well as sodium fluoride, and responded excellently. In February 1975 he was asymptomatic and had no evidence of a monoclonal protein in either serum or urine.

BICLONAL GAMMOPATHIES

In occasional cases, the serum of a patient with multiple myeloma contains two different monoclonal proteins. Most often these are formed by IgG and IgA heavy chains, but IgG and IgM combinations also may be seen (Rosen et al., 1967a). In a series of 870 IgG monoclonal proteins classified according to their subclass, 12 contained biclonal components (Skvaril et al., 1973). IgG1 was present in all the biclonal components. The other proteins were IgG4 in six cases, IgG2 in four and other IgG1 monoclonal proteins in two. In these last two, one patient had different electrophoretic mobilities of the two IgG1 proteins and the other patient had two IgG1 monoclonal proteins of different light-chain types. The high frequency of IgG4 in this group is unexpected because it constitutes only 4 or 5% of normal IgG immunoglobulins and would be expected much less frequently than IgG2.

Detailed studies of serum in macroglobulinemia have revealed biclonal patterns in a number of instances. Harboe et al. (1972) reported that 14% of 90 macroglobulinemia sera contained more than one monoclonal immunoglobulin. A patient with a large amount of IgG monoclonal protein and a smaller amount of IgM protein was described as having symptoms of Waldenström's macroglobulinemia rather than myeloma (McNutt and Fudenberg, 1973). Pruzanski et al. (1974b) had four patients with a monoclonal IgM protein in their serum and also a monoclonal IgA or monoclonal IgG protein. The literature afforded 26 other examples, and a review of the clinical features in the 30 cases disclosed that patients may present with hyperviscosity syndrome and amyloidosis, polyarthritis, or malignant lymphoma, as well as with solitary plasmacytoma, multiple myeloma, or macroglobulinemia.

It has been estimated that approximately 1% of all myeloma sera contained two monoclonal proteins (Bihrer et al., 1974). Although in most cases with IgA and IgG biclonal proteins both monoclonal proteins have the same type of light chain (Fair et al., 1974), different light-chain types also have been found (Bjerrum and Weeke, 1968). Oriol et al. (1974) reported a case of multiple myeloma in which two abnormal bands were seen on electrophoresis. One consisted of an IgG1 κ monoclonal protein and the other an IgG1 λ monoclonal protein. The heavy chains of each monoclonal protein appeared identical because they belonged to the same class and subclass and shared the same allotype, and only one individual antigenic determinant could be detected in both. Wolfenstein-Todel et al. (1974) also reported a case with IgA and IgG biclonal gammopathy in which the two light chains that were of lambda type had similar amino acid composition and could not be distinguished by subtype mapping. Amino acid sequences of the two proteins were identical for the first 30 residues. In another case with biclonal IgA κ and IgM κ, the kappa chains were found to be identical and substantial portions of the α and μ chains also were identical (Seon et al., 1973).

Multiple anomalous immunoglobulins also have been reported. One patient had IgG, IgA, and IgM monoclonal proteins in the serum and Bence Jones protein in the urine (Sanders et al., 1969). Ottó et al. (1972) reported that 3 of their 10 patients with two or more monoclonal proteins had triclonal gammopathies. At present we have one patient with monoclonal IgM κ, IgA κ, and IgG triclonal gammopathy under observation. In another case, both IgG and IgA proteins were in the serum and immunofluorescent studies demonstrated that single plasma cells produced the heavy chains, which indicated that separate proteins were formed in a single neoplastic clone rather than in separate tumors. The light chains of both proteins were of the kappa type (Costea et al., 1967).

CHAPTER XIII

Multiple Myeloma: Course and Prognosis

MULTIPLE MYELOMA runs a progressive course, and most patients die in 1 to 3 years. In a series of 57 cases reported by Kenny and Moloney (1956), 3 survived more than 9 years. Prior to the introduction of effective chemotherapy, median survival ranged from 3.5 to 8.5 months (Feinleib and MacMahon, 1960; Osgood, 1960; Midwest Cooperative Chemotherapy Group, 1964). More recent reports indicate a median survival of 3 to 5 years for *good risk* patients who *respond* to chemotherapy (Alexanian et al., 1972; Costa et al., 1973). Alexanian et al. (1969) reported median survival of 18 months among 104 myeloma patients treated with melphalan alone and 24 months among 79 treated with melphalan and prednisone. In another study the median survival of 23 months in 236 patients with myeloma receiving melphalan, prednisone, and procarbazine was compared with 21 months in 156 patients receiving only melphalan and prednisone (Alexanian et al., 1972).

Follow-up information was obtained in 866 (99.7%) of our 869 cases. Among the 152 patients alive at latest report, 83 had survived more than 3 years since diagnosis and only 4 of them less than 1 year (Table 45). The 717 deaths amount to 82.5% of the series. The median survival was 20 months. At 1 year the anticipated survivorship was 66%, at 3 years 32%, and at 5 years 18% (Table 46; Fig. 49). Autopsy was performed in 54% of deaths.

The causes of death are listed in Table 47. Infection was the most common specific cause, followed next by renal insufficiency. In 44% of cases only multiple myeloma was reported as a cause of death: replies to letters and even death certificates gave this as the only cause. However, we are sure that many of these patients

156

TABLE 45

MULTIPLE MYELOMA: CURRENT STATUS AND FOLLOW-UP
INFORMATION (MAYO CLINIC CASES)

Status			Patients, No. (and %)	
Alive			152	(17.5)
Follow-up period, yr.				
< 1	4	(0.5)		
1-2	38	(4.4)		
2-3	24	(2.8)		
3-5	44	(5.0)		
> 5	39	(4.5)		
No follow-up	3	(0.3)		
Dead			717	(82.5)
Total			869	(100.0)

Modified from Kyle, R. A.: Multiple myeloma: review of 869 cases. *Mayo Clin Proc, 50*:29-40, 1975.

died of septicemia, pneumonia, or renal insufficiency. Bergsagel and Pruzanski (1975) reported that a third of their patients dying of myeloma underwent an acute terminal phase of myeloma characterized by rapidly progressive disease with fever, pancytopenia, and hypercellularity of bone marrow. This may have occurred in some of our patients dying elsewhere. Among our miscellaneous category, two-thirds died from hemorrhage (13 cases), pulmonary embolus (6 cases), and suicide (3 cases).

The great variation in survival—from a few months to more than 5 years—makes prognosis in individual cases a challenge. It

TABLE 46

MULTIPLE MYELOMA: SURVIVORSHIP, PERCENTAGES BY PERIOD
OF DIAGNOSIS (MAYO CLINIC)

Survival Period, Yr.	1960-1964 (N = 327)	1965-1969 (N = 365)	Total* (1960-1971) (N = 869)
1	60	69	66
2	39	50	45
3	25	39	32
5	13	19	18
(Median, mo.)	(18)	(24)	(20)

* Includes 177 cases diagnosed in 1970 and 1971.

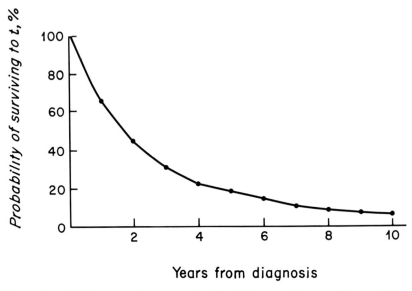

Years from diagnosis

Figure 49. Multiple myeloma: survival in 869 cases diagnosed from 1960-1971.

has been noted that survival in myeloma is longer when the hemoglobin concentration is more than 9 g/dl, the blood urea nitrogen concentration less than 30 mg/dl, the serum calcium concentration less than 12 mg/dl, and the performance status good (Carbone et al., 1967). The Medical Research Council (1973) noted an unfavorable effect on survival in patients with myeloma whose blood urea value was increased and whose hemoglobin and serum albumin concentrations were low. Hoogstraten et al. (1967a) reported that, for 243 patients with myeloma, hypercalcemia and severe azotemia were the best indicators of a poor prognosis. They also noted that hemoglobin less than 9 g/dl, serum calcium greater than 12 mg/dl, blood urea nitrogen (BUN) more than 20 mg/dl, serum albumin less than 3.5 g/dl, and serum globulin more than 7.5 g/dl were findings often associated with poor survival. In a review of 189 patients with myeloma, Costa et al. (1969) reported that hemoglobin concentration, BUN value, clinical performance, proteinuria, serum calcium concentration, and percentage of plasma cells in the marrow were prognos-

TABLE 47

MULTIPLE MYELOMA: CAUSES OF DEATH
(MAYO CLINIC CASES)

Cause	Cases, No. (and %)	
"Myeloma"	232	(44)
Infection	105	(20)
Renal	77	(14)
Cardiac	45	(8)
Stroke	18	(3)
Cachexia	17	(3)
Other malignancy	8	(2)
Miscellaneous	33	(6)
Total	535*	(100)

* Cause was unknown in 182 cases.

Modified from Kyle, R. A.: Multiple myeloma: review of 869 patients. *Mayo Clin Proc, 50:*29-40, 1975.

tically important. Others have emphasized a poorer prognosis with elevated blood urea (Dawson and Ogston, 1971).

Despite their abundance and variety, the morphologic aberrations have virtually no prognostic implications. Before the era of chemotherapy, a study (Bayrd, 1948) showed that survival has a relationship to the degree of differentiation of the myeloma cells. Of the seven patients with most differentiation, four were living 2 to 6 years after diagnosis and three had survived $3\frac{1}{2}$ to nearly 6 years before death. Conversely, none of the 10 patients in the poorly differentiated class survived a year. In a recent study of long-term survivors (> 5 years), we classified the condition of their bone marrows generally as favorable. Although we have found some reason to believe that morphologically recognizable intrinsic differences of malignancy in myeloma patients can affect survival, we still have not learned how response to specific therapy can be predicted.

LINEAR DISCRIMINANT ANALYSIS

The above-mentioned reports describe the effect of individual factors and do not consider the simultaneous effect of multiple parameters in prognosis. Because the several prognostic factors are generally correlated with each other, multivariant analysis is necessary to assess them adequately. We have utilized linear discriminant analysis in an attempt to arrive at a schema of prognostic scoring.

We studied the records of all our patients with the diagnosis of multiple myeloma who had had all laboratory parameters measured initially and who had been followed up until death or for at least 2 years. They were divided into two groups: those who died within 2 years and those who survived for 2 years or longer. Linear discriminant analysis programs (BMD 07M and BMD 04M) were used to discriminate between these two groups. The variables included were the following: initial serum creatinine, serum calcium, serum albumin, abnormal serum globulin peak, hemoglobin, leukocyte count, palpability of liver or spleen, presence of pain, and age. Data for all of these variables were

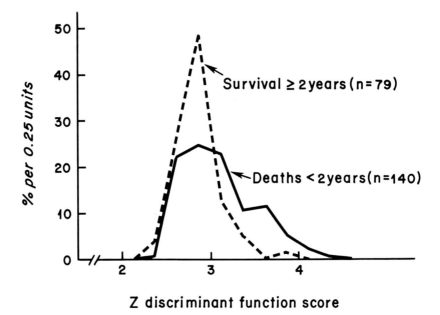

Z discriminant function score
for creatinine, calcium, liver and age

Figure 50. Distributions of discriminant function scores for 2-year survivors and non-survivors (serum creatinine, serum calcium, liver palpability, and age).

obtained within 1 month of the diagnosis of multiple myeloma in 219 cases.

In the stepwise discriminant procedure (BMD 07M) the significant variables at the first step were serum creatinine, serum calcium, liver palpability, hemoglobin level, and leukocyte level. After creatinine had been selected, both hemoglobin and leukocytes dropped out as significant variables, because of their correlation with creatinine. After calcium and liver had been selected, age made the only significant contribution. At no point in the stepwise discriminant procedure did the size of the serum globulin peak approach significance.

The linear discriminant score (Z) was determined for each patient with the BMD 04M program.

$Z = .05234 \times$ creatinine $+ .16229 \times$ calcium $+ .31898 \times$ liver $+ .01347 \times$ age. The distributions of patients who died within 2 years and those who survived 2 years show almost complete overlap (Fig. 50). If we chose to classify all patients with a $Z \geq 3$ as dead, 53% of the dead and 81% of the survivors—or 61% of the total—would be classified correctly. Of the 89 patients classified as dead, 15 (17%) were actually 2-year survivors. Among the 130 classified as survivors, 66 (51%) actually died within 2 years.

Both the classification by survivorship at 2 years and the discriminant classification rule discussed above are quite arbitrary. The method serves to identify the important variables, but the distribution of discriminant scores, with 95% of the 219 patients falling within the overlap, indicates the great importance of

TABLE 48

MULTIPLE MYELOMA: MEAN VALUES FOR FIVE VARIABLES IN 2-YEAR
SURVIVORS AND NON-SURVIVORS (MAYO CLINIC CASES)

Parameter	Dead (N = 140)	Alive (N = 79)
Serum creatinine, mg/dl	2.9	1.4*
Serum calcium, mg/dl	10.3	9.6*
Hemoglobin, g/dl	10.4	11.2*
Serum albumin, g/dl	2.9	2.9
Serum globulin peak, g/dl	3.6	3.5

* $P < 0.05$.

variables not included among the 10 used in the stepwise procedure.

Mean values of several parameters for patients who died in less than 2 years and those who survived for 2 years or longer are given in Table 48. Serum creatinine, calcium, and hemoglobin levels differed significantly between the surviving and non-surviving groups. Interestingly, the size of the serum globulin peak and the serum albumin values did not differ between the groups and were not helpful in prognosis.

An additional 170 patients were eligible for the discriminant analysis except that urea rather than creatinine had been measured. By converting both creatinine and urea to relative values about the appropriate sex-specific regression on age for healthy persons, we were able to consider creatinine and urea as a single variable (CU) indicative of renal function. The second analysis then was based on 389 patients (162 who survived 2 years and 227 who did not). The four variables (urea or creatinine, calcium, hemoglobin, and age) plus serum albumin were selected for discrimination; and thus the results were similar to those from the group with only creatinine levels available.

Discriminant analysis of patients with IgG and IgA myeloma, using the variables listed above, showed no significant differences in correctly classifying the deaths and the survivors.

Table 49 summarizes the joint distribution of initial serum creatinine and calcium values from the patients who died within 2 years and from those who survived. Calcium values were less than 10 mg/dl and creatinine values less than 2 mg/dl in 46% of those who died and 70% of those who survived. But with initial creatinine values of 4 mg/dl or more, only 2 of 28 patients survived 2 years; and with initial creatinine of 2.0 mg/dl or more, only 6 of 61 survived 2 years. And with initial serum calcium of 12 mg/dl or more, only 2 of 23 lived 2 years.

Renal Insufficiency: All patients with multiple myeloma whose creatinine or urea was measured initially were divided into two groups on the basis of normal renal function or insufficiency (creatinine greater than 1.2 mg/dl for males and greater than 0.9 mg/dl for females, or blood urea greather than 50 mg/dl for both

TABLE 49

MULTIPLE MYELOMA: JOINT PERCENTAGE DISTRIBUTION OF INITIAL
SERUM CALCIUM AND CREATININE VALUES FROM 79 PATIENTS WHO
SURVIVED 2 YEARS AND 140 WHO DIED (MAYO CLINIC CASES)

| Creatinine, mg/dl | | Calcium, mg/dl | | | | Total |
		< 10	10-11.9	12-13.9	≥ 14	
< 2	S	70	21		1	92
	D	46	12	1	2	61
2-3.9	S	1	3	1	1	6
	D	5	6	6	2	19
4-5.9	S	1				1
	D	1	4	1		6
6-9.9	S					
	D	5	2	1	1	9
≥ 10	S	1				1
	D	3	1	1		5
Total	S	73	24	1	2	100
	D	60	25	10	5	100

S = Surviving at 2 years.
D = Dead at 2 years.

TABLE 50

MULTIPLE MYELOMA: SERUM CALCIUM AND CREATININE (WITHIN
1 MONTH OF DIAGNOSIS) AND FREQUENCY OF BENCE JONES
PROTEINURIA IN RENAL INSUFFICIENCY AND WITH NORMAL RENAL
FUNCTION (MAYO CLINIC CASES)

| Parameters | Renal Function | |
	Insufficiency	Normal
Serum calcium, mg/dl	(N = 266)	(N = 327)
Mean	10.7	9.5
≥ 10.5	39%	10%
≥ 12.0	24%	1%
Bence Jones protein	(N = 299)	(N = 317)
Positive	58%	43%
Urine, monoclonal protein	(N = 80)	(N = 79)
Kappa	54%	63%
Lambda	46%	37%
Serum creatinine, mg/dl	(N = 225)	(N = 182)
Mean	3.5	0.9
> 1.3	80%	0%
> 2.0	50%	0%

males and females). The number of patients is greater than those utilized in the discriminant function determinations because all parameters had to be measured for the latter studies.

The mean of initial serum calcium values from 266 patients with renal insufficiency was significantly higher than that from the 327 patients with normal renal function (10.7 vs. 9.5 mg/dl; $P < 0.01$) (Table 50). Hypercalcemia with > 10.5 mg/dl of calcium was found in 39% of those with renal insufficiency but only 10% of those with normal renal function, and with 12 mg/dl or more of calcium in 24% of those with renal insufficiency but only 1% of those with normal renal function. Bence Jones proteinuria was revealed (by heat test) in 58% of patients with renal insufficiency and 43% of those with normal renal function. This is of borderline significance.

Of the patients with renal insufficiency, 80 had a monoclonal light chain in the urine—kappa in 54% and lambda in 46%. Of the patients with normal renal function, 79 had a monoclonal light chain in the urine, which was kappa in 63% (Table 50). Hence the presence of a single light chain class was not associated with an excessive incidence of renal insufficiency.

Kappa and Lambda Light Chains in Urine: The 64 patients with kappa monoclonal protein in the urine and those with lambda did not differ significantly in mean creatinine values or in

TABLE 51

MULTIPLE MYELOMA: SERUM CREATININE AND URINARY GLOBULIN
WITHIN ONE MONTH OF DIAGNOSIS IN PATIENTS WITH
MONOCLONAL LIGHT CHAINS IN URINE
(MAYO CLINIC CASES)

Parameters	Urinary Protein	
	Kappa	Lambda
Serum creatinine, mg/dl	(N = 64)	(N = 55)
Mean	1.9	2.3
≥ 2.0	20%	29%
Urinary globulin, g/24 h	(N = 60)	(N = 53)
Mean	3.8	4.2
≥ 2.0	45%	55%
≥ 4	32%	32%
≥ 6	20%	25%
≥ 10	10%	11%

amount of urinary globulin excretion (Table 51). Serum creatinine was 2 mg/dl or more in 20% of the 64 patients with a kappa monoclonal protein in the urine and in 29% of the 55 with a lambda monoclonal protein. We found no evidence that monoclonal lambda protein was significantly more nephrotoxic than kappa.

SURVIVORSHIP

In our study the actuarial method was used to determine survivorship (Elveback, 1958). Survival time was measured in months from the date of diagnosis to the date of death or latest follow-up. Survival in cases diagnosed during the first 5 years of the study (1960-1964) was compared with that in cases diagnosed in the next 5 years (1965-1969) (Fig. 51). The second group had significantly better 3-year survivorship ($P < 0.01$) and a slightly better 5-year survivorship. Median survival was 18 months in the first group, 24 months in the second, and 20 months in the entire

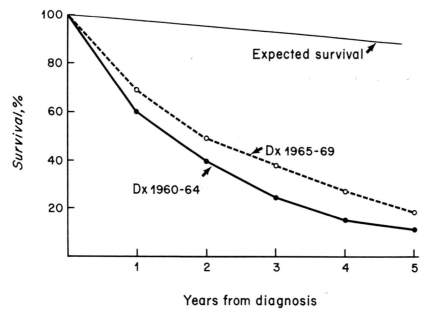

Figure 51. Multiple myeloma: survival in 327 cases diagnosed 1960-1964 and in 365 cases diagnosed 1965-1969, with survival normally expected. At 3 years, survival of later group was significantly better ($P < 0.01$).

series. This modest improvement in survival during the second
5-year period may reflect improved chemotherapy as well as earlier diagnosis and improvement in supportive care.

Whether the prognosis is related to the type of immunoglobulin abnormality is not clear. A report that patients producing
only the lambda type of Bence Jones protein did not respond to
melphalan, whereas those producing only kappa Bence Jones proteins did respond (Bergsagel et al., 1965), was later refuted (Lee
et al., 1965; Osserman, 1965b). It has been said that patients with
lambda light chains had briefer survival than those with kappa
light chains and that those producing only Bence Jones proteins
survived for the shortest period (Alexanian et al., 1969). And in
a reported study (Cooperative Study by Acute Leukemia Group
B, 1975), patients with lambda Bence Jones proteins did not survive as long as those with kappa. Hansen and associates (1973)
reported a median survival with IgA myeloma of 15 months as
compared to 37 months with IgG myeloma.

However, Murphy and Deodhar (1973) reported that survival
of myeloma patients with IgA monoclonal proteins was greater
than that for IgG (27 versus 20 months). Carbone and associates
(1967) found no differences of survival on the basis of immunologic types of protein; Hobbs (1969a) noted no difference in
survival of patients producing IgG or IgA monoclonal proteins.
Bernard et al. (1974) reported median survival of 33 months
with IgG myeloma, 31 months with IgA myeloma, and 23 months
with Bence Jones myeloma. Their patients with renal insufficiency had a median survival of 12.5 months. Median survival of
their group responding to chemotherapy was considerably longer
than that of the entire series.

We found no significant difference in survival of patients with
IgG myeloma and those with IgA myeloma (Fig. 52), nor of
those with monoclonal light chains of either kappa or lambda
type in the urine and those without (Table 52). Three-year survival was 47% among our patients with IgG κ myeloma and 27%
among those with IgA λ myeloma; but the significance of this
difference is borderline because the number of cases is small. Median survival was 31 months with IgG myeloma and 28 months

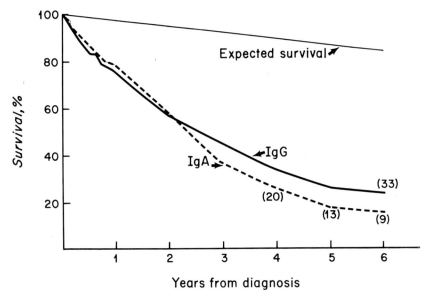

Figure 52. Multiple myeloma: survival in 308 IgG cases and in 123 IgA cases, with survival normally expected. Difference between myeloma groups was not significant. In parentheses are numbers of patients alive and under observation at times plotted.

TABLE 52

MULTIPLE MYELOMA: SURVIVORSHIP BY IMMUNOGLOBULIN TYPE
(MAYO CLINIC CASES)

Protein	*No. Pts.*	*1 Yr.*	*% Surviving at* *3 Yr.*	*5 Yr.*	*Median* *Survival*
IgG κ	223	77	47	27	
λ	85	73	39	25	31 mo.
Total	308*	76	45	26	
IgA κ	79	84	40	20	
λ	44	70	27	16	28 mo.
Total	123*	79	36	18	
Urinary light chains (κ or λ) of patients with IgG or IgA in serum	95	82	43	18	

* Not including patients with IgG and IgA whose light chains were not typed.

with IgA myeloma. This difference is not significant. These median survivals are greater than those for our overall group, but immunologic typing was not done in the early part of this study when survival was shorter.

The rate of response to chemotherapy also appears to affect survival. Hansen et al. (1973) reported that those patients whose monoclonal serum protein decreased by 0.6 g/dl or more within 2 months of institution of therapy had a median survival of 13 months, whereas those who responded slowly had a median of 62 months. It appears that prognosis is poorer in patients who respond to treatment rapidly, and this most likely is due to greater activity of the tumor.

Kiang and associates (1974) evaluated 138 patients with mul-

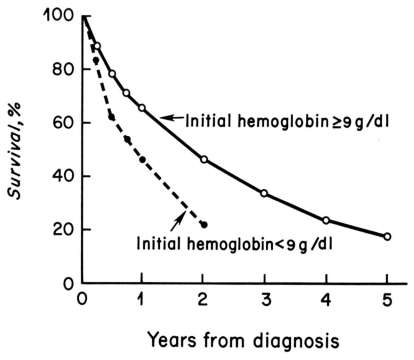

Years from diagnosis

Figure 53. Multiple myeloma: survival in 116 cases with initial hemoglobin < 9 g/dl and in 625 cases with 9+ g. Difference at 6 months was significant (*P* < 0.01).

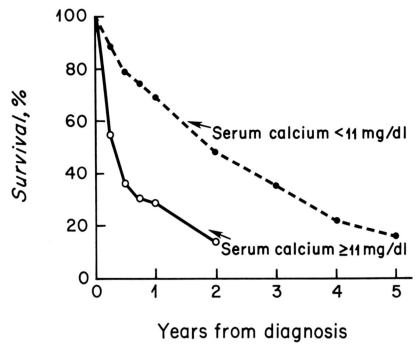

Figure 54. Multiple myeloma: survival in 114 cases with initial serum calcium $\geq$ 11 mg/dl and in 497 cases with less. Difference at 6 months was significant (P $<$ 0.01).

tiple myeloma by means of multiple regression analysis. They found that the sequence of importance of the nine most significant factors was as follows: hemoglobin concentration, age, serum calcium concentration, sex, plasma-cell morphology, Bence Jones protein, serum albumin concentration, BUN value, and presence of osteolytic lesions.

Gompels et al. (1972) reported that myeloma patients whose roentgenographic appearance was normal had a poorer prognosis than those with osteoporosis or circumscribed lytic lesions.

In an attempt to classify myeloma patients on the basis of extent of their disease, Salmon and Durie (1975) analyzed 85 cases and divided them into three categories based on myeloma cell mass. Those patients with a large cell mass ($> 1.2 \times 10^{12}/\text{m}^2$) had

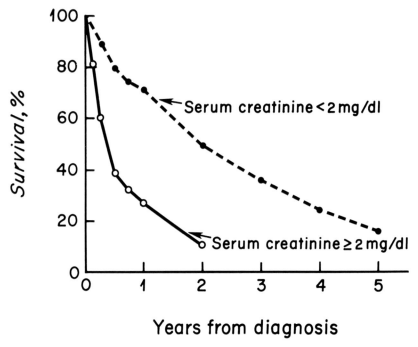

Years from diagnosis

Figure 55. Multiple myeloma: survival in 269 cases with initial serum creatinine < 2 mg/dl and in 120 cases with 2+ mg. Difference at 6 months was significant ($P < 0.01$).

at least one of the following: hemoglobin < 8.5 g/dl, serum calcium levels > 12 mg/dl, IgG monoclonal component > 7 g/dl, IgA > 5 g/dl, Bence Jones proteinuria > 12 g/day, or advanced lytic bone lesions. Those with the low cell mass ($< 0.6 \times 10^{12}/m^2$) had all of the following characteristics: hemoglobin > 10.5 g/dl; serum calcium normal; serum IgG monoclonal component < 5 g/dl or IgA < 3 g/dl or Bence Jones proteinuria < 4 g/day; and no lytic lesions on a skeletal survey. Those patients whose cell mass was between the limits specified were included as intermediate.

Six-month survivorship was significantly less ($P < 0.01$) among our patients if, at diagnosis, the hemoglobin value was less than 9 g/dl, calcium 11 mg/dl or more, or creatinine 2 mg/dl or more (Figs. 53, 54, and 55; Table 53).

In occasional instances, myeloma may progress rapidly after

TABLE 53

MULTIPLE MYELOMA: SURVIVORSHIP BY INITIAL VALUES FOR
HEMOGLOBIN, SERUM CALCIUM, OR SERUM CREATININE
(MAYO CLINIC CASES)

Parameter	No. Pts.	% Surviving at		
		6 Mo.	1 Yr.	2 Yr.
Hemoglobin, g/dl				
≥ 9	625	75*	66	47
< 9	116	58*	47	22
Calcium, mg/dl				
≥ 11	114	36*	29	14
< 11	497	79*	69	48
Creatinine, mg/dl				
≥ 2	120	39*	27	11
< 2	269	79*	71	49

* $P < 0.01$.

several years of little change in the myeloma protein peak or in
the plasma cells of the bone marrow (Stevens, 1965). The patient with plasma-cell leukemia or multiple myeloma has a poorer
prognosis than the patient with a solitary lesion, the shorter
course reflecting the greater generalized involvement.

CHAPTER XIV

Multiple Myeloma: Therapy

MOST PATIENTS WITH multiple myeloma have symptoms or laboratory evidence of significant disease at the time of diagnosis and clearly need to be treated (Kyle, 1973). But some patients have no symptoms and only moderate laboratory abnormalities, and in these cases it may be difficult to distinguish multiple myeloma from benign monoclonal gammopathy (see page 286). This presents a dilemma to the clinician, because the greater the myeloma cell mass in a patient, the less likely a satisfactory response to chemotherapy. Conversely, if the patient is tolerating his disease well, one does not wish to burden him with the inconvenience, expense, and possible untoward side effects of chemotherapy. Furthermore, it conceivably could increase the activity of the myeloma. Hobbs (1975) reported a case in which a monoclonal gammopathy remained static for 5 years while it was untreated but then, when cytotoxic drugs were given, the protein abnormality increased and the patient showed clear evidence of rapidly advancing malignancy.

We believe that patients in whom it is difficult to distinguish between multiple myeloma and benign monoclonal gammopathy and those who have a low-grade, smoldering, or indolent myeloma should be reevaluated at 3- to 6-month intervals without therapy. Conklin and Alexanian (1975) noted that 3% of their myeloma cases had an indolent course. If clinical and laboratory examinations show no progression of the disease, continued observation with repeated evaluation is indicated. We have followed up one patient without therapy for more than 10 years. In this case, an unequivocal diagnosis of myeloma had been made on the basis of bone-marrow morphology and a monoclonal serum protein concentration of 3 g/dl; but these findings have not changed and other features of myeloma have not developed during the 10-year observation period.

Irradiation: Ionizing radiation is a valuable agent for local therapy (Mill, 1975). For a solitary plasmacytoma or localized extramedullary plasmacytoma, the preferred treatment is a tumoricidal dose of 4,000 to 5,000 rads. In multiple myeloma, since it is generalized at the time of diagnosis, radiation therapy should not be used unless pain is severe and localized. Palliative irradiation in a dosage of 2,000 to 2,500 R is usually effective. If patients with multiple myeloma are to be irradiated, it is best to complete the palliative radiation therapy 3 weeks before starting chemotherapy; leukocyte and platelet counts should be repeated at that time because the myelosuppressive effects of radiation therapy and chemotherapy are cumulative.

But although radiation therapy effectively relieves pain in most instances, the patient frequently returns in a short time with pain elsewhere. Radiation therapy may be repeated, but is ultimately limited by the development of leukopenia or thrombocytopenia, which in turn restricts the use of chemotherapy. Thus, irradiation in multiple myeloma is adjunctive and limited, and it should be used only for discrete lesions.

Surgery: The usefulness of surgery in treatment for a solitary myeloma is doubtful. There is no proof that surgical extirpation of this lesion can cure any better than tumoricidal radiation; instead there is every reason to believe that in many patients the disease eventually will become disseminated anyway. However, in patients with acute extradural cord compression, surgery may be a critical factor (see page 191). Surgical biopsy may be necessary for the diagnosis of a solitary or extramedullary plasmacytoma, although needle biopsy sometimes is sufficient.

CHEMOTHERAPY

We believe that chemotherapy is the best initial treatment for generalized myeloma, unless there is disabling pain which is clearly the result of a well-defined focal process. If analgesics together with chemotherapy can control the pain, chemotherapy is preferred to repeated local irradiation because the bone-marrow reserve of many myeloma patients is limited and irradiation does not benefit systemic disease.

Alkylating Agents. *Melphalan:* Melphalan (L-phenylalanine mustard, L-sarcolysin, Alkeran) is an alkylating agent with an active nitrogen mustard radical attached to the amino acid, L-phenylalanine (Fig. 56). Synthesized in 1953 and introduced 5 years later (Blokhin et al., 1958), melphalan has become well established in chemotherapy for multiple myeloma (Bergsagel et al., 1962; Brook et al., 1964; Speed et al., 1964; Hoogstraten et al., 1967b; Alexanian et al., 1968). Good results have been obtained with intermittent courses (Alexanian et al., 1972).

At present, we consider melphalan the drug of choice in treatment for myeloma (Kyle, 1973). We prefer to give it intermittently because the benefits seem to be equivalent to those obtained with the daily oral schedule and fewer blood counts and patient visits are necessary to maintain it. We give 0.15 mg/kg orally each day for 7 days. This is equivalent to 8 to 10 mg daily, or a total dose of 56 to 70 mg for an average-sized person. The addition of prednisone in a dosage of 15 mg 4 times daily for the same period of 7 days increases the favorable response to approximately 70% of patients. While prednisone is being given, the patient should have a bland diet and take antacids. The patient is reevaluated at 6-week intervals for consideration of successive 7-day courses of melphalan and prednisone. Leukocyte and platelet counts must be obtained prior to therapy, as leukopenia and thrombocytopenia commonly occur.

The subsequent courses of melphalan may need to be altered: If the leukocyte and platelet counts have not decreased, the daily dose of melphalan may be increased by 2 mg daily for the next 7-day course; whereas if the counts have decreased, the dose of melphalan should be lessened accordingly. Renal insufficiency may be an indication for using a smaller dose and being cautious,

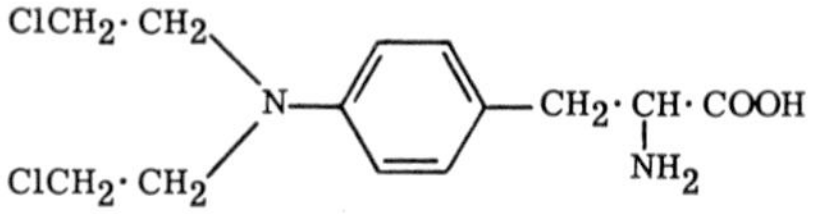

$$ClCH_2 \cdot CH_2 \diagdown N \diagup \text{—} \diagup ClCH_2 \cdot CH_2 \diagup \bigcirc \text{—} CH_2 \cdot \underset{NH_2}{CH} \cdot COOH$$

Figure 56. Structural formula of melphalan (Alkeran®).

for melphalan is excreted by the kidneys. However, we have not been impressed with excessive hematologic toxicity of melphalan in the presence of significant degrees of renal insufficiency. The dose of prednisone ordinarily would not be altered unless the patient has an active peptic ulcer, severe hypertension, or uncontrolled diabetes. Occasionally a patient has withdrawal symptoms; if so, we reduce the prednisone to 0 over a period of 4 to 5 days rather than stop it abruptly at the end of the 7-day course.

The patient should be given at least three 7-day courses before this schedule is abandoned, unless therapy causes significant toxic reactions or the disease progresses rapidly in spite of clearly adequate therapy. Maximal improvement may not be achieved for several months. If there is a response, courses of melphalan and prednisone should be repeated indefinitely at 6-week intervals. Although a recent report indicated that maintenance chemotherapy following good response made no difference in the frequency of relapse, duration of remission, or survival (Southwest Oncology Group Study, 1975), we would recommend continued chemotherapy until this finding is confirmed.

Two other melphalan schedules have been employed. In one, the drug can be given in a loading dose, together with prednisone, as described above. After 6 weeks, the leukocyte and platelet counts are determined; and then melphalan is given orally in a daily dose of 0.05 mg/kg according to hematologic tolerance (Costa et al., 1973). Leukocyte and platelet counts must be done at approximately 2-week intervals during the daily program and the dose of melphalan adjusted to keep the leukocytes between 3,000 and 4,000/mm^3 and the platelets between 100,000 and 150,000. The other schedule involves the administration of 6 to 10 mg daily for the first 8 to 10 days (adjusted to the patient's weight and hematologic status) and then continuous maintenance therapy, usually 2 mg daily, started immediately after completion of the loading dose (Farhangi and Osserman, 1973). Others have also reported satisfactory results with daily oral administration of melphalan (McArthur et al., 1970; Brook et al., 1973). It should be continued for at least 4 months before discontinuance unless toxic reactions are severe or the disease progresses.

Both daily oral and intermittent therapy have advocates, a situation suggesting that the value of the schedule may be a reflection of the diligence and care taken in its use (Alexanian et al., 1969; Hoogstraten et al., 1969; George et al., 1972). It is likely that the therapeutic response to the intermittent and daily oral melphalan schedules is not significantly different.

The major *side effect* of melphalan therapy is hematologic; that is, bone-marrow suppression. Nausea, vomiting, pruritus, and skin rash, which develop occasionally, are seldom significant. Pulmonary fibrosis has been reported in a single instance (Codling and Chakera, 1972).

Cyclophosphamide: If there is no response to melphalan, or if the patient responds to it and then becomes resistant, cyclophosphamide (Cytoxan) may be effective. Cyclophosphamide is an alkylating agent, a cyclic phosphoric acid ester derivative of nitrogen mustard (Fig. 57). It may be given intravenously in a dose of 15 mg/kg every 4 weeks. The amount should be adjusted to the leukocyte and platelet counts taken prior to each dose in this regimen. An alternative is oral administration of 100 to 150 mg (2 mg/kg body weight) daily for long periods, which has brought improvement in at least 25% of patients with myeloma (Korst et al., 1964). Because leukopenia and thrombocytopenia occur frequently, the dose is adjusted according to the leukocyte and platelet counts, which should be determined every 1 to 3 weeks.

Bergsagel et al. (1972) reported good or partial responses to intermittent intravenous administration of large doses of cyclophosphamide in 11 of 19 myeloma patients who had developed resistance to melphalan. Our experience with intravenous administration of cyclophosphamide in cases of that kind has been less encouraging: Good or limited responses were obtained in only 16 of 38 (Kyle et al., 1975c). A number of factors—including

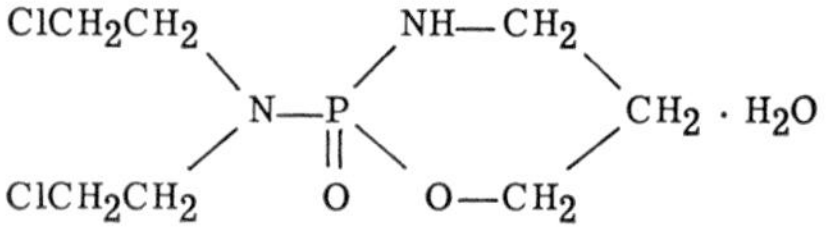

$$ClCH_2CH_2 \diagdown \diagup NH\!-\!CH_2 \diagdown$$
$$N\!-\!P \diagup \diagdown CH_2 \cdot H_2O$$
$$ClCH_2CH_2 \diagup \overset{||}{O} \diagdown O\!-\!CH_2 \diagup$$

Figure 57. Structural formula of cyclophosphamide (Cytoxan®).

smaller doses of cyclophosphamide in our patients, the difficulties in defining resistance to melphalan, and evaluation of response—make direct comparison of series difficult. In addition to leukopenia and thrombocytopenia, *side effects* of cyclophosphamide include nausea, alopecia, hemorrhagic cystitis, urinary-bladder fibrosis (Johnson and Meadows, 1971), carcinoma of the urinary bladder (Wall and Clausen, 1975), and depression of ovarian (Warne et al., 1973) or testicular function (Fairley et al., 1972).

In two separate studies the survival of patients treated with melphalan and others treated with cyclophosphamide has not differed appreciably (Rivers and Patno, 1969; Medical Research Council, 1971).

BCNU: BCNU (1,3-bis[2-chloroethyl]-1-nitrosourea) has proved to be beneficial and appears to be almost as effective as melphalan (Acute Leukemia Group B, unpublished data); but it is not yet available for general use. This drug is given intravenously every 6 weeks, and the patient needs to be seen only at 6-week intervals. Its major side effects include nausea, vomiting, and bone-marrow depression.

Complications With Use of Alkylating Agents: Rapidly fatal *acute myelomonocytic leukemia* has developed in more than 35 patients with multiple myeloma who were treated with an alkylating agent for 15 to 108 months (Andersen and Videbaek, 1970; Kyle et al., 1970c, 1975b). Most of them had been given melphalan, usually on a daily schedule; but some received it intermittently and a few received cyclophosphamide or radiation. No predominance of IgG or IgA monoclonal proteins was noted. More kappa light chains than expected were found, but this is of questionable significance. Evidence favoring acute myelomonocytic rather than plasma-cell leukemia includes the appearance of the leukemic cells (Fig. 58), the increase in plasma muramidase concentration, and the minimal evidence of myeloma at autopsy.

Is the development of acute leukemia analogous to that of polycythemia vera, in which it is unclear whether the increased incidence of acute leukemia is due to therapy with radioactive phosphorus or to the natural course of the disease? A case of

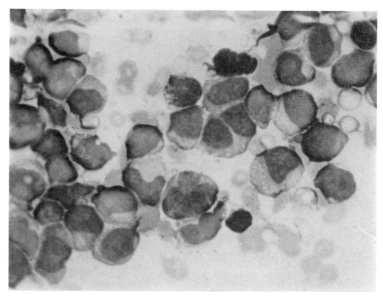

Figure 58. Bone-marrow aspirate showing monocytoid myeloblasts. (Wright's stain; ×1,000.) (From Kyle, R. A., Pierre, R. V., and Bayrd, E. D.: Multiple myeloma and acute leukemia associated with alkylating agents. *Arch Intern Med, 135*:185-192, 1975. By permission of the American Medical Association.)

acute leukemia and myeloma prompted a retrospective review of 133 patients with acute leukemia and 177 patients with myeloma seen at Malmö, Sweden, between 1951 and 1970. This revealed no other patient with both acute leukemia and multiple myeloma (Marcović et al., 1974). We reviewed our records from 1950 to 1970 and did not find any additional cases of coexistent myeloma and acute leukemia. Karchmer et al. (1974) found 5 cases of myeloma and acute leukemia in a population of 1.2 million persons over a 7-year period, where one would expect to find only 0.17 cases. We believe that the association of acute leukemia and myeloma represents a new finding rather than a previously unrecognized aspect of multiple myeloma.

Not all patients with acute leukemia and myeloma have acute myelocytic or myelomonocytic leukemia. Acute erythroleukemia has been reported in multiple myeloma following therapy with alkylating agents (Cardamone et al., 1974). The development of sideroblastic anemia with ring sideroblasts in the bone marrow may be followed by acute myelomonocytic leukemia (Khaleeli et al., 1973). One of our patients would fit in this group.

The occasional development of acute leukemia has been noted with a number of other diseases treated with chemotherapy. This includes primary amyloidosis (Kyle et al., 1974b), carcinoma of the ovaries (Allan, 1970b; Smit and Meyler, 1970; Kaslow et al., 1972; Greenspan and Tung, 1974), carcinoma of the breast (Davis et al., 1973; Meytes and Katz, 1973; Perlman and Walker, 1973), macroglobulinemia (Forbes, 1972; Petersen, 1973a), chronic lymphocytic leukemia (McPhedran and Heath, 1970; Catovsky and Galton, 1971; Castro et al., 1973a), carcinoma of the lung (Garfield, 1970), scleroderma (Tulliez et al., 1974), and cold agglutinin disease (Stavem and Harboe, 1971). The development of reticulum-cell sarcoma has been reported in patients with myeloma treated with alkylating agents (Holt and Robb-Smith, 1973; Mundy and Baikie, 1973).

Simultaneous multiple myeloma and acute myeloblastic leukemia in patients without previous chemotherapy has been reported (Taddeini and Schrader, 1972; Tursz et al., 1974). We have also seen two similar cases. The acute leukemia was the predominating feature in both and it is difficult to be certain the patients had typical multiple myeloma. In another previously untreated patient, therapy for his acute leukemia was followed by an increase of plasma cells in the marrow, which reached 40%; and osteolytic bone lesions were noted at autopsy (Parker, 1973).

Although the cause of acute leukemia in multiple myeloma is unknown, there are elements in the relationship that should be considered. Radiation could be a contributor in some cases, but this is not likely in the majority.

We believe, however, that the alkylating agents, melphalan and cyclophosphamide, did have a part in the development of acute leukemia in these patients. Alkylating agents damage DNA by cross-linking it during the resting phase, thus producing a radiomimetic effect. The acute granulocytic type of leukemia that developed in these patients is the type that would be expected from radiomimetic agents. Alkylating agents that affect bone marrow directly often produce hypoplasia and may cause mutations resulting in an abnormal clone of leukocytes. In mouse myeloma cells melphalan has been very effective in producing mutations that cause stable and heritable changes in immunoglobulin production (Preud'homme et al., 1973). Immunosuppression from these alkylating agents might be regarded as a factor because the incidence of neoplasms (though not of acute leukemia) has been increased in recipients of organ transplants who have been treated with immunosuppressive drugs (Penn et al., 1971; Schneck and Penn, 1971). Cyclophosphamide is a well-known immunosuppressive agent, and melphalan also has this power in both mouse and man (Santos, 1967). Rosner and Grünwald (1974) noted that only three of their patients with myeloma terminating in acute leukemia had not received melphalan.

Although development of acute leukemia in myeloma is probably related to the alkylating agent, it happens rarely (incidence $< 1\%$) and only after a significant period of treatment. During this time the patient is often in a remission which he otherwise would not have had. The median survival for patients with myeloma treated with a placebo is 12 months (Holland et al., 1966), as compared to the median survival of 53 months for good-risk patients who respond to melphalan and prednisone (Costa et al., 1973). Obviously the period of more than 4 years during which melphalan-treated patients with myeloma are relatively symptom-free can hardly be compared to a survival period of only 1 year with increasing disability for the untreated patients. There can be little question that the treatment of myeloma with alkylating agents is justified, despite the small risk of acute leukemia.

The possibility of *clonal mutation* as a complication of therapy with alkylating agents was raised by Hobbs (1972), who reported that during relapse from an initial response to treatment with cyclophosphamide or melphalan the tumor growth pattern changed in 45% of 155 patients. This usually resulted in faster growth, and in many instances Bence Jones proteinuria developed or a new monoclonal protein emerged. Hobbs believed that the chemotherapy, which alters DNA, may have induced mutation;

and he concluded that cytotoxic agents were best reserved for otherwise fatal diseases.

Appearance of a second monoclonal protein, representing a different clone and thus suggesting mutation, has been reported in two most unusual cases. In one, the patient had an IgD λ protein in the serum and a λ monoclonal protein in the urine. During several months of treatment with cyclophosphamide the IgD λ protein disappeared and an IgG1 κ monoclonal protein appeared. Later the IgD λ protein recurred while the IgG κ protein persisted (Oxelius, 1971). The report of the other case (Spengler et al., 1972), though it did not mention chemotherapy, reinforces the likelihood of mutation. The patient had a monoclonal IgG4 κ protein, and 5 years later had an IgG λ protein also (biclonal gammopathy suggesting development of a second malignant clone of plasma cells), and then the next year developed a symptomatic myeloma with increase of the IgG1 λ protein but disappearance of the IgG4 κ.

Different Chemotherapeutic Agents. *Urethan:* First reported to be of benefit by Alwall in 1947, urethan was the only chemotherapeutic agent for several years. Subsequent results have been less impressive than the first, and one controlled study showed that orally administered urethan was not superior to placebo therapy statistically and that in patients treated with urethan the survival was actually shorter (Holland et al., 1966). However, there is no doubt that occasional patients did respond to urethan. Urethan given intravenously may be of some benefit, but the results are not impressive and the toxic effects are significant (Seibert et al., 1966).

Other: Other agents include tryptophan mustard (Kyle et al., 1967), 6-thioguanine (Carbone et al., 1964), a combination of 6-thioguanine and azaserine (Hayes et al., 1967), azathioprine (Imuran®) (Southeastern Cancer Study Group, 1975), streptonigrin, procarbazine (Matulane®) (Moon and Edmonson, 1970), mechlorethamine (nitrogen mustard), triethylenemelamine (TEM), 6-mercaptopurine, chlorambucil (Southeastern Cancer Study Group, 1975), and aniline mustard (Kyle et al., 1973a). Although possessing some activity, these agents are inferior to either melphalan or cyclophosphamide. Adriamycin has been used in a few cases of multiple myeloma but has not produced encouraging results, at least as a single agent (O'Bryan et al., 1973). In one study, doses of 25 to 45 mg/m² of adriamycin produced benefit in three of nine patients who had failed to respond to intermittent treatment with melphalan and prednisone. However, bone-marrow suppression was significant and the remissions were short. Perhaps adriamycin may be more useful in combinations with other chemotherapeutic agents than alone (Alberts and Salmon, 1975). A promising new agent of treatment for myeloma is CCNU, which has the additional advantage of oral administration. Prednisone, in a single dose of 200 mg every other morning, was reported to produce benefit in 8 of 10 patients with myeloma and toxic reactions were minimal (Salmon et al., 1967); and it benefits some patients with anemia (Hoogstraten, 1973). In our opinion prednisone used as a single agent is not a major factor in the management of myeloma, and it is best employed as an adjuvant agent.

Combinations of Chemotherapeutic Agents: Combinations of melphalan, cyclophosphamide, BCNU, and prednisone given intermittently produced an impressive response in one group of 20 patients (Harley et al., 1972a); and melphalan, cyclophosphamide, prednisone, BCNU, and vincristine produced a response in 90% of another group of 36 patients (Lee et al., 1974). Azam and Delamore (1974) also reported encouraging preliminary results from giving BCNU, cyclophosphamide, melphalan, and prednisone to myeloma patients who had ceased to respond to single-agent therapy or who had not been treated previously. We have been unable to demonstrate significant benefit in responses from melphalan, BCNU, cyclophosphamide, and prednisone together when compared in a prospective, randomized study with responses to only melphalan and prednisone given orally. However, survival differences may become apparent (Acute Leukemia Group B, unpublished data). Further evaluation of these combinations of drugs is necessary.

The addition of procarbazine to melphalan and prednisone increased the response to 59% from 48%. The survival time of all patients was similar in the two regimens, as was the duration of remission of responding patients. Moderate nausea and skin eruptions were more frequent in the group given procarbazine (Alexanian et al., 1972). Thus this agent adds little to the management of multiple myeloma.

Chemotherapy often produces cytopenia and is usually the cause of low leukocyte and platelet values obtained during its use. However, progressive invasion of the bone marrow by plasma cells may produce pancytopenia; and in such cases a bone marrow aspiration is necessary to distinguish between the effect of chemotherapy and that of bone-marrow invasion by plasma cells.

Criteria for Response: The effects of therapy should be assessed at regular intervals by determining the hemoglobin and serum and urinary protein concentrations, examining the bone marrow, and evaluating skeletal roentgenograms. Favorable response to therapy can be judged by the following criteria: (1) an increase in the hemoglobin concentration by 2.0 g/dl (without transfusion in a period of at least 4 weeks) from an initial value of less than 11.0 g/dl; (2) a decrease in the monoclonal serum protein to 50% or less of the initial value; (3) a decrease in the monoclonal urinary globulin to 50% or less—if the initial value was 1.0 g/24 h or more; (4) a decrease in the number of plasma cells in bone marrow by 50% or more on the basis of repeated marrow aspirations; (5) recalcification of skeletal lesions and absence of new osseous lesions.

Subjective improvement, to be recognized as significant, should reflect an increase of performance by two grades or more on the following scale of activity: patient is (1) normal; (2) ambulatory, has symptoms, but spends less than 50% of waking time in bed; (3) symptomatic and spends more than 50% of waking time in bed; and (4) completely bedridden. The severity of pain may be graded from 0 to 4 (none to incapacitating; again, improvement by two grades to be significant). Increase in the concentration of the normal (uninvolved) immunoglobulin components has been reported as another useful indicator of response (Alexanian and Migliore, 1970). A proposed guideline for protocol studies for myeloma has recently been published by a Committee of the Chronic Leukemia-Myeloma Task Force of the National Cancer Institute (1973).

BASIS FOR NEW APPROACHES

Although significant advances have been made in the therapy of myeloma, new approaches are necessary.

Plasma-Cell Kinetics: Salmon and Smith (1970) determined that the average plasma cell secreted 10 to 20 pg of immunoglobulins per day. Repeated studies have shown that these values are surprisingly constant for individual patients. If a patient's measured or calculated rate of total-body synthesis of monoclonal protein (M-component) is divided by the mean cellular rate, one may estimate the total number of plasma cells in the body.

$$\frac{\text{Total number of}}{\text{myeloma cells}} = \frac{\text{Total body M-component synthetic rate}}{\text{Cellular M-component synthetic rate}}$$

The total body M-component synthetic rate = FCR (fractional catabolic rate × PV (plasma volume) × PPL (serum M-component concentration). It should be appreciated that the patient with an IgG3 subclass has a T$\frac{1}{2}$ of 7 to 8 days compared with 23 days for IgG1, IgG2, and IgG4. One must also allow for the concentration-dependent changes in the fractional catabolic rate, because catabolism is increased when the serum level is increased. A nomogram may be used for the correction of IgG1, IgG2, and IgG4. The fractional catabolic rate of IgG3 is not influenced by concentration.

In patients with clinically diagnosed myeloma the number of myeloma cells in the body is at least 0.2×10^{12} (about 200 g) and usually more than 1×10^{12} (1 kg). A lethal burden of myeloma cells is found to be in the range of 5 to 7% of body weight (assuming that 10^{12} myeloma cells = 1 kg). In individual cases of myeloma, the myeloma cell number does not usually correlate directly with the serum concentration of a monoclonal component, its total body synthetic rate, or its cellular synthetic rate. Patients with large concentrations of monoclonal protein (in the range of 8 g/dl) generally had far-advanced myeloma. The reverse was not true, however, as some myeloma cells had a very low synthetic rate (2 pg/cell per day), producing only small spikes of serum monoclonal protein; but other evidence indicated extensive myeloma. Patients with benign monoclonal gammopathies usually have at least 100 g of plasma cells. Monoclonal proteins cannot be detected by electrophoresis unless the tumor mass exceeds 20 g. In this situation a serum electrophoretic spike of about 0.2 g/dl can be obscured easily by the normal beta or gamma bands.

During the clinical course from "early diagnosis" to death from far-advanced disease, the number of tumor cells was calculated to have doubled approximately four times, indicating a doubling time of 6 months in a patient with a 2-year survival. If clonal doubling had occurred at a constant exponential rate from its initiation, one would calculate, depending on the tumor type, that the tumor had been present from 11 to 33 years before clinical diagnosis (Hobbs, 1969b, 1971).

However, tumor growth is not exponential in animals; and indeed, it slows as the tumor enlarges. This phenomenon can be described with a gompertzian growth equation, which contains terms not only for the growth rate at any given time *(A)*—a function of the number of tumor cells—but also a constant *(a)* that sets the degree of slowing of tumor growth (Sullivan and Salmon, 1972). With the aid of a precise computer program, Salmon (1973) showed that in man myelomas do indeed grow in gompertzian fashion and that the exponential models grossly overestimate the duration of the disease. The tumor grows quickly at first: The initial doubling of the clone of plasma cells occurs at 1 to 3 days. One must remember that in myeloma cells DNA synthesis takes only 12 to 24 hours and the generation time is 48 to 60 hours (Queisser et al., 1973). This rapid initial growth is consistent with observations of transient monoclonal gammopathies following certain infections (see page 33). Although tumor cell proliferation occurs indetectably and asymptomatically at first, probably only 1 to 2 years elapse before diagnosis becomes possible in the usual case.

With a good response to chemotherapy, the number of myeloma cells in the body generally decreases by a factor of 1 to 2 logs.

This regression of the tumor during treatment with melphalan and prednisone may be described with the gompertzian equation. Accordingly, tumor size decreases rapidly at first, then slows and reaches a plateau that may be stable for months or years, even though treatment is continued. One may predict the eventual plateau level of tumor in the body from a series of measurements made during the initial 6 to 8 weeks of treatment, though the plateau may not be reached for more than 6 to 8 months (Salmon, 1973).

Effects of Therapy on Plasma-Cell Kinetics: The labeling index of myeloma cells indicates the fraction of cells in DNA synthesis and provides an estimate of the growth fraction of the cell population. Salmon determined the labeling index of myeloma cells with tritiated thymidine and found that it increased after each course of melphalan and prednisone. By the time the plateau had been reached in 6 to 8 months, the labeling index increased from an initial value of 3% to as high as 30%. Others have noted a sixfold increase in the median labeling index when the myeloma tumor cell mass was reduced by more than 50% (Drewinko et al., 1974). Recently a technique for high-speed scintillation autoradiography (HSARG) has been described that determines the labeling index within 5 hours as compared to the usual period of 6 to 7 days (Durie and Salmon, 1974). Incubation of myeloma cells after chemotherapy revealed a high tritiated thymidine labeling index, indicating that an increased proportion of myeloma cells were proliferating during apparent remission. Treatment of the myeloma cells with S-phase specific agents such as cytosine arabinoside or hydroxyurea before exposure to tritiated thymidine inhibited the thymidine uptake, indicating that prereplication and not repair DNA synthesis is the basic mechanism underlying the high labeling indices. The concentrations of cytosine arabinoside and hydroxyurea that block DNA synthesis by myeloma cells in vitro are in the range attainable in vivo (Alberts and Golde, 1974). Thus S-phase specific agents may be potentially effective in myeloma patients when the tumor-cell labeling index is elevated after successful chemotherapy. Indeed, Salmon (1975) reported further decrease of myeloma tumor cells following vincristine therapy. In another attempt to design a chemotherapeutic program to take advantage of plasma-cell kinetics, 13 patients were treated with methotrexate followed in 16 hours by vincristine, and 24 hours later by melphalan, whose daily administration was continued for 12 days. However, the results were not impressively different from those achieved in 13 other cases by high-dose intermittent administration of melphalan and prednisone (Western Cancer Study Group, 1975).

Other Approaches: Recent work indicates that chloroquine or caffeine inhibits the repair of DNA in cyclophosphamide-resistant plasmacytomas in hamsters, so that these tumors become responsive to cyclophosphamide, nitrogen mustard, or irradiation (Gaudin and Yielding, 1969). This suggests that one mechanism of resistance to alkylating agents may be an enhanced ability to repair the damage they inflict on DNA.

We performed a prospective randomized study to determine the effects of two different therapeutic regimens in 41 patients with multiple myeloma resistant to melphalan. One therapeutic combination was cyclophosphamide plus prednisone, the other cyclophosphamide, prednisone, and chloroquine. Cyclophosphamide was administered in a dosage of 600 mg/m² intravenously every 6 weeks while prednisone was given in a dosage of 0.5 mg/kg daily for 7 days with each course. Chloroquine, 250 mg, was given twice daily for 7 days before the injection of cyclophosphamide and continued for 3 days afterward to provide a maximal tissue level. The patients given chloroquine were encouraged to drink at least 6 cups of tea and coffee or cola drinks daily, while those on the other regimen were told to avoid caffeine. We could detect no difference between the patients randomized to the cyclophosphamide-prednisone-chloroquine regimen and those who received only cyclophosphamide and prednisone (Kyle et al., 1975c).

In another approach, after initial reduction of the tumor-cell burden, a patient might be given an immunotherapeutic agent such as BCG or MER (methanol extractable residue of BCG).

Use of idiotypic antisera to the patient's myeloma protein may be helpful in following the course of the patient's response to chemotherapy. For measuring serum monoclonal protein, radio-immunoassay utilizing an idiotypic antiserum to a patient's my-eloma protein is more sensitive than conventional techniques by a factor of 10^4. This assay could be used for detecting early re-lapse and thus indicating a change in chemotherapy for multiple myeloma (Ricks et al., 1975). However, the development of an idiotypic antiserum for every myeloma patient is not practical at present.

Plasmacytomas of BALB/c mice may be inhibited by anti-idio-typic antibody. Both prevention of tumor growth and regression of plasmacytomas may be seen after injection of anti-idiotypic antibodies (Chen et al., 1975). It is conceivable that injection of anti-idiotypic antisera might be beneficial in myeloma.

Chemotherapeutic agents might be delivered by carriers such as radioisotopes.

Recently it was reported that idiotypic immunoglobulins on lymphocytes of human patients with myeloma decreased after chemotherapy (Abdou and Abdou, 1975). These findings require confirmation.

In mice with MOPC 104E myeloma, prednisone and melphalan had therapeutic effect; and BCNU, cyclophosphamide, and pred-nisone in combination had significant therapeutic effect but also significant toxicity (Hiramoto et al., 1975). The use of this tu-mor system in evaluating other drug combinations may be help-ful.

Total-body irradiation has been suggested as treatment for myeloma. It has been estimated that a single dose of 225 to 300 rads should reduce the tumor cell burden by approximately 1 log (Bergsagel, 1971). In a trial, 11 patients with myeloma were given 100 R total-body radiation while 10 others received a con-ventional course of melphalan orally. The melphalan produced better therapeutic results with less toxic reaction than the total-body irradiation (Horvath et al., 1974).

MANAGEMENT OF SPECIAL PROBLEMS

Hypercalcemia: Hypercalcemia (Deftos and Neer, 1974; New-mark and Himathongkam, 1974) occurs in at least one-third of patients with multiple myeloma. To be recognized, it must first be considered; and it must be excluded in the presence of anorexia, nausea, vomiting, polyuria, increased constipation, weakness, confusion, stupor, or coma. For hypercalcemia in a symptomatic stage, treatment is urgent. Hypercalcemia has been reported as the most common course of acute renal failure in myeloma (De-Fronzo et al., 1975). Further, hypercalcemia often leads to chronic renal insufficiency and is a major cause of renal failure in myeloma.

Because dehydration is a common accompaniment, the patient with hypercalcemia should be hydrated. Saline is the agent of choice, since sodium promotes the renal excretion of calcium. The addition of furosemide (Lasix®), 40 mg every 4 hours, may be beneficial. Ethacrynic acid may be used as a diuretic, but thiazide diuretics are contraindicated because they decrease urinary excretion of calcium and can aggravate the hypercalcemia. During diuretic therapy, urinary loss of electrolytes must be monitored closely. Hypocalcemia must be avoided, particularly if the patient is taking digitalis. In addition to hydration and diuresis, we recommend prednisone in an initial dose of 100 mg daily. This must be reduced after a few days and discontinued as quickly as possible. Inorganic phosphate (Neutra-Phos®) may be given with or instead of prednisone. We prescribe 150 ml orally 4 times daily (equivalent to 2.0 g of phosphorus daily). If the patient is comatose, the inorganic phosphate solution can be given via gastric tube. If the patient is comatose and critically ill, inorganic phosphorus can be given slowly in doses of 1,000 to 1,500 mg intravenously over 6 to 8 hours. Diarrhea has not been a troublesome side effect (Goldsmith et al., 1968). Extravascular calcification has followed administration of inorganic phosphorus orally for long periods to both hypercalcemic and normocalcemic patients (Dudley and Blackburn, 1970). Fulmer et al. (1972) considered inorganic phosphate more effective than sodium sulphate or hydrocortisone in 22 cases of hypercalcemia with neoplastic diseases. These authors found no more soft-tissue calcification on light microscopy in patients treated with inorganic phosphate than would be expected in patients with hypercalcemia. When using either inorganic phosphate or sodium sulfate, the clinician must be careful not to precipitate congestive heart failure. Neutra-Phos is contraindicated in the presence of hyper-phosphatemia.

If these measures fail, mithramycin may be given intravenous-ly in a dosage of 25 μg/kg body weight. It produces its effect within 24 to 48 hours, but the hypercalcemia can recur after 2 or 3 days. Thrombocytopenia may follow, so depression of bone-marrow function is a relative contraindication to the use of mithramycin. Calcitonin may prove helpful in treatment for hypercalcemia, since it reduces calcium levels in blood and is rela-tively free of toxicity. But it is still an experimental drug and not yet available commercially except for use in Paget's disease.

Occasionally, hypercalcemia may occur in myeloma but pro-duce no symptoms because of a calcium-binding myeloma globu-lin. In this situation the serum ionized calcium is normal (Lind-gärde and Zettervall, 1973). One must also be aware that hypo-albuminemia is common in myeloma and causes serum calcium values to be spuriously low (Payne et al., 1973).

Renal Insufficiency: More than 50% of patients with myeloma have renal insufficiency (creatinine > 1.2 in males and > 0.9 in females); moreover, it is one of the major causes of death (see page 156). Hypercalcemia is one of the most treat-able causes of renal insufficiency and has been discussed above. If hyperuricemia occurs, allopurinol provides effective therapy. If the patient is allergic to this agent, alkalinization of the urine with sodium bicarbonate 0.6 to 0.9 g 3 or 4 times daily and aceta-zolamide (Diamox®) 250 mg at bedtime is effective. Urinary volume should be maintained at a minimum of 3 liters per day. Polycitra® syrup (Willen Drug Co., Baltimore, MD) also may be used to alkalinize the urine.

A trial of hemodialysis is certainly indicated in acute renal in-sufficiency and myeloma (Cohen and Rundles, 1975). We have had occasional patients who regained adequate renal function.

Long-term hemodialysis also has been used (Leech et al., 1972; Lock et al., 1973), but this is subject to availability and other local circumstances. For dialysis to be considered on a long-term basis, the patient must have no other debilitating complications; his myeloma must be responding to chemotherapy; and he must have significant rehabilitation potential. A possible problem in long-term dialysis is deposition of light chains in multiple organs, producing functional impairment. This has been reported as occurring in two patients with plasmacytosis of the marrow who were in a sustained program of hemodialysis (Randall et al., 1972).

Infections: Bacterial infections are frequent in myeloma and sometimes fatal (see page 111). Significant fever is an indication for appropriate cultures, roentgenography, and consideration of antibiotic therapy. This therapy can be made more specific once the results of the cultures are known. One double-blind study has shown that prophylactic injections of gamma globulin failed to alter the rate or type of infections from those in a control group; there is thus considerable doubt as to the efficacy of gamma globulin injections (Salmon et al., 1967). Occasionally we have used penicillin prophylactically with good results in cases of multiple recurrent, severe bacterial infections. Use of gentamicin for infections in patients with multiple myeloma must be carefully monitored, as we have seen an occasional patient have a marked decrease in renal function following small doses of gentamicin.

Neurologic Complications: Extradural extension of myeloma may compress the spinal cord or cauda equina and produce progressive weakness and sensory loss leading to complete and permanent paraplegia. Although irradiation may be the best therapy (Martin and Heller, 1965; Garrett, 1970), the effect of ionizing radiation is rather slow; and if the neurologic deficit progresses during radiation therapy, surgical decompression is essential. Consultation and cooperation of the hematologist, neurologist, neurosurgeon, and radiotherapist are most helpful in the management of these cases. Hall and Mackay (1973) reported satisfactory response to laminectomy in 4 of 10 cases of extradural myeloma.

One should not abandon consideration of therapy, even for the patient who is paraplegic from spinal-cord compression. We have seen a patient who had had symptoms of cord compression for more than 2 weeks prior to surgery, and had been unable to walk for 4 days, recover the function of his lower extremities after surgical decompression and radiation therapy. The ultimate prognosis should not unduly affect the decision to operate; patients generally prefer survival for only a year as an ambulatory patient rather than permanent paraplegia.

Skeletal Lesions: Skeletal lesions with pain and fracture are a major problem in patients with myeloma. Although bone lesions are reported to heal with chemotherapy (Rodriguez et al., 1972), we have been disappointed in this regard. Frequently a brace or supporting garment is helpful; but avoidance of trauma is more important, because even mild injury may result in multiple fractures. Nevertheless, the patient should be encouraged to be as active as possible, because confinement to bed increases demineralization of the skeleton. Analgesics should be given to control pain so that the patient can be ambulatory. Physical therapy also may be beneficial. Fixation of fractures of the long bones with an intramedullary rod and methyl methacrylate has given very satisfactory results in our experience. Rib fractures may be of considerable concern to the patient, but they usually respond to analgesics and rarely require any focal radiation therapy. Older patients, in particular, must be compelled to be active lest they become permanently bedridden. Patients useless to themselves and others tend to think of death as a means of escape.

It has been reported that mithramycin relieved bone pain and abolished hypercalcemia and hypercalcinuria in two patients with multiple myeloma (Stamp et al., 1975). This observation requires confirmation. Caution is necessary because of the potential toxicity of mithramycin.

The combination of sodium fluoride, calcium lactate, and androgens was reported to produce skeletal fluorosis in patients with myeloma (Cohen and Gardner, 1964; Cohen et al., 1969). Carbone et al. (1968) also described coarsening of the bony trabeculae in five patients with myeloma who were treated with sodium fluoride for 7 to 32 months. Yet, another study by Harley and coworkers (1972b) suggested that fluoride had no beneficial effect. They conducted a prospective randomized study of 150 patients with myeloma who were given a placebo or 100 mg of sodium fluoride or 200 mg of sodium fluoride daily, and they concluded there was no improvement in the clinical course or survival of the fluoride treated groups. However, they did note fluorosis in seven patients who received fluoride.

The lack of agreement among these studies and the knowledge that sodium fluoride, calcium, and vitamin D were beneficial in treatment for osteoporosis (Jowsey et al., 1972) prompted us to undertake a prospective trial to compare the effect of sodium fluoride and calcium carbonate with that of placebo treatment for bone disease in myeloma. All of our patients received melphalan plus prednisone for 7 days every 6 weeks as basic treatment for their myeloma. Complete roentgenographic skeletal surveys, bone scans with ^{99m}Tc-SN-EHDP, and a bone specimen for microradiography were obtained prior to randomization between two regimens. One was sodium fluoride, 50 mg twice daily with meals, and calcium carbonate, 1 g 4 times daily 1 hour after meals and at bedtime; the other consisted of identical-appearing placebo capsules.

At the end of 1 year, the studies—including bone biopsy—were repeated and the code was broken. Bone morphology data before

TABLE 54

BONE CHANGES IN MYELOMA PATIENTS TREATED WITH
FLUORIDE-CALCIUM OR PLACEBO
(MAYO CLINIC)

	No.	Before Treatment, Mean	No.	After Treatment, Mean
Fluoride-calcium				
Formation, %	10	3.6	12	9.0*
Resorption, %	5	8.1	4	2.4
Cortical thickness, mm	10	0.6	13	0.9†
Trabecular thickness, μm	11	118.0	13	208.6†
Osteoid width, μm	12	11.8	13	14.2‡
Placebo				
Formation, %	10	2.3	9	2.3
Resorption, %	6	5.0	5	2.9
Cortical thickness, mm	10	1.0	10	0.7
Trabecular thickness, μm	10	112.1	10	121.3
Osteoid width, μm	10	11.5	9	12.4

Significance of difference from before treatment: * $P < 0.01$; † $P < 0.02$; ‡ $P < 0.005$.

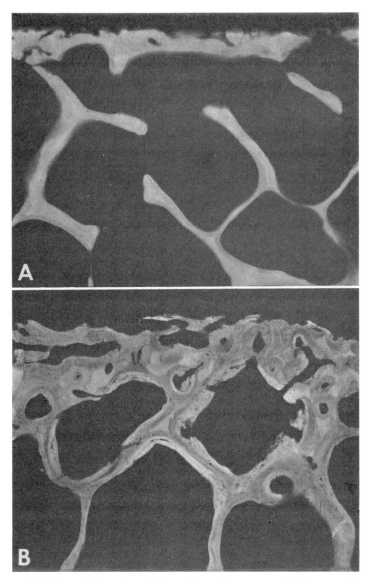

Figure 59. Microradiographs of bone from iliac crest. *A*, Prior to therapy: thin trabeculae and cortical bone. (×40.) *B*, After 1 year of fluoride-calcium treatment: thickening of both cortex and trabeculae, and increased amount of bone. (×40.) *C*, After 1 year of fluoride-calcium treatment: pretreatment bone is surrounded by bone formed during treatment, which is highly calcified and contains some large osteocyte lacunae. (×100.) (From Kyle, R. A., Jowsey, J., Kelly, P. J., and Taves, D. R.: Multiple-myeloma bone disease: the comparative effect of sodium fluoride and calcium carbonate or placebo. *N Engl J Med, 293*:1334-1338, 1975a. By permission of The Massachusetts Medical Society.)

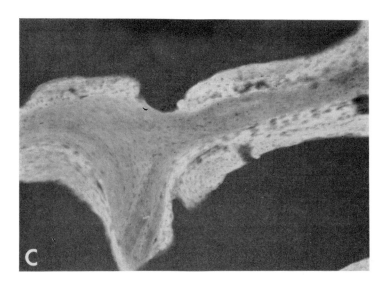

and after fluoride-calcium or placebo therapy were available in
22 cases. Microradiography studies of the bone specimens showed
that bone formation was significantly increased in patients who
had received fluoride and calcium, whereas there was no change
in bone formation in the other group (Table 54). Significant increases of the cortical and trabecular thickness and less resorption occurred in the fluoride-calcium group (Fig. 59). Increased
prominence and thickening of the trabeculae of the vertebral
bodies of the thoracic and lumbar vertebrae and often the pelvis
were seen in the roentgenograms of 6 of the 13 cases from the
fluoride-calcium group but in none of the placebo group. Hypercalcemia developed in two fluoride-calcium patients and in one
who received placebo, but in each instance the hypercalcemia was
thought to be due to progression of the myeloma. Alkaline phosphatase values tended to increase in the fluoride-calcium group
and were above normal in seven of them. Modest elevation in
serum creatinine (to 1.5 mg/dl, or less) occurred in two fluoride
cases and in three placebo cases. Two patients receiving fluoride
and calcium experienced mild nausea; no other side effects were
noted.

The combination of fluoride and calcium resulted in increased bone mass. The bone appeared relatively normal and there was no evidence that it had poor mechanical properties. We concluded that sodium fluoride and calcium supplementation may be a useful adjunct in treatment for myeloma bone disease (Kyle et al., 1975a).

Anemia: Anemia is a common finding, occurring eventually in almost every patient with myeloma. Transfusion of packed red cells remains the cornerstone of therapy. A hemoglobin concentration of 8 to 10 g/dl is adequate in most cases unless there is significant coronary-artery disease or cerebrovascular insufficiency. Successful treatment for the primary disease with alkylating agents and corticosteroids may restore erythropoiesis. Androgens may raise the hemoglobin levels in some patients (Schilling and Finkel, 1975). In efforts to raise the hemoglobin concentration and reduce transfusion requirements, one can give fluoxymestrone (Halotestin®) 10 mg 3 times daily or testosterone enanthate (Delatestryl®) 400 mg intramuscularly every 4 weeks. Androgens usually have been disappointing in our experience.

Psychologic Problems: Any patient with a serious disease such as multiple myeloma needs substantial, continuing emotional support. The approach must be positive. The physician must have confidence in his ability to cope with the patient's problems, and the patient should be able to sense this confidence. Potential benefits of therapy should be emphasized. It reassures the patient to know that some persons survive for 5 or more years while receiving treatment. It is vital that the physicians caring for the myeloma patient have the interest and capacity to deal with incurable disease over a span of months to years with assurance, sympathy, and resourcefulness.

CHAPTER XV

Waldenström's Macroglobulinemia (Primary Macroglobulinemia)

In 1944, WALDENSTRÖM described two patients with oronasal bleeding, severe normocytic normochromic anemia, high erythrocyte sedimentation rates, lymphadenopathy, and low serum fibrinogen values. Both had an abnormally large amount of a homogeneous gamma globulin with a sedimentation coefficient of 19 to 20S, corresponding to a molecular weight of more than 1,000,000. (The description of a third patient does not permit a definite diagnosis of macroglobulinemia.) Waldenström postulated that the protein consisted of a giant molecule rather than an aggregation of gamma globulin. Subsequently the serum globulin was identified as an immunoglobulin and was designated IgM. As an entity, macroglobulinemia bears similarities to multiple myeloma, lymphoma, and chronic lymphocytic leukemia. It should be considered as a malignant lymphoplasmoproliferative disorder (Ritzmann et al., 1960; McCallister et al., 1967; Martin, 1968; MacKenzie and Fudenberg, 1972).

ETIOLOGY AND PATHOGENESIS

Although the cause of Waldenström's macroglobulinemia is unknown, the disease may be more frequent in certain families. In one, two brothers had macroglobulinemia with a very similar clinical pattern and protein abnormality; and serum from their mother also showed a narrow band on electrophoresis and increased IgM on immunoelectrophoresis (Massari et al., 1962). Yet in another, no protein or chromosomal abnormalities appeared in the monozygotic twin sister of a macroglobulinemia patient who had a large extra group A chromosome in both the peripheral blood and bone marrow. This suggests that the macro-globulinemia and chromosomal abnormality were acquired (Spengler et al., 1966). Two studies of relatives of other patients with Waldenström's macroglobulinemia revealed an increased frequency of IgM monoclonal proteins as well as quantitative abnormalities (Seligmann et al., 1967; Kalff and Hijmans, 1969). Fine et al. (1973c) reported a monoclonal IgG κ protein in a sister and a polyclonal increase of IgM immunoglobulin in a brother of a patient with Waldenström's macroglobulinemia. It is of interest that the patient also had a polyclonal increase in IgG. But these are only isolated instances, and the vast majority of patients with macroglobulinemia have no familial history of the disease or other protein abnormality.

Most patients with macroglobulinemia have chromosomal abnormalities, though these are not specific. A large median or submedian marker chromosome commonly may be found both in cultures of leukocytes in the peripheral blood and in direct marrow preparations (Elves and Israëls, 1963; Goh and Swisher, 1970). There may be structural abnormalities and too few or too many chromosomes (Houston et al., 1967). Chromosomal abnormalities may be found also in relatives of patients with Waldenström's macroglobulinemia, but in most of these subjects no excess of gamma globulin has been demonstrated (Brown et al., 1967; Elves and Brown, 1968).

The basic abnormality in macroglobulinemia is uncontrolled proliferation of cells with lymphoplasmocellular characteristics. Their morphology varies, ranging from small lymphocytes to frank plasma cells. The cytoplasm is frequently ragged. Some of the cells contain intranuclear and intracytoplasmic PAS-positive material that is probably identical with circulating macroglobulin (Dutcher and Fahey, 1959). Electron microscopic features include a well-developed endoplasmic reticulum with rough and dilated areas filled with protein (Brecher et al., 1964; Wanebo and Clarkson, 1965). The lymphoplasma cells appear to be the site of production of the macroglobulin, which can be demonstrated by immunofluorescence in cells from lymph-node imprints, bone marrow, and buffy-coat smears. IgM staining was noted in large and medium-sized lymphocytes and in lymphoblasts (Zucker-Franklin et al., 1962).

To the unwary observer, the histology of lymph nodes in macroglobulinemia is very difficult to distinguish by light microscopy from lymphosarcoma or chronic lymphocytic leukemia. The lymph nodes are usually normal in size or only slightly enlarged and show capsular, hilar, and trabecular invasion. Retention of a surprisingly normal reticulum pattern, scarcity of peripheral follicles, scantiness of mitotic figures, excess of clearly recognizable plasma cells, presence of PAS-positive intranuclear inclusions, and increased numbers of mast cells should suggest the diagnosis of macroglobulinemia (Harrison, 1972).

CLINICAL MANIFESTATIONS AND RELATED FEATURES

Age and Sex; Symptoms and Physical Signs: Macroglobulinemia of Waldenström has a predilection for older men. In several series about two-thirds of the patients were males, with ages ranging from 32 to 92 and averaging about 60 years. It rarely occurs in those aged 40 or less.

As a rule, the onset is insidious. Weakness, fatigue, and bleeding (especially oozing from the oronasal areas) are not uncommon presenting symptoms. Blurring or other impairment of vision affects about one-third of the patients and may be the major complaint. Recurrent infections, dyspnea, congestive heart failure, weight loss, and neurologic symptoms occur. Bone pain is virtually nonexistent, a contrast to multiple myeloma. Pallor, mild splenomegaly, hepatomegaly, and peripheral lymphadenopathy are the most common physical findings. Retinal lesions, including hemorrhages, exudates, and venous congestion with vascular segmentation (sausage formation), may be the most impressive feature (Fig. 60); but they can be due to hyperviscosity from other causes. Occlusion of the central vein of the retina may be seen. In a series of 34 patients with macroglobulinemia, MacKenzie and Babcock (1975) found relative serum viscosity greater than 6 in 38%. This was usually associated with IgM values greater than 5 g/dl. Rarely, there may be subcutaneous tumors consisting of collections of lymphoid cells (Silva et al.,

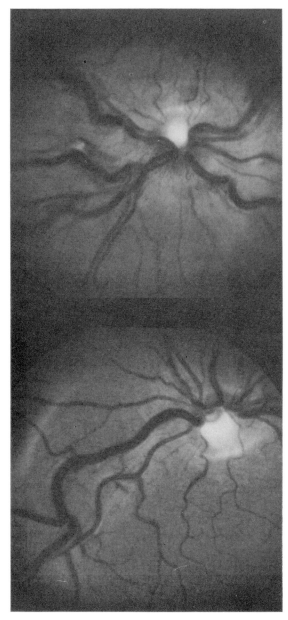

Figure 60. Ocular fundi of patient with macroglobulinemia of Waldenström.

1969). Rupture of the spleen with minimal trauma has been reported in macroglobulinemia (Karakousis and Elias, 1974).

Neurologic Manifestations: With macroglobulinemia of Waldenström, 25% of patients have neurologic abnormalities. These include peripheral neuropathy, a syndrome that resembles the Guillain-Barré syndrome, encephalopathy, and subarachnoid hemorrhage (Logothetis et al., 1960). Neurologic symptoms ordinarily associated with hyperviscosity, such as headache, dizziness, vertigo, ataxia, and altered sensorium, have been referred to as the Bing-Neel syndrome. Whether the first two cases reported by Bing and Neel (1936) were macroglobulinemia is doubtful, but another case which they thought to be chronic lymphocytic leukemia was most likely macroglobulinemia (Bichel et al., 1950).

Peripheral neuropathy may be the initial symptom in macroglobulinemia. It almost always involves both sensory and motor modalities and may affect all extremities. Biopsy of the sural nerve reveals myelin degeneration but no significant infiltration by lymphocytes or plasma cells (Darnley, 1962; Dayan and Lewis, 1966). Amorphous hyaline, PAS-positive material in the perineurium, endoneurium, and blood vessel walls has been reported in polyneuropathy with macroglobulinemia. Immunofluorescent studies showed this substance contained IgM but not amyloid (Iwashita et al., 1974). Peripheral neuropathy may progress and produce neuropathic joint disease (Charcot joints) (Scott et al., 1973). Amyloidosis may be associated with macroglobulinemia and peripheral neuropathy (see page 277). A combination of peripheral neuropathy, macroglobulinemia, amyloidosis, and macroglobulinemia with low-molecular-weight IgM has been noted (Bigner et al., 1971). The sensorimotor peripheral neuropathy seen in macroglobulinemia seems no different from that of multiple myeloma or carcinoma. The presence of peripheral neuropathy in an older patient should always bring these entities to mind, because peripheral neuropathy may precede and dominate other manifestations of the disease.

Multifocal leukoencephalopathy has been reported in macroglobulinemia (Lyon et al., 1971). Progressive spinal muscular atrophy responding to chlorambucil was reported in one case

(Peters and Clatanoff, 1968). Tinnitus and vertigo masquerading as labyrinthitis may be the presenting symptom of macroglobulinemia (Afifi and Tawfeek, 1971). Sudden deafness, first in one ear and then in the other, has been noted in a case of macroglobulinemia (Ruben et al., 1969). Waldenström's macroglobulinemia should be considered in the differential diagnosis of sudden sensorineural hearing loss or vestibular symptoms of sudden onset (Ronis et al., 1966).

Other Clinical Features: The incidence of infection is twice normal (Fahey et al., 1963). Antibody production may be reduced, as suggested by one study wherein IgM antibody production was decreased when stimulated by a weak antigen (sheep cell stroma) but not when a more potent antigen (brucellin) was used (Pitts and McDuffie, 1967). *Pneumocystis carinii* and cytomegalic inclusion disease were found at postmortem examination in a patient with macroglobulinemia who died of pneumonitis (Font and Zimmerman, 1970). These entities should always be considered when a patient who has been given chemotherapy for macroglobulinemia develops unexplained fever or a pulmonary infection.

A bleeding diathesis in macroglobulinemia is not uncommon. Perkins et al. (1970) reported bleeding in 5 of 14 cases and stressed prolongation of the bleeding time, abnormalities in platelet adhesiveness, prothrombin time, and thromboplastin generation, and decreased levels of Factor VIII. Castaldi and Penny (1970) described a patient with a large amount of monoclonal IgM λ (5.4 g/dl) that had specific activity against Factor VIII, thus producing a hemophilia-like condition. Thrombocytopenia or hyperviscosity also may contribute to the bleeding diathesis.

Abnormalities of Other Organs: Renal failure occurs ultimately in one-third of patients with macroglobulinemia. Deposits of IgM on the endothelial aspect of the basement membrane may become large enough to occlude the capillary lumen and resemble thrombi. Presumably they result from passive deposition of circulating IgM. Lymphocytic or plasma-cell infiltration identical to that found in the bone marrow has been reported in two-thirds of the cases. Deposition of amyloid in the glomerulus was noted in 3 of 16 patients. Although Bence Jones proteinuria may be present in macroglobulinemia, tubular casts surrounded by giant cells as in myeloma do not develop (Morel-Maroger et al., 1970).

Intramembranous electron-dense deposits in the outer margin of the lamina densa on electron micrographs of the kidney were seen in a case of Waldenström's macroglobulinemia and nephrotic syndrome. No abnormalities appeared on light microscopy. Immunofluorescent staining of the kidney biopsy tissue showed IgM, IgG, and complement in the capillary loops of the glomeruli. The glomerular deposits consisted of IgM, IgG, and C3. The IgM was not complexed to the IgG, but IgG was present in an aggregated form. The authors believed that IgG, IgM, and complement all contributed to the patient's nephrotic syndrome (Martelo et al., 1975).

Precipitation of acute renal failure by dehydration in macroglobulinemia has been reported (Argani and Kipkie, 1964). Approximately 25% of our patients have had Bence Jones proteinuria (McCallister et al., 1967).

Pulmonary involvement—manifested by progressive pulmonary infiltration, pleural effusion, and plasma-lymphocytoid infiltrations of the lung and pleura—has been seen (Strunge, 1969). Pleural effusion may be the presenting finding in macroglobulinemia (Schur and Appel, 1961). Nodular pulmonary lesions (Furgerson et al., 1963) and miliary infiltrations (Moeschlin, 1966) which biopsy showed to be plasmacytoid cells have been reported. In both instances, the lesions responded to chlorambucil. A large right-upper-lobe tumor was found at presentation in typical macroglobulinema of Waldenström (Major et al., 1973). Recurrent pneumonia may be a manifestation of the entity (Neiman et al., 1973).

Winterbauer et al. (1974) reported that 5 of 20 patients with macroglobulinemia had pulmonary involvement. Four had multiple asymmetric nodular infiltrates in both lungs and the fifth had a unilateral pleural effusion. Chest roentgenograms showed abnormality in four at the time of diagnosis, and in two cases had done so for more than 2 years. In four cases, pulmonary biopsy or autopsy specimens revealed infiltration with lymphocytes and plasmacytoid cells. Chlorambucil produced significant roentgenographic improvement in three of four patients. The authors provided an excellent review of the literature of pleural and pulmonary involvement in macroglobulinemia.

An IgM κ protein measured as 3.3 g/dl, hilar enlargement, and lymphocytic infiltration of the bronchus have been reported as the only manifestations of macroglobulinemia (Rabiner et al., 1972), as has a large monoclonal IgM protein in association with a lymphosarcoma of the lung (Ward et al., 1971). We have seen a similar case: A mass in the right lung had enlarged progressively over a 15-year period, during which time the patient had refused any diagnostic procedures. Biopsy of the lesion showed a malignant lymphoid proliferative process, and electrophoresis of the patient's serum showed a large monoclonal IgM spike. There was no evidence of macroglobulinemia in the marrow. Irradiation of the mass and a short course of chlorambucil resulted in significant reduction of the pulmonary mass and the monoclonal protein concentration.

Diarrhea and steatorrhea may be prominent features complicating macroglobulinemia (Cabrera et al., 1964; Bradley et al., 1968; Khilnani et al., 1969; Beker et al., 1971; Bedine et al., 1973). In many of these cases, deposits of an amorphous hyalinelike material appeared in the small intestine. A patient with such abnormalities and severe malabsorption had extracellular amorphous material in the lamina propria and in the dilated mucosal lymphatics of the upper duodenum and jejunum. The material was PAS-positive and no amyloid was found. Moderate numbers of plasma cells, small lymphocytes, and eosinophils were present in the deeper layers of the lamina propria. Immunofluorescent studies showed strong specific staining for IgM and lambda light chains, confirming the presence of a monoclonal immunoglobulin (Pruzanski et al., 1973). Obstructive jaundice secondary to bleeding into the biliary tract has been reported in two patients with macroglobulinemia (Elias et al., 1972).

Lymphocytes, plasmacytoid cells, and intranuclear PAS-positive material may invade the lacrimal gland (Little, 1967), and orbital tumors also have been noted (Godeau et al., 1972). Bilateral diffuse corneal degeneration has been observed in macroglobulinemia (Gloor, 1968).

Association With Other Diseases: Macroglobulinemia of Waldenström has been reported in association with various other diseases. However, one must be cautious in linking macroglobulinemia with any other entity unless one has an adequate control population to exclude fortuitous association. The combination of macroglobulinemia and amyloidosis is well known (see page 277). Combination with chronic lymphocytic leukemia (Zlotnick and Robinson, 1970) and with lymphoma (Carter, 1974) has been reported, but to distinguish between these closely related entities is difficult.

An increased incidence of non-lymphoid malignancies was noted by MacKenzie and Fudenberg (1972), who reported carcinoma in 8 of 40 patients with macroglobulinemia. Three additional patients had a well-localized basal-cell carcinoma. In contrast, Yamaguchi (1973) found only 1 carcinoma (gastric) in 35 autopsies of macroglobulinemia. It is impossible to know whether there is an increased incidence of carcinoma in macroglobulinemia or not.

Rheumatoid arthritis (Gothoni et al., 1965), polycythemia vera (Franzén et al., 1966), xanthomatosis and hypercholesterolemia (Petersen, 1973b), discoid lupus erythematosus, and chronic lymphocytic leukemia (Abdou and Abdou, 1974) have been reported with macroglobulinemia. Plane xanthomatosis (Millard, 1973) also has been reported, but the elevation of IgG, the absence of anemia and bone-marrow abnormalities, and the lack of progression despite absence of therapy raise serious questions about the diagnosis of macroglobulinemia. It is likely that this is a case of benign monoclonal gammopathy of the IgM type.

Sjögren's syndrome has been associated with macroglobulinemia (Talal et al., 1967). Acute myelomonocytic leukemia, Bence Jones proteinuria, and hypercalcemia in one instance (Allen et al., 1973) and carcinoma of the breast, chronic lymphocytic leukemia, eosinophilic chloroma, and myelosclerosis of the marrow in another (Benvenisti and DeBellis, 1969) were associated with moderate amounts of monoclonal IgM protein but not with the other features of macroglobulinemia. Probably it was benign monoclonal gammopathy of the IgM type. Another instance of "macroglobulinemia" (IgM κ with Bence Jones proteinuria) was reported in a child with acute leukemia. The amount of IgM protein was about 1.0 g/dl, which is below the range seen in macroglobulinemia of Waldenström (Čejka et al., 1974).

LABORATORY FINDINGS

Peripheral Blood and Bone Marrow: Almost every patient with Waldenström's macroglobulinemia has moderate to severe degrees of normocytic, normochromic anemia. Depression of erythropoiesis (presumably due to the abnormal proliferation in the marrow) and excessive destruction or loss of red cells are the usual causes. In one study, erythrocyte survival was shortened in 80% of patients and 60% gave some evidence of iron-deficiency anemia that was usually related to external blood loss (Cline et al., 1963). Occasionally one sees Coombs-positive hemolytic anemia (McCallister et al., 1967). The plasma volume may be greatly increased—thus lessening the hemoglobin and hematocrit values independently of change in the red cell mass (Kopp et al., 1969)— so the anemia may be more apparent than real. Rouleau formation is striking and may be the first clue to the diagnosis. The erythrocyte sedimentation rate usually is greatly increased, though occasionally it may be recorded as 0 because of the excessive gelation of the protein. The leukocyte count usually is normal, but mild leukocytosis or leukopenia occurs in some cases. Mild degrees of lymphocytosis or monocytosis are common. The number of platelets usually is normal but may be decreased even before chemotherapy is begun.

The serum cholesterol concentration is low in many cases of macroglobulinemia, particularly if the amount of protein is large. Strisower and Galleto (1962) found that all four low-density serum lipoprotein classes were reduced in a patient with macroglobulinemia. The serum uric acid concentration may be modestly increased.

Usually the bone marrow aspirate is hypocellular. However,

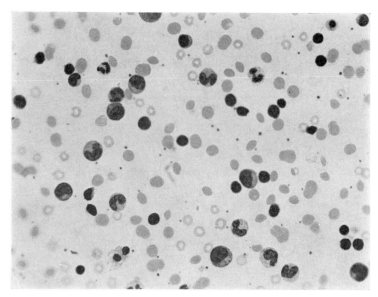

Figure 61. Bone-marrow aspirate showing hypocellularity and increased numbers of small, cytoplasm-poor lymphocytes. (Wright's stain; ×850.)

fixed sections of the same marrows are very cellular and extensively infiltrated with lymphoid cells; they may suggest lymphoma. The lymphocytes tend to be small, are often basophilic, and have plasma-cell characteristics. The number of plasma cells is always greater than normal. Marrow smears, in typical cases, are of poor cellularity and display an increase of cytoplasm-poor small lymphocytes and plasma cells (Fig. 61), with lymphoplasma cells having cytologic characteristics as an intermediate type. Naked nuclei are common, and small ragged lymphocytes with so-called cytoplasmic shedding may be evident. Normal marrow elements are correspondingly decreased. Mast cells increase in macroglobulinemia and may help to differentiate it from myeloma or lymphoma (MacKenzie and Fudenberg, 1972); macroglobulinemia has been associated with urticaria pigmentosa (Nixon, 1966).

Serum Proteins: The serum-protein electrophoretic pattern of Waldenström's macroglobulinemia is indistinguishable from that of multiple myeloma: a sharp, narrow peak or dense band migrating with gamma- or beta-globulin mobility. The response to the Sia water test ordinarily is positive, but this nonspecific test may elicit a positive response in myeloma or other conditions with hyperglobulinemia (see page 53). Analysis of serum by immunoelectrophoresis with a specific antiserum to IgM reveals a localized dense precipitin arc (Fig. 19). Approximately 80% of monoclonal IgM proteins are of the kappa type, though this was true of only two-thirds of a series reported from Japan (Yamaguchi, 1973). Ultracentrifugational analysis may be used in identifying serum macroglobulins (which sediment as a 19S peak), but it is no longer necessary for diagnosis and would fail to detect the IgM monomer. Frequently, low-molecular-weight IgM (7S) is present; and it may account for as much as 40% of the excess of this immunoglobulin (see page 27). About 10% of macroglobulins have cryoprecipitable properties and are designated macrocryoglobulins (see page 216). Whereas IgM normally constitutes 10% or less of the immunoglobulins, in macroglobulinemia IgM may amount to more than 90% of them.

Roentgenographic Features: The bones most often appear normal, but diffuse osteoporosis may be seen. Bone destruction with lytic lesions is rare (Welton et al., 1968); Vermess et al. (1972) reported that roentgenography among their 41 cases of macroglobulinemia revealed osteolytic lesions in 8 which were not distinguishable roentgenologically from those of multiple myeloma. The osteolytic lesions were multiple in four cases and single in the other four. They noted cyst-like symmetric lesions in the iliac bone of 3 of their 41 patients and thought that this might point toward the diagnosis of macroglobulinemia. We have seen two patients with osteolytic bone lesions. Each of them had a large monoclonal IgM spike in the serum and an excess of plasma cells in the bone marrow. Stanley et al. (1971) described a patient with an IgM monoclonal protein who had thickened but fewer bony trabeculae as well as patchy sclerosis. This roentgenographic picture resembled fibrogenesis imperfecta ossium. Lymphangiography in Waldenström's macroglobulinemia often shows enlarged nodes with areas of lymph node replacement, but many nodes have normal lymphatic channels (Whitehouse et al., 1974) and are indistinguishable from lymphosarcoma. The same picture was reported in a case of macroglobulinemia with amyloidosis (Bottomley et al., 1974).

DIAGNOSIS

A combination of typical symptoms and physical findings, demonstration of more than 2 g/dl of monoclonal IgM protein, and appropriate abnormalities of the bone marrow provide the diagnosis of Waldenström's macroglobulinemia. Major problems in differential diagnosis center around the distinction from multiple myeloma, chronic lymphocytic leukemia, lymphoma, and benign monoclonal gammopathy of the IgM type. These diseases are closely related, and some patients actually have characteristics of more than one disorder.

We have seen several patients who had clinical evidence of macroglobulinemia (weakness, fatigue, and anemia), as well as large numbers of lymphoid cells in the bone marrow and no lytic bone lesions, but who had a large concentration of monoclonal IgG protein in the serum and decreased concentrations of IgM (Vladutiu and Sielski, 1973). We classify such cases as IgG myeloma despite the lymphoid cells in the marrow suggesting macroglobulinemia. But conversely, we have seen patients who had large amounts of monoclonal IgM proteins in the serum, anemia, oronasal bleeding, and blurred vision—but who also had lytic bone lesions and typical immature plasma cells in the bone marrow, characteristic of myeloma. Others also have described patients with a monoclonal IgM protein, lytic bone lesions, and abnormal plasma cells in the bone marrow (Adner et al., 1960; Waldenström, 1962; Welton et al., 1968; Case Records of the Massachusetts General Hospital, 1972; Berman, 1975). For the present we prefer to classify these cases as macroglobulinemia rather than IgM myeloma. Though the problem is insoluble at present, future knowledge, including etiology, may show how to combine or separate these entities correctly.

It is also difficult to distinguish Waldenström's macroglobulinemia from lymphoma and benign monoclonal gammopathy of the IgM type; and in some instances the distinction is arbitrary. Nodal biopsy may fail to rule out lymphoma, leaving the diagnosis dependent upon the clinical and laboratory findings. Yet some of our patients with the typical features of lymphocytic lymphosarcoma or chronic lymphocytic leukemia have been found to have a large concentration of monoclonal IgM protein. In such cases it may be impossible to tell whether one is facing an association of lymphoma with macroglobulinemia or an association of Waldenström's macroglobulinemia with prominent hepatosplenomegaly and lymphadenopathy (see page 199).

Even more difficult than the distinction between IgG and IgA benign monoclonal gammopathy and multiple myeloma is the distinction between IgM benign monoclonal gammopathy and Waldenström's macroglobulinemia. Rywlin et al. (1975) emphasized the difficulty in separating Waldenström's macroglobulinemia from benign monoclonal gammopathy and other lymphoproliferative processes. A monoclonal IgM protein concentration of less than 1.0 g/dl, the lack of anemia, the absence of organomegaly, mild lymphocytosis of the bone marrow, and the lack of clinical symptoms or hyperviscosity suggest benign monoclonal gammopathy rather than macroglobulinemia. Carter and Hobbs (1971) reported that low-molecular-weight IgM (7S) was present in sera of many patients with macroglobulinemia or lymphoma but absent from sera of patients with benign monoclonal gammopathy of the IgM type. This may prove to be helpful in differentiating the two entities, but careful observation must be continued for several years before the diagnosis is final.

This is well illustrated by a patient of ours who presented in December 1971 with a large concentration of IgM monoclonal protein (5.6 g/dl), severe anemia (9.4 g after 3 units of blood), and hyperviscosity syndrome (7.6). A question of macroglobulinemia had been raised by his home physician 9 months before. A review of his record revealed that he had been here in 1958 and serum protein electrophoresis had showed a small gamma spike. Immunoelectrophoresis had not been done at that time, of course; and no serum is available currently; but it seems reasonable to assume that the electrophoretic abnormality represented a small monoclonal IgM protein. In another case, serum electrophoresis produced a gamma globulin peak in 1955. Ten years later the patient developed anemia; and subsequently the abnormal band (1.6 g) was identified as an IgM κ monoclonal protein. Lymphadenopathy appeared, his clinical course deteriorated, and he died 2 years later. The autopsy findings were consistent with Waldenström's macroglobulinemia (Clinicopathological Conference, 1968). Both of these cases could well be classified as benign monoclonal gammopathy of the IgM type initially, with subsequent development of Waldenström's macroglobulinemia.

IgM may be increased in a variety of disorders, among them rheumatoid arthritis, Sjögren's syndrome, lupus erythematosus, cirrhosis, recurrent infections, parasitic infestations, and sarcoidosis (Rosen, 1962). In these conditions, the macroglobulins usually are polyclonal and their concentration in the serum generally is lower than in Waldenström's macroglobulinemia, in which the IgM is monoclonal.

COURSE AND THERAPY

Survival: Cohen et al. (1966) reported that survival from the estimated date of clinical onset of Waldenström's macroglobulinemia varied from 23 to 152 months (average, 55 months), and the duration of survival from the date of diagnosis averaged 34 months. MacKenzie and Fudenberg (1972) reported mean post-diagnosis survival of 49.2 months in those patients responding to chemotherapy and 24.1 months in the nonresponders. McCallister et al. (1967) noted that their 23 patients with macroglobulinemia who had significant symptoms and complications early in the course of their disease had an average survival of 5.3 years from the onset of symptoms and 3.2 years from the time of diagnosis. It is evident that this disease is slowly progressive and at times almost benign. The patients who survive longest probably have either so-called benign monoclonal gammopathy of the IgM type or low-grade (indolent, smoldering) macroglobulinemia.

Occasionally the course of macroglobulinemia is most unusual: Wolf et al. (1972) reported a case of Waldenström's macroglobulinemia with hyperviscosity syndrome and severe anemia in which an episode of severe serum hepatitis was followed by a remission that lasted 3½ years. Some patients tolerate macroglobulinemia well; in others the process is more malignant. Sometimes macroglobulinemia having a typical course for several years develops into a rapidly progressive reticulum-cell sarcoma (Wanebo and Clarkson, 1965; Österberg and Rausing, 1970) or lymphoblastic lymphosarcoma (Wood and Frenkel, 1967). The development of acute leukemia in patients with macroglobulinemia treated with alkylating agents also has been observed (see page 179).

Treatment: Specific therapy should be directed toward suppressing the abnormal proliferation. A number of therapeutic agents have been used with varying success. Continued administration of small doses of chlorambucil has proved beneficial (Bayrd, 1961; Clatanoff and Meyer, 1963; McCallister et al., 1967). We ordinarily recommend that patients take chlorambucil in a dosage of 6 to 8 mg daily. In the rare instances where such an amount is not readily tolerated, it can be given in divided doses. Leukocyte and platelet counts should be determined every 2 weeks and the dosage adjusted so that the leukocytes remain about $3,000/mm^3$ and the platelets more than $100,000/mm^3$. Treatment should be continued indefinitely unless it brings no response or its side effects are significant. In view of development of acute leukemia in some instances, it might be advisable to discontinue administration of chlorambucil after the patient has been treated for 2 years or so and has obtained a satisfactory response. No prospective randomized studies of this situation have been performed, and experience is limited, so definite advice cannot be given concerning duration of chemotherapy.

Favorable subjective and objective responses have been achieved with cyclophosphamide given orally for prolonged periods (Bouroncle et al., 1964). Response to procarbazine may occur (Mitrou et al., 1972). Chemotherapy with a combination of alkylating agents including cyclophosphamide, BCNU, melphalan, vincristine, and prednisone has been reported to be beneficial (Lee et al., 1974). A patient with atypical macroglobulinemia (chronic lymphocytic leukemia with an IgM spike) who had not responded to chlorambucil, betamethasone, and cyclophosphamide responded to a combination of azathioprine, prednisone, and folic acid (Heading et al., 1970).

Since many of the clinical features of primary macroglobulinemia are attributable directly to the quantity of protein in the plasma, attempts have been made to diminish the amount of macroglobulin by repeated plasmapheresis (Solomon and Fahey, 1963). This need be done only when hyperviscosity causes significant symptoms. When undertaken as treatment, plasmapheresis should be vigorous, 1 or 2 units of plasma being removed each day for 7 to 10 days. Use of an NCI-IBM continuous-flow blood-cell separator or Haemonetics blood processor, if available, may alleviate the symptoms of hyperviscosity (Powles et al., 1971) (see page 222). Such a program can significantly ameliorate retinopathy and visual abnormalities, diminish the tendency to hemorrhage, increase the survival of red cells, and lower the incidence of auditory and vestibular disturbances. Although its effect is transient, plasmapheresis is useful in modifying symptoms during the induction phase of cytotoxic therapy. Some have advocated the use of a combination of plasmapheresis and alkylating agents (Sakalová et al., 1973) but we have found that repeated plasmapheresis is usually not necessary.

Corticosteroids can relieve symptoms in some cases, but these drugs should be reserved for use when resistance to alkylating agents has developed. They may be of benefit when anemia is a problem, particularly if it is hemolytic (Hoogstraten, 1973). Penicillamine, although used in the past because of its ability to depolymerize IgM in vitro, has not proved valuable clinically.

CHAPTER XVI

Cryoglobulinemia and Pyroglobulinemia

C RYOGLOBULINS ARE PROTEINS that precipitate or gel when cooled and dissolve when heated (see page 54). They may be classified simply in the following categories: monoclonal cryoglobulins—IgG, IgM, IgA, or monoclonal light chains (Bence Jones proteins); mixed cryoglobulins in which two or more immunoglobulins are found and one is monoclonal; and polyclonal cryoglobulins in which no monoclonal protein is found. The third kind do not reach high concentrations (Grey and Kohler, 1973) and will not be discussed further in this review.

Monoclonal Cryoglobulins: Monoclonal cryoglobulins are most commonly IgM or IgG, but IgA and Bence Jones cryoglobulins have been reported. Patients with monoclonal cryoglobulinemia may have symptoms of cold intolerance such as Raynaud's phenomenon, purpura, cold urticaria, neuropathy, leg ulcers, and gangrene of the extremities. On the other hand, we have been impressed with a number of patients who have 4 to 5 g of a monoclonal IgG or IgM cryoprotein in their serum but who have no symptoms whatever upon exposure to the cold. IgG monoclonal cryoglobulins are most often associated with multiple myeloma. Five percent of our patients with myeloma had a cryoglobulin, and Brouet et al. (1974) found 6% in their series. In some instances there is no evidence of myeloma, and these are termed "idiopathic" or "essential" cryoglobulinemia (Farmer et al., 1960; Meltzer and Franklin, 1966). Three patients with an apparently idiopathic or essential IgG cryoglobulin have developed typical multiple myeloma 4, 5, and 15 years later (Gordon-Smith et al., 1968; Grey and Kohler, 1973). One of our patients with essential

cryoglobulinemia of the IgG κ type died 9 years later of generalized amyloidosis (Maldonado et al., 1973).

We have also seen vasculitis in a patient with myeloma and a
large amount (5.0 g/dl) of IgG monoclonal cryoglobulin (Fig.
62). In another instance, a patient with 2.9 g/dl of monoclonal

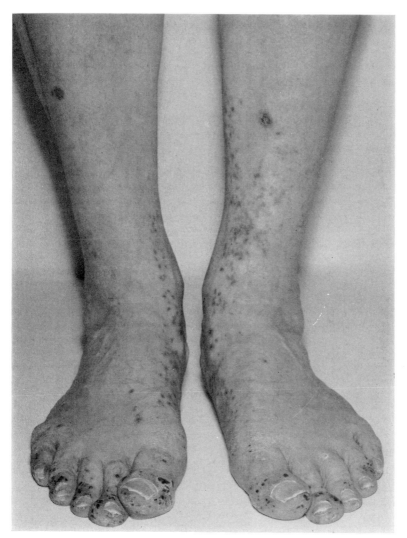

Figure 62. Vasculitis of feet and legs in multiple myeloma and cryoglobulinemia.

IgG κ cryoprotein and recurrent incapacitating necrotic ulceration of her legs responded to melphalan and prednisone (Brody and Samitz, 1973). A patient with a monoclonal IgG3 κ protein that spontaneously formed crystals had recurrent purpura and necrotic ulcerations of her skin (Grossman et al., 1972). The predominance of IgG3 subclass in cryoimmunoglobulinemia is suggested by the finding that 8 of 21 cryoglobulins were of this type (Grey et al., 1968b; Virella and Hobbs, 1971).

Cryoprecipitation is a result of a variety of noncovalent interactions, including hydrogen bonding and hydrophobic interactions. These interactions are very weak, which is why small chemical modification of the protein results in a loss of cryoprecipitability (Grey and Kohler, 1973).

Between 5 and 10% of patients with macroglobulinemia of Waldenström have an IgM monoclonal protein that will either gel or precipitate upon exposure to the cold. Approximately 95% of these proteins are of the kappa type (Grey and Kohler, 1973), whereas only 35% of IgG cryoproteins are kappa. It should be noted that approximately 80% of all monoclonal IgM proteins are kappa.

IgA cryoglobulins have been reported (Slavin et al., 1971; Sugai, 1972; Watanabe et al., 1974). In one such case (Watanabe et al., 1974), the protein consisted mainly of a polymer of IgA with a sedimentation coefficient of 16.1S. This protein, in addition to its cryoglobulin properties, also precipitated when heated to 56°C. Neither the unusual cold nor heat properties were retained when the protein was reduced to its 6.7S component.

Monoclonal light chains (Bence Jones protein) also may have cryoglobulin properties (Harris and Kohn, 1974).

The presence of cryoglobulinemia may cause spurious elevation of the leukocyte count by the model S Coulter counter. It is thought that this may be due to particle formation between the cryoglobulin and fibrinogen (Emori et al., 1973).

Mixed Cryoglobulins: Mixed cryoglobulins most commonly consist of IgM-IgG, but IgG-IgG and IgA-IgG have been reported (Brouet et al., 1974). Usually the quantity of the cold-precipitating protein is less than 0.2 g/dl and the serum protein electrophoretic pattern indicates normality or diffuse hypergammaglobulinemia. In the 11 mixed cryoglobulin cases of Meltzer et al. (1966) the IgM component was essential for cryoprecipitation while IgG could be derived from any source. Six of the seven IgM proteins that were studied contained both kappa and lambda light chains and thus were polyclonal. Nine of these 11 cases of mixed IgG-IgM cryoglobulin had a rather characteristic clinical pattern consisting of purpura, arthralgias, and weakness; in some, acute renal failure secondary to diffuse glomerulonephritis developed. Mixed IgA and IgG cryoglobulins also have been reported (Wager et al., 1968). One patient had cold urticaria, intermittent purpura, and cold-sensitive arthralgias; one had toxoplasmosis and had been treated with sulfonamides for 5 years; and the third had latent lues and a long history of cold urticaria. Mixed cryoglobulinemias may be seen in many infections and in lupus erythematosus and glomerulonephritis (Grey and Kohler, 1973).

Treatment: The treatment for cryoglobulinemia depends on the circumstances of the case. Protection from cold is important. If the abnormality is associated with myeloma or macroglobulinemia, the treatment for both cryoglobulinemia and the underlying disease is the same. Reduction of the quantity of the cryoglobulin by plasmapheresis may alleviate the severity of symptoms associated with cold intolerance. Chlorambucil and corticosteroids have been tried in cases of mixed IgM-IgG cryoglobulinemia, but usually without significant effect. In one reported case of mixed IgM-IgG syndrome, splenectomy and cyclophosphamide reduced the amount of cryoglobulin and stabilized the clinical course (Mathison et al., 1971).

Cryofibrinogen: Cryofibrinogen becomes apparent when plasma is cooled to 0°C. Its presence was first recognized in a case of bronchogenic carcinoma (Korst and Kratochvil, 1955). Cryofibrinogens have been reported in 3% of blood samples in a large laboratory (Smith and Arkin, 1972). Most cases have been associated with metastatic carcinoma, connective-tissue diseases, myocardial infarction, or pregnancy; but in some, no underlying disease was found (Zlotnick and Landau, 1966). An increased incidence of cryofibrinogen has been reported in females who were taking oral contraceptives (Pindyck et al., 1970). Many patients have no clinical manifestations, but extensive necrosis and gangrene of the extremities have been noted (Zlotnick and Landau, 1966); and necrotizing skin lesions developed in one patient treated with a hypothermic blanket (Waxman and Dove, 1969). Streptokinase-streptodornase (Varidase) has been reported to produce clinical improvement in patients with serious vascular symptoms (Rachmilewitz et al., 1970).

Pyroglobulinemia: Monoclonal proteins that precipitate when serum is heated to 56°C are called pyroglobulins (Martin and Mathieson, 1953; Solomon and Steinfeld, 1965; Patterson et al., 1968; Invernizzi et al., 1973). These proteins precipitate irreversibly and do not dissolve when cooled. And in contrast to Bence Jones proteins, they do not dissolve when heated to boiling. They usually are discovered when serum is inactivated for the VDRL serologic test.

In most cases pyroglobulinemia is associated with multiple myeloma (Martin et al., 1959); but it may also occur in macroglobulinemia, lymphoproliferative syndromes, and other neoplastic diseases. Occasionally the presence of a pyroglobulin is the initial finding in myeloma (Lipman, 1964). Of our patients with myeloma, 1% had a pyroglobulin. However, pyroglobulinemia is not associated with specific clinical effects and may be regarded as a laboratory curiosity. Again it must be emphasized that Bence Jones proteinemia should not be confused with pyroglobulinemia and can be distinguished from it by immunoelectrophoresis utilizing specific antisera. Pyroglobulins of the IgM class (19S) have been reported (Patterson et al., 1968; Stefanini et al., 1970; Invernizzi et al., 1973). Rarely, IgA pyroglobulins have been seen (Sugai, 1972; Invernizzi et al., 1973).

CHAPTER XVII

Hyperviscosity Syndrome

A LTHOUGH HYPERVISCOSITY of serum has been noted since 1929 (Bannick and Greene), its significance was not appreciated by clinicians until the review by Fahey et al. appeared in 1965. Bleeding is the most common symptom. Chronic nasal bleeding and oozing from the gums are the most common; but this disorder may cause postsurgical hemorrhage also, and possibly gastrointestinal bleeding, including hematemesis or rectal bleeding. Flame-shaped retinal hemorrhages are common, and papilledema may be seen. Patients may complain of blurring or loss of vision. Neurologic symptoms include dizziness, headaches, vertigo, nystagmus, decreased hearing, ataxia, paresthesias, or diplopia. Hyperviscosity can precipitate or aggravate congestive heart failure. Somnolence, stupor, coma, and cerebral hemorrhages develop in some cases. Somer (1966, 1975) has made an excellent review of viscosity studies in multiple myeloma and Waldenström's macroglobulinemia.

Most patients have symptoms when the relative serum viscosity reaches 6 or 7, but the relation between serum viscosity and clinical manifestations is not precise. We have seen a patient with serum viscosity of 15 but no symptoms of the hyperviscosity syndrome. Symptoms are not attributable to hyperviscosity when the relative viscosity is below 4 (normal less than 1.8) (see page 53). It should be emphasized that the viscosity/protein-concentration curve for monoclonal IgM is not linear. At low serum IgM concentrations, an addition of 1 to 2 g/dl makes only a small increase in the serum viscosity; but at higher serum levels (e.g., 4 to 5 g/dl), a similar increment increases the relative viscosity much more (Fahey et al., 1965). It is likely that the specific viscosity level at which clinical symptoms occur is affected not only by the serum protein concentration, molecular characteristics of the pro-

219

tein, or aggregation of protein molecules, but also by a combination of other factors, including the presence of primary diseases of the microvasculature, hematocrit level, cardiac status, local pH, and ionic strength (Bloch and Maki, 1973). MacKenzie et al. (1970) noted that the plasma volume increased beyond what was required to compensate for the decreased red cell mass. Aldosterone excretion was normal to low, and the increase of plasma volume was correlated with serum viscosity and mediated by sodium retention mechanisms not involving modification of aldosterone secretion.

The viscosity of blood is affected by both the hematocrit and the macroglobulin concentration, and in patients with macroglobulinemia it is increased. Presumably the protein causes increased red-cell aggregation and rouleau formation, which adds to hyperviscosity (Mannik, 1974).

Next to macroglobulinemia of Waldenström, IgA myeloma is the most common cause of hyperviscosity syndrome (Bloch and Maki, 1973). This is due to the propensity of IgA to form polymers. In one instance (Freel et al., 1972) a major portion of the patient's IgA protein had a sedimentation coefficient of 9S, while in another patient with hyperviscosity the IgA consisted mainly of 11S polymers (Dine et al., 1972). An IgA monoclonal protein with pyroglobulin properties was found to have hyperviscosity (Sugai, 1972). The serum viscosity was decreased when the monoclonal protein was reduced from its original 15.5S sedimentation coefficient to 6.7S. Tuddenham et al. (1974) also emphasized the frequency of hyperviscosity in IgA myeloma in a report of four cases. They noted an increase of viscosity at lower temperatures in three of them. The importance of IgA polymers and their molecular configuration was emphasized in the report of two cases of hyperviscosity syndrome (Virella et al., 1975).

The incidence of hyperviscosity syndrome was 4.2% in a series of 238 patients with IgG myeloma. It increased to 22% among those with more than 5 g/dl of IgG monoclonal protein (Pruzanski and Watt, 1972).

Either the aggregation of IgG molecules or very high concentrations of proteins may produce the hyperviscosity syndrome.

Aggregation of IgG molecules was thought to be the cause of hyperviscosity syndrome in two patients with myeloma (Smith et al., 1965). In another instance, aggregates of an IgG1 κ monoclonal protein containing as many as 10 protein molecules or more produced the hyperviscosity syndrome (Lindsley et al., 1973). Capra and Kunkel (1970) presumed the tendency of IgG3 monoclonal proteins to form aggregates was the cause of hyperviscosity in three cases, and believed marked excess of IgG1 monoclonal proteins was necessary for the development of hyperviscosity in a fourth. In a larger series (Virella and Hobbs, 1971) there did not appear to be a predominance of IgG3 monoclonal proteins in patients with hyperviscosity. It is of interest in this regard that the monoclonal protein in all 10 of Pruzanski and Watt's (1972) patients with IgG myeloma who had hyperviscosity was of the IgG1 class. In addition to the concentration of the IgG protein, the molecular configuration may be an important determinant of the presence or absence of hyperviscosity (MacKenzie et al., 1970; Rubies-Prat et al., 1974).

It should be pointed out that hyperviscosity is not limited to cases of myeloma or macroglobulinemia. Elevated serum viscosity was reported in 32 of 37 patients with rheumatoid arthritis who had a high titer of rheumatoid factor and in 13 of 18 patients with lupus erythematosus (Shearn et al., 1963). Hyperviscosity in rheumatoid arthritis appears to be related to the formation of polymers of IgG (intermediate complexes) in the serum (Pope et al., 1975). The hyperviscosity syndrome in Sjögren's syndrome has been reported recently (Alarcón-Segovia et al., 1974; Blaylock et al., 1974).

IgM-producing plasma-cell tumors in mice provide a model for the study of the pathogenesis of the hyperviscosity syndrome (McIntire et al., 1965). In this model, hyperviscosity was found to be a function of both the plasma concentration of macroglobulin and the hematocrit. The macroglobulin produced aggregation of the erythrocytes, which further elevated the viscosity (Rosenblum and Asofsky, 1968). These erythrocyte aggregates may cause vasoconstriction to occlude the microcirculation further (Rosenblum, 1969). IgM-producing plasma-cell tumors have been reported in more than 30% of NZB-NZW F1 mice older than 11 months (Sugai et al., 1973). Macroglobulins with hyperviscosity were found in a dog that bled excessively following dental surgery (Hurvitz et al., 1970).

Treatment for the hyperviscosity syndrome per se consists of plasmapheresis, as introduced by Adams et al. in 1952. Satisfactory results may be obtained with a Sorvall RC3 centrifuge and plasmapheresis sets from Fenwal Laboratories. A large intravenous needle is inserted and 500 ml of blood is withdrawn into the blood-donor pack. The needle is kept open with a slow drip of normal saline. The pack contains ACD anticoagulant and has an attached 300-ml plasma pack. The blood is centrifuged at 5,000 rpm (Sorvall RC3 centrifuge) for 5 minutes and the plasma separated into the plasma pack. Red cells are returned to the patient after resuspension in saline and the plasma is discarded. One or two or more units may be withdrawn each day, depending upon the patient's symptoms. Dramatic improvement in symptoms may occur; retinopathy resolves, neurologic symptoms disappear, and bleeding ceases. Plasmapheresis usually is well tolerated, but side effects may include syncope, nausea, or dizziness.

Rapid plasmapheresis has been reported to be facilitated by the installation of an arteriovenous shunt (Loughrey and Meyer, 1974). A more effective method is the use of an NCI-IBM continuous-flow blood-cell separator (Powles et al., 1971) (see page 213). We have found the Haemonetics blood processor (Haemonetics Corp., Natick, MA) effective and more economical than the NCI-IBM separator. Plasmapheresis is effective in the treatment of the hyperviscosity syndrome from macroglobulinemia because three-fourths of IgM is in the intravascular space and therefore readily available for removal. Obviously, plasmapheresis is more effective with polymers of IgA and aggregates of IgG than with the monomer forms of these immunoglobulins.

CHAPTER XVIII

Heavy-Chain Diseases

HEAVY-CHAIN DISEASES are characterized by the presence of monoclonal proteins comprising a portion of the immunoglobulin heavy chain in the serum or urine, or both. In the first report of γ heavy-chain disease, Franklin et al. (1964) postulated the existence of two additional heavy-chain diseases, α and μ—a prophecy fulfilled.

γ **Heavy-Chain Disease (γHCD):** Osserman and Takatsuki (1964) described the features of four additional cases of γ heavy-chain disease in the same journal issue as the first report. The abnormal protein is the heavy chain of IgG (γ), mainly the Fc fragment of it, for the monoclonal protein does not include all of the variable portion of the heavy chain. Approximately two-thirds of the patients are male, and most are beyond the age of 40. The onset is insidious in about half of the cases. Weakness, fatigue, and lymphadenopathy are common initially. The lymphadenopathy usually is cervical or axillary but may be generalized. In some cases the nodes enlarge and shrink. Fever, not attributed to infection, is present in about half of the patients. Hepatosplenomegaly is found in almost half initially and in a majority at some time during the illness. Edema of the uvula and palate has been seen in a number of instances and is presumably due to involvement of Waldeyer's ring of lymph nodes with resulting lymphatic obstruction.

Anemia, usually normocytic and normochromic, develops in virtually all patients. Leukopenia and relative lymphocytosis are common. The lymphocytes are atypical and plasma cells may be seen in the peripheral blood. In fact, two instances of plasma-cell leukemia have been reported (Frangione and Franklin, 1973). Thrombocytopenia is not uncommon and eosinophilia has been noted often. The bone-marrow aspirate contains increased numbers of plasma cells and lymphocytes and occasionally manifests eosinophilia. Roentgenologically the skeleton appears normal, and only one case with osteolytic bone lesions has been reported (Bloch et al., 1973). Thus the clinical pattern suggests an atypical lymphoma. Indeed, nodal biopsy in one case suggested Hodgkin's disease because of the presence of several reticulum cells resembling Reed-Sternberg cells (Ellman and Bloch, 1968).

The most significant laboratory feature is formation of a dense globulin band or spike on electrophoresis of the urine, a negative response to the Bence Jones heat test, and lack of light-chain identity on immunoelectrophoresis. In such cases, immunoelectrophoresis of the concentrated urine will reveal a γ heavy chain. The urinary excretion of γ heavy chain has varied from trace amounts to 20 g/day, but in more than half of instances it has been less than 1 g/day. Consequently, careful study of concentrated urine samples may be necessary. The serum electrophoretic pattern usually reveals a band in the beta-gamma region, but often the band is broad and looks heterogeneous and more suggestive of a polyclonal than a monoclonal protein. The size of the serum spike ranges from several grams to instances in which no discrete band can be seen, again illustrating the need for immunoelectrophoresis with appropriate antisera.

Therapy has been disappointing. Most patients follow a downhill course and die in a few months, but some survive for 5 years or longer. Local radiation may be beneficial temporarily by reducing the size of the spleen or lymph nodes. Alkylating agents have accomplished little. Occasional responses to prednisone, vinblastine, or a combination of nitrogen mustard, vincristine, prednisone, and procarbazine have been recorded (Bloch et al., 1973). In one case, pulsed administration of cyclophosphamide and prednisone produced a complete remission lasting more than 2 years (Lyons et al., 1975). At autopsy one usually finds lymphadenopathy and increases in lymphocytes, plasma cells, plasmacytoid lymphocytes, reticulum cells, and eosinophils. Malignant lymphoma has been diagnosed definitively in some cases, but in others the histologic evidence has been considered benign. Two patients have had amyloid infiltrates at autopsy.

The etiology of γ heavy-chain disease is unknown, but association with rheumatoid arthritis in two cases has been reported (Zawadzki et al., 1969; Kretschmer et al., 1974). Interestingly, a γ chain resembling that in γ heavy-chain disease has been isolated from normal human plasma; this is the counterpart of an "abnormal protein" in normal humans (Lam and Stevenson, 1973).

The heavy chain is usually present as a dimer and has a sedimentation coefficient of 3.5 to 4S and a molecular weight generally between 45,000 and 55,000. The majority of cases have belonged to the IgG1 subclass, in accord with the known incidence of the subclasses. The chain in γ heavy-chain disease is not complete, and significant amino acid deletions have been found in all instances. Frangione and Franklin (1973) have classified the γ heavy-chain proteins into four types: type 1—partial deletion of the Fd fragment with resumption of normal synthesis at position 216; type 2—deletion of the hinge region; type 3—partial deletion of the Fd fragment and the hinge region; and type 4—perhaps derived enzymatically from a large H chain. The heavy-chain sequence begins in the hinge region and probably represents degradation of a heavy-chain disease protein rather than an intact product of a gene.

Originally the γ heavy chain was presumed to be a structure synthesized de novo and not a degradation product of a normal IgG molecule (Franklin et al., 1964), and this has been confirmed by Buxbaum and Preud'homme (1972), who found no evidence of post-ribosomal intracellular degradation of the γ chain.

Bence Jones proteinuria is not a feature of γ heavy-chain disease. However, small quantities of free light chains in the urine have been recorded (Kretschmer et al., 1974).

One patient with γ heavy-chain disease had a benign, stable course characterized by splenomegaly and moderate plasmacytosis in the bone marrow and spleen (Westin et al., 1972). This is analogous to benign monoclonal gammopathy of the heavy-chain type.

α **Heavy-Chain Disease (α HCD):** First described in 1968 (Seligmann et al., 1968, 1971), α heavy-chain disease has become the most frequently reported type, having 59 cases in the literature (Seligmann, 1975a, b). This entity is characterized by severe malabsorption with weight loss, diarrhea, and steatorrhea. It is most common in the second and third decades of life, and about 60% of the patients are men. Most cases have been reported from the Mediterranean region, but it occurs elsewhere too. Pittman et al. (1975) described a patient from South America with severe malabsorption from malignant lymphoma of the jejunum and ileum and a monoclonal α heavy chain in the serum. Florin-Christensen et al. (1974) described a patient with α-chain disease and dyspnea and the roentgenographic pattern of diffuse interstitial pulmonary fibrosis. At autopsy no lymphoma was found. The authors reviewed the published reports of α-chain disease involving the lung and emphasized absence of lymphoma in the pulmonary form of α-chain disease.

Rarely has the digestive tract been spared; and when it has, the respiratory system was involved. In a review of 25 cases of primary intestinal lymphoma, Shahid et al. (1975) reported that 4 (16%) had α-chain disease. They suggested that α heavy-chain disease is a variant of primary intestinal lymphoma and not a separate disease entity.

Abdominal pain is common and abdominal masses have been palpable, particularly late in the course of the disease. Hepatosplenomegaly and peripheral lymphadenopathy are not seen or occur only in an advanced stage.

Radiologic studies and biopsies indicate that the entire length of the small intestine and rectum is involved. There is diffuse and extensive infiltration of the lamina propria by lymphoid cells with plasmacytoid features. Osteolytic bone lesions have not been reported, and the bone marrow is rarely involved. Occasional plasma cells have been detected in the peripheral blood.

The serum protein electrophoretic pattern is normal in half the cases, and in the remainder an unimpressive broad band may appear in the alpha-2 or beta regions. The characteristic sharp band or peak suggestive of a monoclonal protein is never seen. Consequently, immunoelectrophoresis with antisera to IgA or α chain is necessary. One must be careful in diagnosis, because in some cases a complete monoclonal IgA protein will not type with light-chain antisera. Hypogammaglobulinemia is common. The amount of a chain in the urine is small, and the urine must be concentrated before it can be detected. Bence Jones proteinuria has never been reported.

All monoclonal a chains have been of the a_1 subclass. They tend to polymerize, and J chain has been found in all instances. The molecular weight ranges from 29,000 to 34,000 and represents 50 to 75% of a complete a_1 heavy chain. The Fd segment of the a chain is missing, but the hinge structure is present. There is no evidence that degradation of the a chain occurs after its release from the ribosomes.

Not all young persons with diffuse lymphoid infiltration of the small intestine have a-chain disease. An 18-year-old patient with lymphocytic infiltration of the gastrointestinal tract and an IgG3 κ monoclonal protein (Kopéc et al., 1974) and a 30-year-old woman with malabsorption had massive mature plasma-cell infiltration of the lamina propria of the small intestine and mesenteric lymph nodes and a monoclonal IgA κ protein in the serum (Chantar et al., 1974).

Most often, a-chain disease is progressive and fatal; yet remissions in response to melphalan or cyclophosphamide and prednisone (Doe, 1975), and, surprisingly, to antibiotics, have been recorded (Seligmann, 1975a, b). The latter finding suggests that the causative agent might be an infectious agent.

μ **Heavy-Chain Disease** (μ **HCD**): A case of μ heavy-chain disease associated with chronic lymphocytic leukemia and amyloidosis was reported in 1970 (Ballard et al., 1970; Forte et al., 1970). Seven cases of this disease were described by Franklin (1975); and chronic lymphocytic leukemia was associated in all but one. The lack of peripheral lymphadenopathy, the presence of vacuolated plasma cells in the bone marrow, and the large amounts of Bence Jones protein excreted in the urine distinguished these from the usual cases of chronic lymphocytic leukemia. Hepatosplenomegaly is common. All patients have been more than 40 years of age. The serum-protein electrophoretic pattern usually appears normal, and the presence of a dense band is exceptional. Hypogammaglobulinemia is common. The diagnosis is made by immunoelectrophoresis. Only one patient excreted the μ-chain fragment in the urine.

But not all μ HCD cases have the features described above. Bonhomme et al. (1974) reported one that did not include chronic lymphocytic leukemia and differed from the others in having massive splenomegaly, no vacuoles in the bone-marrow plasma cells, a dense band in the serum-protein electrophoretic pattern, and no Bence Jones proteinuria. They mentioned that they had seen a second case of μ HCD with splenomegaly but no chronic lymphocytic leukemia. Biserte et al. (1973) described a patient with μ HCD who had an abnormal band in the alpha-1 area of the serum electrophoretic pattern, but no evidence of chronic lymphocytic leukemia, Bence Jones proteinuria, or vacuolated plasma cells in the bone marrow.

Although μ-chain disease is rare in chronic lymphocytic leukemia, it is worthwhile to screen the sera of chronic lymphocytic leukemia patients with immunoelectrophoresis, particularly if Bence Jones proteinuria or other features not typical of lymphocytic leukemia are present.

Both μ and κ chains have been demonstrated in the same cell. This suggests that both heavy and light chains are synthesized. It appears likely that the portion of the μ chain that contains the cystine residue involved in attachment of the light chain to the heavy chain is deleted, thus preventing excretion of a complete IgM molecule (Zucker-Franklin and Franklin, 1971).

CHAPTER XIX

Amyloidosis

A MYLOIDOSIS WAS PROBABLY first noted in the 17th century by Bonet, who described a patient with a liver abscess whose enormous spleen contained innumerable white "stones." This presumably was the sago spleen of amyloidosis. Rokitansky, in 1842, described waxy liver with lardaceous degeneration and found it occurred in tuberculosis, syphilis, and rickets (Schwartz, 1970).

The term *amyloid* was coined by Schleiden to describe a normal amylaceous constituent of plants. Using the iodine and the iodine-sulfuric acid tests, Virchow misnamed the substance "amyloid" because he thought that it resembled starch or cellulose. Meckel discovered that the lardaceous changes were present not only in the liver, spleen, and kidney but also in the aorta, arteries, and intestinal wall—the distribution of amyloid that we recognize today. Budd stated that the waxiness of the liver was attributable to an albuminous rather than a fatty substance. Friedreich and Kekulé also believed that amyloid was actually "albuminoid" and thus protein, but they suggested that the term *amyloid* should not be abandoned (Schwartz, 1970).

Primary amyloidosis was probably first reported in 1856, when Wilks described a 51-year-old man with "lardaceous viscera" in whom the changes were unrelated to syphilis, osteomyelitis or other osseous disease, or tuberculosis. Another case, that of a woman in whom the findings were compatible with multiple myeloma and amyloidosis, was presented in 1872 by Adams. Even so, the first case report of primary amyloidosis is generally credited to Wild, in 1886. In 1903, Weber described a patient with myeloma and amyloidosis; and in the following year Askanazy-Königsberg (1904) gave an excellent description of amyloid in myeloma. Lubarsch, in 1929, described three cases of primary amyloidosis and presented criteria for differentiating primary from secondary amyloidosis; the only criterion that has been strictly adhered to, however, is the absence of preexisting or coexisting etiologic disease.

The subject of primary amyloidosis has been reviewed comprehensively by Koletsky and Stecher (1939), Eisen (1946), Dahlin (1949), Higgins and Higgins (1950), Mathews (1954), Rukavina et al. (1956), Symmers (1956), Kyle and Bayrd (1961, 1975), Osserman et al. (1964), Engle and Wallis (1966), Brandt and colleagues (1968), and—in a superb study—by Cohen (1967).

MICROSCOPIC APPEARANCE AND PATHOGENESIS

Microscopic Features: Amyloid, a substance that appears homogeneous and amorphous under the light microscope, stains pink with hematoxylin and eosin and metachromatically with methyl violet or crystal violet. Thioflavine T produces an intense yellow-green fluorescence with amyloid; but false-positives occur, and it is not completely satisfactory as a test (Rogers, 1965). Congo red is widely used for staining, though it stains collagen and elastic tissue in addition to amyloid. Under the polarizing microscope, however, Congo red produces a green birefringence of amyloid; and it is the most specific stain for the detection of amyloid. Romhányi (1971), who modified the Congo red method by treating the tissue with proteolytic enzymes, facilitated the distinction of the birefringence of amyloid from that of collagen tissues.

The amorphous, hyaline-like appearance of amyloid is misleading, because amyloid is a fibrous protein (Cohen and Calkins, 1959). Under the electron microscope, it is seen to consist of rigid, non-branching fibrils approximately 50 to 150 Å in width. The length of the fibrils has not been determined because a single fibril cannot be seen in its entirety; but it has been estimated as of the order of 8,000 Å.

Primary amyloid, compared with secondary amyloid, is said to stain atypically. It has also been said that primary amyloid involves the heart, tongue, gastrointestinal tract, nerves, and skin, whereas secondary amyloid mainly involves the liver, kidney, and spleen; but it must be emphasized that no consistent differences between primary and secondary amyloid have been demonstrated by staining characteristics, organ distribution, or even electron microscopy (Cohen and Shirahama, 1973).

Amyloid fibrils are arranged in an antiparallel relation and β-pleated sheet conformation as is revealed by low-angle x-ray diffraction—which is the third major technique (after light and electron microscopy) for specifically recognizing amyloid substance. Amyloid fibrils are insoluble, generally resist proteolytic digestion, and are components of the amyloid deposits that replace and destroy normal cardiac, renal, and other tissues.

Another structure in all amyloid tissue that has been described is the "doughnut," "rod," or "P" (plasma or pentagonal) component (Bladen et al., 1966). This is a glycoprotein, migrating as an a_1-globulin. Its presence is not limited to amyloid and its part in the pathogenesis of amyloid is unexplained. The P component has a molecular weight of 180,000 but can be reduced to 36,000, suggesting that it is composed of five subunits. Preliminary amino acid sequencing shows that it is different from all other protein sequences known to date (Skinner et al., 1974). The polysaccharide portion usually reported in amyloid deposits probably represents an accumulation as a secondary phenomenon (Glenner et al., 1973).

Pathogenesis: The cause of amyloidosis is not known. Casein injections have long been used for experimental induction of amyloidosis in mice. It has been postulated that the endotoxin of *Escherichia coli,* an endotoxin that frequently contaminates casein, may be the factor that causes the induction (Barth et al., 1968a, b). The morphologic, histochemical, and serologic abnormalities produced in mice by casein injection or by reticulum-cell sarcoma in mice did not appear fundamentally different from those seen in amyloidosis (Christensen and Rask-Nielsen, 1962). Tolerance to casein, but not to other antigens, has developed during induction of experimental amyloidosis in guinea pigs; and this may be important in pathogenesis (Cathcart et al., 1970). Moesner et al. (1974) reported that tolerance to casein was not a prerequisite for amyloid development; but the two groups of investigators were not using the same casein preparation, and this may account for some of the differences.

Although abnormalities of immunoglobulins are common in amyloidosis, the functional response of the lymphocytes to phytohemagglutinin stimulation has shown no distinct abnormality (Briccetti et al., 1973). Scheinberg and Cathcart (1974) showed a depression of T-cell function in CBA/J mice during administration of casein. This occurred just before amyloid was seen and at a time when B-cell function was normal. However, similar T-cell abnormalities are seen in other animals that do not develop amyloid; and this observation suggests an additional mechanism in the development of amyloidosis. The same investigators reported an increase in B-cell proliferation of spleen cells of CBA/J mice before and during amyloid deposition (Scheinberg and Cathcart, 1975).

Repeated casein injections can induce amyloidosis in mice with congenital aplasia of the thymus, but the number of casein injections necessary is greater than in C3H mice. Spleen grafts from C3H mice accelerated amyloid induction, but similar grafts from casein-sensitized nude mice did not. The absence of acceleration of amyloid deposition may be due to poorer trapping of donor spleen cells in the nude mouse spleens than in the normal C3H spleens (Hardt and Claësson, 1974).

An amyloid-inducing factor from spleen cells of animals tolerant to casein produced amyloid at an accelerated rate (Cathcart et al., 1972b). Keizman et al. (1972) reported finding a glycopeptide with a molecular weight of 10,000 that produced increased amounts of amyloid in mice given casein. An influence of the immune apparatus in production of amyloidosis in mice is also suggested by the finding of increased amyloid deposition after casein injections when various immunosuppressive agents were given (Hardt, 1971). In another study, however, deposition of amyloid did not increase when cortisone acetate was given during induction of amyloid with Freund's adjuvant (Polliack et al., 1973). What immunosuppressive agents do, if anything, in the production of amyloidosis remains to be elucidated. Decrease of immunoglobulin production may affect the development of amyloidosis in laboratory animals, because spontaneous amyloidosis is more common in germ-free mice than in normal ones (Anderson, 1971).

The relationship of Bence Jones protein to amyloid was first postulated by Magnus-Levy (1931, 1952) more than 40 years ago. Osserman and associates (1964) emphasized the association of Bence Jones protein and amyloidosis and proposed that Bence Jones proteins were directly involved in the production of amyloid. Glenner and associates (1971b) demonstrated that amyloid fibrils in a patient with amyloidosis were virtually identical to the variable portion of a monoclonal light chain (Bence Jones protein)—a major advance. This development culminated in the demonstration of identical sequences for the 27 amino-terminal residues of the amyloid fibril protein isolated from the small intestine of a patient and kappa Bence Jones protein isolated from the urine of the same patient (Terry et al., 1973).

Furthermore, Glenner and associates (1971a) used pepsin (pH 3.5, 37°C) to digest monoclonal human Bence Jones proteins and created amyloid fibrils. These amyloid fibrils had both the electron microscopic appearance and the characteristic staining reactions of amyloid; thus the place of Bence Jones protein in the pathogenesis of amyloid was confirmed. But although other investigators also have produced amyloid fibrils from Bence Jones protein, many monoclonal Bence Jones proteins do not produce amyloid fibrils under these conditions (Linke et al., 1973b; Shirahama et al., 1973). In one study, amyloid fibrils formed from the Bence Jones proteins of eight of nine patients were of the $V_{\lambda I}$ subclass (Linke et al., 1973a).

Tan and Epstein (1972) found that lysosomes of normal human kidney would degrade monoclonal light chains and thus produce an insoluble polymer. Although this insoluble polymer was not stained for amyloid, a similar process might form amyloid fibrils *in vivo*. Recently Epstein et al. (1974) reported that kappa and lambda monoclonal light chains formed fibrils with the appearance and size of naturally occurring human amyloid fibrils. Congo red showed a variable degree of green birefringence under polarized light.

Lambda light chains are more commonly associated with amyloidosis than are kappa chains. This is unexpected because, under normal circumstances and in patients with myeloma, kappa chains are more common than lambda. Lambda light chains have a β-pleated sheet conformation as do some kappa light chains (Epp et al., 1974). In addition, lambda light chains may be more likely than kappa chains to form polymers that might produce amyloid rather than be excreted (Glenner and Terry, 1974).

Osserman and associates (1964) reported that Bence Jones protein from patients with amyloidosis had a greater tendency to bind to certain normal tissues than did other Bence Jones proteins—so evidencing a greater tissue affinity. Perhaps, therefore, these could be called amyloidogenic. This difference, if confirmed, would be most important. It is likely that the amyloidogenic characteristics would be found in the variable portion of the light chain.

Thus, light chains or light-chain fragments may be secreted by the plasma cell and react with tissue components or receptors to form amyloid fibrils. The amyloid fibrils may be produced within cells or the light chains, after being secreted, may form fibrils outside the cell (Franklin and Zucker-Franklin, 1972).

In rare instances, heavy chains apparently produce amyloidosis. Pepsin digestion of an IgG3 heavy chain from a patient with amyloidosis and γ HCD produced a precipitate that gave a green birefringence under polarized light after Congo red staining. An electron micrograph of the pepsin digest showed amyloid fibrils (Pruzanski et al., 1974a).

Besides recognition of the immunoglobulin nature of some patients' amyloid, another major advance has been the recognition that in patients with familial and secondary amyloidosis, much of the amyloid consists of a component termed protein A (Benditt and Eriksen, 1971), ASF (acid-soluble fraction) (Levin et al., 1972), amyloid of unknown origin (AUO) (Glenner et al., 1973), or amyloid subunit (AS) (Husby et al., 1973). This protein has a molecular weight of 8,500 and does not resemble any known immunoglobulin.

Husby and Natvig (1974), using an antiserum to protein AS, demonstrated a specific precipitin band (protein AS-related component, protein ASC) in sera from 48 of 55 patients with various types of amyloidosis. Using a more sensitive technique, they found protein ASC in normal sera. Apparently, therefore, it may be a precursor or a component of some forms of amyloid; but its biochemical relationship to the two major forms of amyloid discussed above remains to be clarified.

Utilizing a radioimmunoassay, Rosenthal and Franklin (1975) confirmed and extended the previous findings by detecting the amyloid-related component of the human serum (SAA) in all of 228 normal sera. The SAA level was elevated in all cases of amyloidosis except those associated with nephrotic syndrome, as well as in many patients with myeloma, macroglobulinemia, lymphoma, rheumatoid arthritis, and tuberculosis. The SAA concentration increased with age and reached very high levels in the eighth and ninth decades. Marked increases of SAA were found in early stages of acute inflammatory and infectious states. Benson et al. (1975a) reported that SAA suppressed antibody formation.

Recently, Husby et al. (1974) reported another serum component (ARC) related to amyloid protein AR that was derived from a patient with primary amyloidosis. Among 352 sera with monoclonal components, ARC was detected in 16 and ASC in 149. Only 1 of the 16 sera with protein ARC contained protein ASC, indicating a high degree of mutual exclusion between the two serum components.

There may be additional components or forms of amyloid yet to be described biochemically.

Although amyloidosis can be separated into two major groups —i.e., the fibrils consist mainly of light chains or of protein A— there may be common components or factors in the production of amyloid fibrils in the various forms of amyloidosis. Benson et al. (1975c) produced antisera to amyloid fibrils from patients with primary amyloidosis, amyloidosis associated with myeloma, and secondary amyloidosis. There was a high degree of cross reactivity among the three types of amyloid. One antiserum directed against protein A induced a reaction in several of the secondary cases, as expected, but in two primary cases also.

Furthermore, the metabolism or breakdown of amyloid fibrils may be an important pathogenetic factor. Recently, one heat-stable component in normal human serum has been shown to degrade amyloid from a patient with familial Mediterranean fever; and another has had the same effect on amyloid from a patient with Hodgkin's disease (Kedar et al., 1974). This degradation, possibly proteolytic, may be related to the phenomenon of sensitivity to proteolytic digestion as described by Romhányi (1972), which seems to affect chiefly the amyloid not related to immunoglobulin. Excellent reviews of the pathogenesis of amyloidosis have been published by Franklin and Zucker-Franklin (1972), Glenner et al. (1973, 1974), and Cohen and Cathcart (1974).

CLASSIFICATION

There is no truly satisfactory classification of amyloidosis. Reimann and associates (1935) classified amyloidosis as primary when there was no underlying disease, as secondary when there was an associated chronic disease, as tumor-forming when small localized masses of amyloid were found, and as associated with multiple myeloma when that disease was present. Missmahl (1968) and Aly and associates (1969) divided amyloidosis into two types: perireticular, including hereditary and secondary types; and pericollangenic, comprising primary amyloidosis and amyloidosis associated with myeloma. This classification, based on the initial deposition of amyloid along the reticulum fibers or among collagen fibers, has not been generally accepted. Recently Isobe and Osserman (1974a) have suggested a new classification based on the predominant clinical patterns of amyloid distribution; this will be discussed in detail separately.

We prefer the following classification, which is very similar to that of Reimann et al. (1935) and has the advantage of exploiting what is currently known about the biochemistry of the amyloid fibril.

Classification	*Major Protein Component**
1. Primary amyloidosis: no evidence of preceding or coexisting disease	Ig-V_L
2. Amyloidosis with multiple myeloma	Ig-V_L
3. Secondary amyloidosis: coexistence of other conditions such as rheumatoid arthritis or chronic infection	AUO
4. Localized amyloid: involvement of a single organ without evidence of generalized involvement	Ig-V_L[†]
5. Familial amyloidosis	AUO

* Ig-V_L = variable portion of light chain; AUO = amyloid of unknown origin.
† Page et al., 1972.

TABLE 55

AMYLOIDOSIS: DISTRIBUTION OF CASES BY TYPE
(MAYO CLINIC)

	Cases	
Type	*No.*	*%*
Primary (group 1)	132	56
With myeloma (group 2)	61	26
Localized	22	9
Secondary	19	8
Familial	2	1
Total	236	100

Much of the following data is based on a review of amyloidosis seen at the Mayo Clinic in the 13-year period 1960 through 1972 (Kyle and Bayrd, 1975). On the basis of the appearance and number of the plasma cells in the bone marrow, the amount of monoclonal protein in the serum and urine, and the presence or absence of skeletal lesions, the patients with systemic amyloidosis were divided into two groups: those with primary amyloidosis (group 1) and those with amyloidosis with multiple myeloma (group 2). In addition, patients with secondary, localized, and familial amyloidosis were categorized. Histologic proof of amyloidosis was found in 236 cases. Their distribution is seen in Table 55. Of the 236 patients, 193 had either primary amyloidosis (group 1) or amyloidosis with myeloma (group 2); there were 132 patients in group 1 and 61 in group 2.

CLINICAL FEATURES

Primary amyloidosis and amyloidosis with myeloma occur more often in men (63 and 56%, respectively) than in women, and each type is rare before the age of 40 years (Table 56). The mean age was virtually identical to that of 869 patients with myeloma seen at the Mayo Clinic. A history of malignancy was obtained in 6% of the cases of primary amyloidosis (group 1) and in 3% of the cases of amyloidosis with myeloma (group 2).

The most common presenting symptoms were fatigue or weakness, weight loss, ankle edema, dyspnea, paresthesias, and light-headedness or syncope (Table 57). Weight loss was a feature in

TABLE 56

AMYLOIDOSIS: AGE AND SEX AT DIAGNOSIS
(MAYO CLINIC)

			Distribution, %			
		Primary			With Myeloma	
Age Group	M	F	Total	M	F	Total
< 40	1	4	2	3	4	3
40-49	10	18	13	3	7	5
50-59	31	33	32	35	37	36
60-69	38	33	36	38	33	36
70-79	12	10	11	21	19	20
≥ 80	8	2	6	0	0	0
No. patients	83	49	132	34	27	61
(% of group)	(63)	(37)	(100)	(56)	(44)	(100)
Mean age, yr.	62.5	57.5	60.6	61.2	61.0	61.1

more than half of our cases and was severe in many, amounting to 22.5 kg (50 lb) in some. Among all who lost weight, the mean amount was 12.2 kg. Light-headedness or syncope, usually associated with orthostatic hypotension, was fairly common; it should always suggest the possibility that amyloidosis is present. Symptoms of the carpal tunnel syndrome, including paresthesias of the hands, were frequent, though often direct questioning was needed to elicit mention of them. Hoarseness or change of the voice to a weak, high-pitched sound—very distinctive and easily

TABLE 57

PRESENTING SYMPTOMS WITH AMYLOIDOSIS
(MAYO CLINIC)

	Distribution and Mean Duration in			
	Primary		With Myeloma	
Symptom	% 132 Pts.	Months	% 61 Pts.	Months
Fatigue	67	14	65	13
Weight loss	55	11	62	9
Ankle edema	46	11	41	7
Dyspnea	30	13	33	10
Paresthesias	26	24	26	12
Light-headedness or syncope	30	9	7	20
"Hoarseness"	12	14	16	4
Bleeding, gross	7	3	11	9
Pain	5	6	34	15

recognized—should alert one to the possibility of amyloidosis. This symptom was noted in approximately 13% of cases, and probably is more common than that. Gross bleeding, usually manifested as purpura, was seen occasionally. The only differences in incidence of symptoms between the two groups are the increased frequency of light-headedness or syncope in those of primary amyloidosis and, as might be expected from the definitions used in our groupings, the infrequent complaint of bone pain in patients of that group.

Most important was the duration of presenting symptoms (Table 57), which for most categories was approximately 1 year, though the mean duration of paresthesias among the patients with primary amyloidosis was 2 years, which thus affords the clinician a period of 1 to 2 years for diagnosis.

The principal initial physical findings included ankle edema, purpura, and enlargement of the liver and tongue (Table 58). The liver was palpable in almost half of patients; and in half of these, its edge was palpable more than 5 cm below the costal margin. Splenomegaly was an initial finding in less than 10% of patients, and when present was usually modest. Lymphadenopathy is not common. Macroglossia, though it appeared in only 26% of group 2 and 12% of group 1, can be extremely impressive (Fig. 63). In occasional cases a portion of the tongue protruded

TABLE 58

AMYLOIDOSIS: INITIAL PHYSICAL FINDINGS
(MAYO CLINIC)

Finding	Incidence, % in	
	Primary	With Myeloma
Liver palpable	45	49
Ankle edema	35	33
Spleen palpable	7	11
Macroglossia	12	26
Lymphadenopathy		
Generalized	8	8
Submandibular	9	11
Purpura	17	15
Hypotension, orthostatic	16	8
Skin lesions (amyloid)	4	8

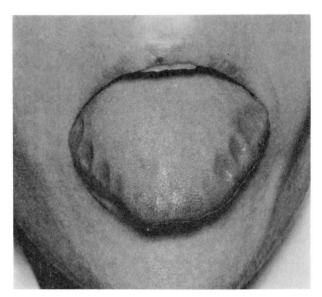

Figure 63. Macroglossia of primary amyloidosis. Note dental indentations. (From Kyle, R. A., and Bayrd, E. D.: Monoclonal gammopathies. In Linman, J. W.: *Hematology: Physiologic, Pathophysiologic, and Clinical Principles*. New York, Macmillan Company, 1975, pp. 753-822. By permission.)

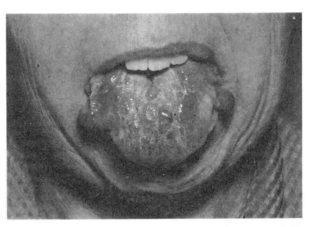

Figure 64. Irregular enlargement of tongue in primary amyloidosis. Some portions of tongue extend through gaps between teeth.

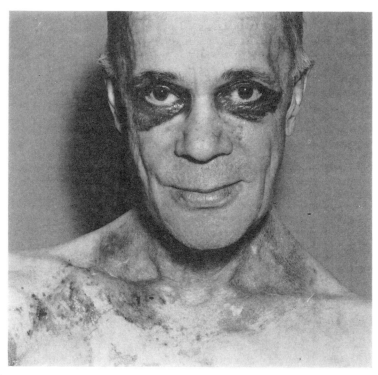

Figure 65. Postproctoscopic periorbital purpura (PPPP) in amyloidosis. Patient also has purpura on neck and upper part of chest. (From Kyle, R. A., and Bayrd, E. D.: Monoclonal gammopathies. In Linman, J. W.: *Hematology: Physiologic, Pathophysiologic, and Clinical Principles.* New York, Macmillan Company, 1975, pp. 753-822. By permission.)

through gaps where teeth were missing to produce a unique deformity (Fig. 64). Enlargement of the submandibular structures, which is almost always associated with macroglossia, occurred in about 10% of patients; this finding, as well as dental indentation, may help in deciding whether the tongue is enlarged.

Purpura was not infrequent and often involved the face and neck, particularly the upper eyelids. Purpura of the eyelids after pinching is a characteristic sign of amyloidosis; periorbital purpura may be striking after proctoscopy (postproctoscopic palpebral purpura; PPPP) (Fig. 65). This can also be seen with

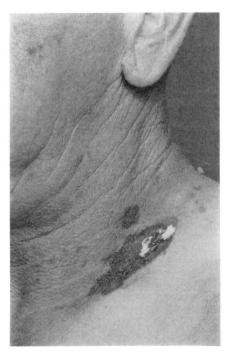

Figure 66. Results of fragility of skin in primary amyloidosis.

vomiting or coughing, or after the Valsalva maneuver. Skin lesions of amyloid, other than purpura, were uncommon. The skin is fragile and occasionally seems virtually to be shed during routine examination (Fig. 66). Pseudohypertrophy of the shoulders and cervical muscles from amyloid infiltration may be prominent (Fig. 67). Edema is common and may be associated with congestive heart failure or the nephrotic syndrome. Orthostatic hypotension may be prominent, and its presence should alert one to the diagnosis of amyloidosis. Specific signs of congestive heart failure, nephrotic syndrome, malabsorption, peripheral neuropathy, and the carpal tunnel syndrome must be sought during the history and physical examination of these patients.

Syndromes: The carpal tunnel syndrome, the nephrotic syndrome, congestive heart failure, sprue, peripheral neuropathy, and orthostatic hypotension all are common with amyloidosis

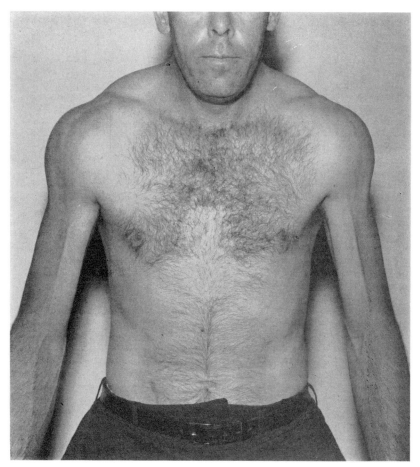

Figure 67. Pseudohypertrophy of muscles in primary amyloidosis. (From Kyle, R. A., and Bayrd, E. D.: Amyloidosis: review of 236 cases. *Medicine* [Baltimore], *54*:271-299, 1975. By permission of Williams & Wilkins Company.)

(Table 59). The nephrotic syndrome was found in 32% of the patients with primary amyloidosis, congestive heart failure in 26%, and the carpal tunnel syndrome, peripheral neuropathy, and orthostatic hypotension each in 16 or 17%. In most patients these abnormalities had existed for 1 to 3 years, thus reflecting the delay in diagnosis of this disease. Among the patients of group 2,

TABLE 59

AMYLOIDOSIS: ASSOCIATION OF OTHER ABNORMALITIES AND SYNDROMES
(MAYO CLINIC)

Syndrome or Other Abnormality	Primary—with Syndrome					With Myeloma—and Syndrome				
	Relation to Diagnosis of Amyloid		After, Cases	In Group (N=132)		Relation to Diagnosis of Amyloid		After, Cases	In Group (N=61)	
	At or Before					At or Before				
	Cases	Months		No.	%	Cases	Months		No.	%
Carpal tunnel	19	34	2	21	16	19	18	1	20	33
Nephrotic	37	10	5	42	32	6	4	1	7	11
Congestive heart failure	28	11	6	34	26	14	9	4	18	30
Sprue	5	29	1	6	5	3	17	0	3	5
Peripheral neuropathy	22	20	1	23	17	3	4	0	3	5
Hypotension Orthostatic	17	17	4	21	16	4	5	1	5	8
Other	4	0.4	4	8	6	0	...	0	0	0

the incidence of the carpal tunnel syndrome and congestive heart failure was high, whereas that of the other syndromes was inconsequential.

LABORATORY FINDINGS

Blood and Urine Studies: Table 60 lists initial findings of blood and urine tests in our series. Initially, anemia was present in less than 50% of our patients and usually was of modest degree. As expected, anemia was more common and more severe in patients with myeloma. The leukocyte count was normal in most patients. The erythrocyte sedimentation rate varied, exceeding 50 mm in 1 hour (Westergren) in approximately 50% of cases. Thrombocytosis has been noted (Selroos, 1973); and the count was greater than 500,000/mm³ in 5% of our cases. The platelet

TABLE 60

AMYLOIDOSIS: INITIAL HEMATOLOGIC AND URINARY FINDINGS
(MAYO CLINIC)

Finding	Primary		With Myeloma	
	Tested Pts., No.	Results Pos., %	Tested Pts., No.	Results Pos., %
Hemoglobin, < 12 g/dl	116	29	56	52
Leukocytes				
< 4,000/mm³	115	3	56	7
Immature	106	13	47	15
ESR, > 50 mm in 1 h	107	54	52	48
Thrombocytes				
< 100,000/mm³	71	4	38	16
> 300,000/mm³	71	34	38	18
Proteinuria	116	90	55	98
Bence Jones protein, positive (heat test)	73	8	46	57
Creatinine, increased	80	51	36	44
Uric acid, increased	32	22	26	31
Calcium, > 10.1 mg/dl	78	4	42	33
Cholesterol				
Decreased	73	11	28	32
Increased	73	34	28	18
(Mean)	(301 mg/dl)		(230 mg/dl)	
Triglycerides				
Decreased	40	8	16	6
Increased	40	42	16	37
(Mean)	(184 mg/dl)		(169 mg/dl)	
Plasma cells (bone-marrow), > 15%	87	0	58	52

TABLE 61

AMYLOIDOSIS: INITIAL SERUM CREATININE VALUES
(MAYO CLINIC)

Creatinine, mg/dl	Primary		With Myeloma	
	% of 51 Males	% of 29 Females	% of 20 Males	% of 16 Females
Normal				
Males, < 1.3	49	. . .	60	. . .
Females, < 1.0	. . .	48	. . .	50
Elevated				
—2.0	18	31	25	19
2.1-5.0	29	7	15	19
5.1-10.0	4	11	0	12
> 10	0	3	0	0
(Mean, mg/dl)	(1.9)	(2.3)	(1.5)	(2.3)

count exceeded 300,000/mm³ in more than 30% of our patients with primary amyloidosis.

Proteinuria (sulfosalicylic acid test) occurred in more than 90% of patients. Bence Jones proteinuria (conventional heat test) was demonstrated in 57% of patients with myeloma and its low incidence—only 8%— in those of group 1 is unexplained, though the smaller amount of protein in the primary cases is a significant factor.

Renal insufficiency was present in approximately half of the

TABLE 62

AMYLOIDOSIS: SERUM AND URINARY ELECTROPHORETIC FINDINGS
(MAYO CLINIC)

Finding	Primary		With Myeloma	
	Serum: % 109 Pts.	Urine: % 72 Pts.	Serum: % 55 Pts.	Urine: % 44 Pts.
Mobility of peak				
Gamma	19	4	25	9
Beta	5	3	5	48
Alpha-2	2	1	0	7
Hypogammaglobulinemia	25	. . .	35	. . .
Mainly albumin	. . .	70	. . .	23
Albumin and globulin peaks	. . .	10	. . .	6
Normal	48	11	33	5
Not available	1	1	2	2

patients at the time of diagnosis (Tables 60 and 61); severe renal insufficiency, however, is often a late manifestation. Elevation of the serum uric acid concentration was found in about one-fourth of patients.

As anticipated, the incidence of hypercalcemia was approximately the same among the patients with amyloid and myeloma as among the 869 patients with myeloma seen from 1960 through 1971 and was rare in primary amyloidosis.

Serum protein electrophoresis (Table 62) among the cases of primary amyloidosis showed a peak in one-fourth, hypogammaglobulinemia in one-fourth, and a normal pattern in almost one-half. Among the cases of group 2 the above three kinds of pattern were almost equally common. As expected, the magnitude of the serum globulin peak was greater in the patients of group 2 than in those of group 1 (mean values, 2.9 and 1.7 g/dl, respectively). In fact, 96% of the patients with primary amyloidosis had a serum peak of 3.0 g/dl or less, while more than half with amyloidosis and myeloma had a peak greater than 3.0 g/dl.

Electrophoresis of the urine (Table 62) in group 1 showed a globulin peak in 8% of cases, an albumin peak in 70%, and both albumin and globulin spikes in 10%. In contrast, a urinary globulin peak appeared in 70% of the cases of amyloidosis and myeloma. As expected, the urinary globulin spike in group 2 was significantly greater than in group 1 (4.1 vs. 2.6 g/24 h). The amount of urinary albumin exceeded 5 g/24 h in almost two-thirds of the patients of group 1, but in less than half of those of group 2 from whom a 24-hour urine specimen was obtained. (The amount of the albumin and globulin peaks in the urine were recorded in fewer cases, because for several cases only single specimens were studied and no 24-hour collection was made.)

Immunoelectrophoresis of the serum disclosed a monoclonal protein in almost 50% of the cases of primary amyloidosis and in 74% of those with amyloidosis and myeloma (the numbers being 24 and 25, respectively). Among the latter group, 10 patients had light chains only in the serum (Bence Jones proteinemia) (Table 63). The results of immunoelectrophoresis of urine are shown in Table 64.

TABLE 63

AMYLOIDOSIS: SERUM IMMUNOELECTROPHORETIC FINDINGS
(MAYO CLINIC)

Immunoglobulin	Primary		With Myeloma		Total	
	No.	%	No.	%	No.	%
IgG	20*	41	10	29.5	30*	36
Kappa	6	12	6	17.5	12	14
Lambda	13	27	4	12	17	21
IgA	1	2	3	9	4	5
Kappa	0	...	2	6	2	2.5
Lambda	1	2	1	3	2	2.5
IgM	1	2	0	...	1	1
Kappa	0		0		0	
Lambda	1	2	0		1	1
IgD	0		2	6	2	2
Kappa	0		0		0	
Lambda	0		2	6	2	2
Free	2	4	10	29.5	12	15
Kappa	0		4	12	4	5
Lambda	2	4	6	17.5	8	10
Negative	25	51	9	26	34	41
Total	49	100	34	100	83	100

* 1 with indeterminate light chain.

TABLE 64

AMYLOIDOSIS: URINARY IMMUNOELECTROPHORETIC FINDINGS
(MAYO CLINIC)

Light Chain	Primary Cases	%	With Myeloma Cases	%	Total Cases	%
Kappa	2	10	8	38	10	24
Lambda	5	25	9	43	14	34
Negative	13	65	4	19	17	42
Total	20	100	21	100	41	100

Only 12% of the cases of primary amyloidosis and none of the secondary cases were without evidence of a monoclonal protein in the serum or urine when both were studied (Table 65). It is certain that more cases would have been positive if the urine had been studied in more. We have seen several cases in which electrophoresis and immunoelectrophoresis of a urine specimen concentrated 50- to 100-fold was negative but a monoclonal protein was detected on immunoelectrophoresis when the urine was concentrated 200-fold or when monospecific antiserum of another source was utilized. The incidence of lambda light chains in the serum of the patients of group 1 was striking, 17 of 23 light chains being of this class; but in patients of group 2 the light chain classes were almost equally divided between kappa and lambda.

Osserman (1965a) reported that Bence Jones proteins were found in all of 14 patients whose amyloidosis was associated with

TABLE 65

AMYLOIDOSIS: INCIDENCE OF MONOCLONAL PROTEIN IN SERUM
AND URINE, BY IMMUNOELECTROPHORESIS (MAYO CLINIC)

Result	Primary Cases	%	With Myeloma Cases	%
Positive				
Serum or urine	29	58	32	89
Negative				
Serum (urine not tested)	15	30	4	11
Serum and urine	6	12	0	...
Total	50	100	36	100

overt myeloma and in 21 of 22 patients with primary amyloidosis. Recently Isobe and Osserman (1974a) reported the presence of a monoclonal protein in either the serum or the urine of 88% of 100 patients with different patterns of amyloidosis. Barth and associates (1969) found a monoclonal protein in the serum of 5 patients and a monoclonal light chain in the urine of 4 others in a group of 15 patients with primary amyloidosis. Cathcart and associates (1972a) detected a monoclonal protein in the serum or urine of 10 of 11 patients with lymphoproliferative disorders (including myeloma) and amyloidosis, and found a monoclonal protein in 7 of 14 patients with primary amyloidosis. They found no monoclonal proteins in the serum or urine of patients with localized amyloidosis, hereditary amyloidosis, or secondary amyloidosis. Parr and associates (1971), in a review of the literature, stated that monoclonal serum proteins were present in 80% of patients with primary amyloidosis. The proteins were IgG in half, Bence Jones protein in one-fourth, and IgA and IgM in equal proportions among the remainder.

Decreases in the amount of IgG are common; IgA and IgM values are generally normal.

Normal to modest increases of plasma cells are seen in primary amyloidosis. Bone-marrow aspirate was available for review in 145 of our cases. None of the patients of group 1 had more than 15% plasma cells in the bone marrow, whereas more than half of those of group 2 did (Table 66).

Involvement of Individual Organ-Systems. *1. Kidney:* Renal involvement is extremely common in amyloidosis and is one of the major causes of death. In the glomerulus, amyloid is first deposited in the mesangium. Early lesions show amyloid fibrils around interstitial capillaries and adjacent fibroblasts (Jao and Pirani, 1972). The basement membrane is thickened and contains amyloid fibrils. Such fibrils have also been seen within the tubular lumen and in the urinary sediment. Jao and Pirani (1972) were unable to detect intracytoplasmic amyloid fibrils in the kidney and suggested that the development of the fibrils was an extracellular phenomenon. Reportedly, the heavier the amyloid deposits in the glomerulus, the more severe the renal disease (Mar-

TABLE 66

AMYLOIDOSIS: INITIAL DISTRIBUTION OF BONE-MARROW
PLASMA CELLS (MAYO CLINIC)

Plasma Cells, %	Primary: % of 87 Pts.	With Myeloma: % of 58 Pts.
0-5.0	76	10
5.1-10.0	19	21
10.1-15.0	5	17
15.1-20.0	0	12
20.1-40.0	0	21
40.1+	0	19
(Mean plasma cells)	(4%)	(23%)

tin et al., 1966). Renal-vein thrombosis has been described in primary amyloidosis (Fraser and Kaye, 1961), but is more common in secondary amyloidosis (Barclay et al., 1960). Angiography of the kidneys has shown narrowing and tortuosity of the intrarenal arteries or irregularity of the interlobar arteries in primary amyloidosis (Ekelund and Lindholm, 1974).

The nephrotic syndrome is common, occurring—as mentioned —in 32% of our patients with primary amyloid and in 11% of those with amyloid and myeloma (Table 59). Maxwell and associates (1964) reported that among 83 adults with the nephrotic syndrome, amyloid was the causative factor in 12%. In a series of 1,500 renal biopsies reported by Triger and Joekes (1973), 3% disclosed evidence of amyloidosis.

Association of the adult Fanconi syndrome, Bence Jones proteinuria, and amyloidosis without evidence of myeloma has been reported (Finkel et al., 1973). We also have seen one such case. Massive urinary excretion of a monoclonal IgG κ protein without free light chains has been noted in a case of multiple myeloma and amyloidosis with renal insufficiency (Ooi et al., 1972). Renal amyloidosis and the nephrotic syndrome have been associated with retroperitoneal fibrosis (Littman, 1971).

2. Cardiovascular System: The heart is frequently affected in amyloidosis. Congestive heart failure is the most common manifestation, occurring in 26% of our patients of group 1 and in 30% of group 2 (Table 59). The cause of death was cardiac in one-third of our cases. Amyloidosis might well be considered in any case of congestive heart failure of indeterminate cause—especially if the condition is refractory to treatment—because in amyloidosis cardiac failure is progressive and usually refractory. Cardiac arrhythmias are common, particularly in patients taking digitalis (Buja et al., 1970); amyloid involvement of the sinus node may produce arrhythmias aggravated by digitalis and lead to sudden death (James, 1966). Decreased voltage of the electrocardiogram is the most common finding, but the tracing also may suggest myocardial infarction. Effects of amyloidosis may resemble those of valvular heart disease (Garcia and Saeed, 1968). Constrictive pericarditis may be difficult to exclude because of the low-voltage QRS complex and other features indicating restricted physiologic function of the heart (Crockett et al., 1972). Angina pectoris and myocardial infarction may result from amyloid deposits in the coronary arteries (Barth et al., 1970; Buja et al., 1970). Rupture of the myocardium in amyloidosis has been reported also (Lindberg, 1971).

Myocardial ischemia and congestive heart failure from nodules of amyloid in the media, adventitia, and intima of intramyocardial arteries has been seen in a patient who also had large amyloid deposits in the media of the arteries supplying the bundle of His (Paulsen, 1974). In addition, she had amyloid in the arteries of the liver, spleen, lungs, and kidneys and 20% plasma cells in the bone marrow.

Intermittent claudication in patients with amyloidosis has been thought to be due to deposition of amyloid in the arterioles, which makes the vessels fixed and non-expansile (Zelis et al., 1969). We have seen patients with intermittent claudication of the jaw as well as of the lower extremities.

Orthostatic hypotension was found in 13% of our current series (Table 59). In another review of 138 patients with primary amyloidosis, we found that 11 had orthostatic hypotension (Table 67). Dizziness, light-headedness, or syncope hampered these patients; 3 of the 11 were so incapacitated by orthostatic hypotension that they were unable to get out of bed. Diarrhea was common, and steatorrhea was documented in two cases. Lack of

TABLE 67

AMYLOIDOSIS: FINDINGS IN 11 CASES OF PRIMARY AMYLOIDOSIS AND
ORTHOSTATIC HYPOTENSION (MAYO CLINIC)

Case	Blood Pressure, mm Hg (Systolic/Diastolic)		Syncope	Diarrhea	Nephrotic Syndrome	Peripheral Neuropathy	Onset of Orthostatic Hypotension	Diagnosis of Amyloidosis
	Recumbent	Standing						
1	120/70	60/?	+	+	0	0	Dec 1961	Jun 1962
2	120/80	80/60	S	+	0	0	Mar 1955	Apr 1956
3	78/60	44/?	+	0	S	0	Sep 1961	Nov 1961
4	96/64	44/34	+	+	0	+	Jan 1950	Aug 1962
5	90/?	50/?	0	+	+	0	May 1960	Feb 1961
6	124/84	60/30	+	+	0	0	Jul 1952	Mar 1953
7	88/70	45/?	+	0	S	0	Dec 1951	Jan 1952
8	100/70	50/36	+	0	0	0	1958	Aug 1959
9	134/100	84/66	+	+	0	+	Jul 1958	Aug 1958
10	100/65	50/40	+	+	0	0	1961	Jun 1964
11	80/60	30/?	S	0	+	0	Mar 1964	Sep 1964

+ = present; 0 = absent; ? = not recorded; S = suspected but inadequate data.
From Kyle, R. A. Kottke, B. A., and Schirger, A.: Orthostatic hypotension as a clue to primary systemic amyloidosis. *Circulation* 34:883-888, 1966. By permission of American Heart Association.

sweating was noted in all cases in which it was tested, and impotence or decrease of libido was reported in two cases. Adrenal insufficiency was considered seriously in the differential diagnosis of more than one-half of this group (Kyle et al., 1966a). Extensive deposits of amyloid have been seen in sympathetic ganglia and nerves and in the peripheral nerves of a patient with postural hypotension and amyloidosis (Gaan et al., 1972). Treatment for orthostatic hypotension associated with amyloidosis is not satisfactory, but we have used 9-α-fludrocortisone (Florinef®) with some benefit. Tranylcypromine and levodopa have been used; but with them, nausea and vomiting may be a problem (Yuill, 1974).

In contrast to orthostatic hypotension, hypertension also has been reported. Bentwich and associates (1971) found hypertension in 3 of their 12 patients with primary amyloidosis and, in a review of several other series, cited a 30% incidence of hypertension in primary amyloidosis.

3. Respiratory Tract: Involvement of the respiratory tract in amyloidosis is also common, but usually produces no symptoms. In our experience, dyspnea is a rare major symptom secondary to extensive amyloid infiltration of the lung in patients with primary amyloidosis. Amyloid deposits may displace alveolar capillaries without significantly hindering gas diffusion (Rajan and Kikkawa, 1970). However, impairment of gas diffusion by amyloid infiltration of the alveolar capillaries in a case of myeloma with generalized amyloidosis has been reported (Crosbie et al., 1972).

4. Alimentary Tract: Disorder of the gastrointestinal tract is common in systemic amyloidosis. Usually there are no symptoms, but widespread dysfunction may occur (Gilat and Spiro, 1968).

In the mouth, macroglossia (Figs. 63 and 64) is the most prominent manifestation; but it occurred in only 17% of our patients. Although partial resection of the tongue has been undertaken (Hicks and Dickie, 1973), it is fraught with potential difficulties and we do not recommend it. Recurrent hemorrhagic bullae of the oral cavity may be seen (Keith, 1972). Primary amyloidosis may present as a swelling in the floor of the mouth (Van der

Waal et al., 1973). Focal amyloidosis has presented as a mass on the soft palate with later multiple involvement of the cervical and axillary lymph nodes (Johner et al., 1972).

Amyloidosis of the esophagus may produce bleeding and perforation; Heitzman and associates (1962) reported such a case in which no systemic amyloidosis was documented, but the patient did have congestive heart failure.

In the gastrointestinal tract proper, amyloid is deposited in the walls of the vessels of the gut and in the submucosa (Gilat et al., 1969). Malabsorption was well documented in 5% of our patients. In the series of Herskovic and associates (1964), the incidence of malabsorption in primary amyloidosis was 8.5%. Ascites was noted in 17% of 59 patients with primary amyloidosis (Gregg et al., 1965). Prepyloric obstruction from amyloid has been reported (Lewis, 1968), and we have seen systemic amyloidosis with partial prepyloric obstruction from amyloid in one patient who also had a mass at the ligament of Treitz that partially obstructed the small bowel. We have seen myeloma patients with a mass that was interpreted roentgenographically as carcinoma of the stomach but was proved by gastroscopy and biopsy to be amyloid. Absence of rugal patterns and decrease of motility have been seen in amyloidosis involving the stomach (Legge et al., 1970a).

Decreased motor activity of the small bowel is not uncommon in amyloidosis. In some instances, apparent mechanical obstruction may in fact be pseudo-obstruction, for which surgical treatment is ineffectual and actually dangerous (Legge et al., 1970b). Perforation of the small bowel from amyloid infiltration has been reported in systemic amyloidosis (Akbarian and Fenton, 1964), and acute intestinal infarction may occur (Brody et al., 1964a). Involvement of the colon in systemic amyloidosis may resemble chronic ulcerative colitis and present as diarrhea and rectal bleeding (Casad and Bocian, 1965; Chernenkoff et al., 1972). One of our patients had extensive involvement of the colon with amyloid, and her major symptom was attributable to prolapse of the rectal mucosa. Williamson (1972) described a patient who presented with rectal bleeding and a large ulcerating rectal mass, which was thought initially to be a carcinoma but actually consisted of amyloid. This patient was said to have primary systemic amyloidosis, but no mention of amyloid in other organs was made. Another patient, who presented with rectal bleeding and malabsorption, was found at exploration to have multiple nodules of amyloid in the jejunum and ileum. No autopsy was done; but the malabsorption, together with evidence of nephrosis, suggested generalized involvement (O'Grady and O'Connell, 1968).

5. *Liver and Spleen:* The liver is frequently affected in amyloidosis. Hepatomegaly was an initial finding in almost half of our patients (Table 68); and it may be the presenting symptom or sign of amyloidosis. Indeed, the liver may be huge; but other physical findings of primary liver disease are uncommon. Alteration of hepatic function is generally considered to be minimal (Levine, 1962), despite the significant amount of amyloid deposition. In contrast to this belief, our patients frequently had abnormalities of liver function. The serum alkaline phosphatase concentration was increased in nearly half of our cases (Table 68); its mean value was 108 U/liter in group 1 and 66 in group 2. The serum glutamic oxaloacetic transaminase (SGOT) value was elevated in more than one-third of cases. BSP retention was increased in more than half, contradicting the statement that hepatomegaly with normal or only slightly abnormal liver function is characteristic of amyloidosis. The presence of congestive heart failure contributes significantly to the BSP retention and

TABLE 68

AMYLOIDOSIS: LIVER FINDINGS (MAYO CLINIC)

| Finding | Primary | | With Myeloma | |
	Tested Pts., No.	Results Pos., %	Tested Pts., No.	Results Pos., %
Liver palpable	114	45	55	49
Alkaline phosphatase, increased	68	49	37	41
SGOT, increased	29	38	13	46
BSP, > 5% in 1 h	66	61	21	62
Bilirubin				
Direct, increased	79	9	25	8
Indirect, increased	79	5	25	12
Albumin, serum				
< 3.0 g/dl	109	76	55	69

may be responsible for the increased incidence in our experience. Approximately 9% of our patients had an increase in the concentration of direct-reacting bilirubin, and approximately 8% had an increase in indirect-reacting bilirubin (Table 68). Seven cases of obstructive jaundice from systemic amyloidosis have been described (Mir-Madjlessi et al., 1972b; Oliai and Koff, 1972). More than two-thirds of our patients had 3.0 g/dl of serum albumin or less.

Portal hypertension with bleeding esophageal varices from amyloid has been reported (Kapp, 1965). A patient who had had significant hepatomegaly for 17 years was found at autopsy to have generalized amyloidosis (Smith, 1971).

Spontaneous rupture of the spleen may occur in amyloidosis (King and Oppenheimer, 1948; Drapiewski et al., 1955; Polliack and Hershko, 1972).

6. *Nervous System:* Peripheral neuropathy is a common feature in primary amyloidosis and was found in 17% of our patients. Neuropathy in amyloidosis has been described well by Chambers and associates (1958). It usually begins with paresthesias or pain, particularly in the legs, which is followed by weakness. Loss of pain and temperature sensations is common in amyloid neuropathy. Thomas and King (1974) found a marked loss of myelinated fibers in two of three cases and severe loss of unmyelinated axons in all three. The amyloid deposits were mainly intrafascicular but also occurred in the perineurium and epineurium. The neuropathy may involve the autonomic nervous system, with consequent diarrhea, lack of sweating, impotence, and orthostatic hypotension. Occasionally, retention or incontinence of urine or feces may be a problem. Amyloid deposits in both the peripheral nerves and autonomic nervous system have been described (French et al., 1965; Davies-Jones and Esiri, 1971).

Benson et al. (1975b) found median-nerve neuropathy (carpal tunnel) or peripheral neuropathy in 20% of patients who had primary amyloid or amyloid with myeloma. Interestingly, all of their patients with neuropathy had a monoclonal protein in either the serum or the urine.

7. *Miscellaneous:* Involvement of the skin with amyloidosis may take the form of papules, plaques, or nodules. Extensive involvement results in purpura from the deposition of amyloid in the walls of the dermal blood vessels (Brownstein and Helwig, 1970b). Xanthoma-like nodules in the skin may be the presenting feature (Chapman et al., 1973), as may bullous lesions involving the skin and the oral mucosa (Northover et al., 1972). We have also seen a patient with a long history of urticaria pigmentosa in whom amyloidosis involving the kidneys and peripheral neuropathy subsequently developed.

Systemic amyloidosis may involve the upper eyelids and serve as a significant clue in the diagnosis of amyloidosis (Natelson et al., 1970). We have one patient whose vision is significantly decreased because massive amyloid infiltration of the eyelids makes it impossible for him to open his eyes adequately. In another case, amyloidosis in the orbit produced proptosis; but it was not certain whether the amyloidosis was systemic (Raab, 1970). One of our patients presented with proptosis from amyloidosis of the orbit but no recurrence or other evidence of systemic amyloidosis appeared in a 4-year follow-up. Extensive deposits of amyloid in the extraocular muscles of a patient with primary systemic amyloidosis have been reported; but interestingly, this patient had no visual symptoms (Goebel and Friedman, 1971).

Involvement of the lacrimal and parotid glands in cases of generalized amyloidosis may produce dryness of the eyes and mouth (Kuczynski et al., 1971).

Amyloid deposits in primary systemic amyloidosis reportedly have occluded both external auditory canals (Noojin and Arrington, 1965).

Primary amyloidosis may present as lymphadenopathy (Mackenzie, 1963).

Rapid enlargement of a goiter from amyloid has been a rare manifestation of primary amyloidosis (Daoud et al., 1967). Shapiro and associates (1971) described a patient with hoarseness and thyroid enlargement from amyloid who subsequently manifested macroglossia. This patient died of an acute cardiac disorder. Panhypopituitarism from destruction of the pituitary by amyloid deposits has been reported (Feinberg and Harlan, 1961).

Involvement of the bones has been reported to produce severe osteoporosis and compression fractures (Axelsson et al., 1970). Occasionally osteolytic lesions may be seen, but it is difficult to exclude myeloma in these instances (Himmelfarb et al., 1974). The roentgenographic appearance of bones was normal in 94% of our cases of primary amyloidosis. Most of the abnormalities consisted of osteoporosis, with an occasional compression fracture, of a degree compatible with the patient's age. Half of our patients with myeloma and amyloidosis had abnormal roentgenographic abnormalities of bone. Amyloidosis may involve periarticular structures and resemble rheumatoid arthritis (Goldberg et al., 1964; Wiernik, 1972; Gordon et al., 1973; Nashel et al., 1973). Amyloid arthritis does not cause joint narrowing that is notable radiographically, and the articular surface is better preserved than in rheumatoid arthritis (Renner and Smith, 1974). Aspirates of synovial fluid may contain a monoclonal protein and small fragments of amyloid, thus establishing the diagnosis (Gordon et al., 1973). Joint symptoms are common manifestations of amyloidosis and present a difficult problem in differential diagnosis: to mistake the disease for rheumatoid arthritis is easy in this situation. Prominence of the shoulders may be striking, and is known as the "shoulder-pad sign" (Katz et al., 1973). We have seen three patients with primary amyloidosis who scarcely could open their mouths, although roentgenograms and examination of the temporal mandibular joints revealed no abnormalities.

In association with systemic amyloidosis, isolated deficiency of Factor X (Bernhardt et al., 1972; Jacobson et al., 1972; Galbraith et al., 1974), disseminated intravascular coagulation with severe gastrointestinal bleeding (Bowie et al., 1969), and fibrinolysis with a severe bleeding diathesis (Redleaf et al., 1963) have been reported.

Diagnosis. *Tissue Biopsy:* The diagnosis of amyloidosis depends on demonstration of amyloid deposits in tissue by means of appropriate staining procedures. The results of biopsy of various tissues in our series are given in Table 69. When systemic

TABLE 69

AMYLOIDOSIS: RESULT OF BIOPSY (MAYO CLINIC)

	Primary		With Myeloma		Total	
	Tested	Results	Tested	Results		
Site	Pts., No.	Pos., %	Pts., No.	Pos., %	Pts.	% Pos.
Rectum	83	82	36	89	119	84
Kidney	31	90	...	...	31	90
Carpal tunnel	8	100	8	88	16	94
Liver	20	95	3	100	23	96
Small intestine	8	75	4	50	12	67
Bone marrow	67	48	36	42	103	46
Skin	10	80	7	86	17	82

TABLE 70

AMYLOIDOSIS: RECTAL BIOPSY AND INVOLVEMENT* OF TISSUE
WITH AMYLOID (MAYO CLINIC)

		Rectal Tissue			Metachromasia
		Muscularis			With Methyl
Case	Mucosa	Mucosae	Submucosa	Vessels	Violet
1	−	++	+++	++	++
2	−	−	+++	+++	++++
3	++	++	+++	+++	++++
4	−	+++	+++	−	++++
5	+	+++	++	+	+
6	+	?	?	?	+
7	?	++	++	++	+++
8	−	++	−	++	++
9	−	++++	++++	+++	+++
10	−	+	++++	+++	+++
11	−	−	++	++	+
12	−	−	+++	+++	++++
13	−	+	+++	+++	++++
14	+	+	++	++	+++
15	−	−	+++	+++	+++
16	−	+++	++++	++	+++
17	−	+	+++	++	+++
18	−	?	−	−	?
19	−	−	−	−	−
20	−	−	−	−	−
Total	4	12	15	15	17

* Degrees of involvement and of metachromasia were graded arbitrarily from + to +++ (least to most).

? means questionable involvement, and − means no involvement.

From Kyle, R. A., Spencer, R. J., and Dahlin, D. C.: Value of rectal biopsy in the diagnosis of primary systemic amyloidosis. *Am J Med Sci, 251*:501-506, 1966. By permission of Lea & Febiger.

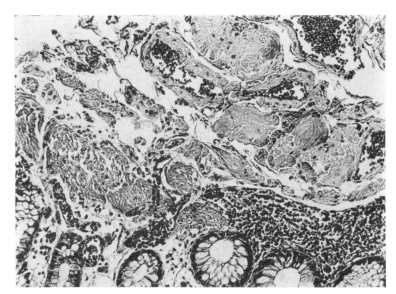

Figure 68. Large clumps of amyloid replacing muscularis mucosae, extending into submucosa and even involving vessels. (Hematoxylin and eosin: ×115.) (From Kyle, R. A., Spencer, R. J., and Dahlin, D. C.: Value of rectal biopsy in the diagnosis of primary systemic amyloidosis. *Am J Med Sci, 251*:501-506, 1966. By permission of Lea & Febiger.)

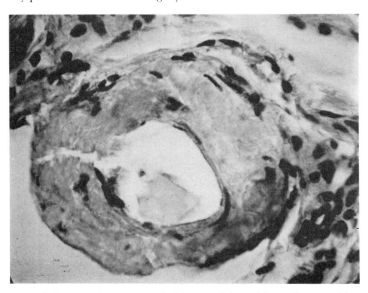

Figure 69. Submucosal vessel, probably arteriole, with wall markedly thickened by amyloid. (Hematoxylin and eosin; ×500.) (From Kyle, R. A., Spencer, R. J., and Dahlin, D. C.: Value of rectal biopsy in the diagnosis of primary systemic amyloidosis. *Am J Med Sci, 251*:501-506, 1966. By permission of Lea & Febiger.)

amyloidosis is suspected, the initial diagnostic procedure should be *rectal biopsy* because it is relatively easy to perform, free of complications, and usually positive if the disease is present. Among our cases, rectal biopsy has given positive results in 84%. To be adequate, the biopsy specimen must contain submucosa, because this tissue is involved more frequently than the mucosa (Kyle et al., 1966c) (Table 70; Figs. 68 and 69).

More often positive than rectal biopsy is *renal biopsy,* but the procedure is more difficult and complications are more frequent (Fig. 70). *Liver biopsy* frequently provides evidence of amyloidosis, but bleeding may result; moreover, rupture of the liver, though rare, has been fatal. *Carpal-tissue biopsy*—tissue being obtained at carpal tunnel decompression—reveals amyloid in more than 90% of cases of amyloidosis with associated carpal-tunnel syndrome. Surgeons should be encouraged to send tissue to be analyzed for it.

Biopsy of the *small intestine* may be helpful, positive findings being obtained in two-thirds of these cases of amyloidosis. Sections of *bone marrow* aspirations or biopsies have shown amyloid deposits in 46% of this group and can be helpful in diagnosis. We have not found gingival biopsy particularly fruitful; but it

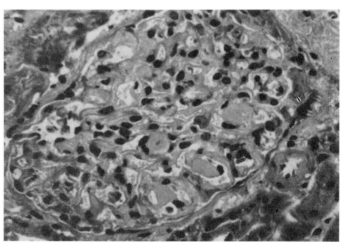

Figure 70. Renal biopsy specimen: glomerulus containing amyloid. (Hematoxylin and eosin; ×400.)

AMYLOIDOSIS: BONE-MARROW AMYLOID* AND PLASMA CELLS

Case	Primary Amyloidosis	Myeloma With Amyloidosis	Source of Tissue Diagnostic of Amyloid	Plasma Cells in Bone Marrow, %	Amyloid in Paraffin Sections			Amyloid in Smear
					Extra-mural	Perivascular	Giant Cell	
1	Yes	No	Rectum	5.0	Yes	No	No	Yes
2	Yes	No	Rectum	7.4	No	Yes	No	No
3	Yes	No	Rectum	13.0	Yes	No	No	Yes
4	Yes	No	Rectum	11.2	Yes	Yes	No	Yes
5	Yes	No	Rectum	8.6	No	Yes	No	No
6	Yes	No	Liver and autopsy	13.0	Yes	Yes	No	Yes
7	Yes	No	Kidney, rectum	3.8	No	Yes	No	No
8	Yes	No	Liver	7.6	Yes	Yes	Yes	Yes
9	Yes	No	Muscle	3.0	Yes	Yes	No	Yes
10	Yes	No	Liver	5.0	No	Yes	No	No
11	Yes	No	Autopsy	5.0	Yes	Yes	No	Yes
12	Yes	No	Tongue	24.4	Yes	Yes	No	Yes
13	Yes	No	Liver	6.4	Yes	No	No	No
14	Yes	No	Lymph node	19.8	Yes	Yes	No	Yes
15	Yes	No	Liver	15.2	Yes	No	Yes	Yes
16	Yes	No	Autopsy	4.8	Yes	No	No	Yes
17	Yes	No	Liver	11.8	Yes	Yes	No	Yes
18	Yes	No	Rectum	8.4	No	Yes	No	No
19	Yes	No	Liver	12.2	Yes	No	Yes	Yes
20	Yes	No	Liver and autopsy	10.8	Yes	Yes	No	No
21	Yes	No	Liver	11.0	Yes	Yes	No	Yes
22	Yes	No	Small bowel	11.8	No	Yes	No	No
23	Yes	No	Liver	20.8	Yes	No	No	Yes
24	Yes	No	Spleen	17.0	Yes	Yes	No	Yes
25	Yes	No	Autopsy	11.6	No	Yes	No	No
26	No	Yes	Skin	32.8	No	Yes	No	No
27	No	Yes	Rectum	43.0	Yes	No	Yes	No
28	No	Yes	Clavicle	79.0	Yes	Yes	Yes	Yes
Total	25	3			19	20	5	16

*Antemortem specimens obtained by aspiration.

From Kyle, R. A., Pease, G. L., Richmond, H., and Sullivan, L.: Bone marrow aspiration in the antemortem diagnosis of primary systemic amyloidosis. *Am J Clin Pathol, 45:252-257,* 1966. By permission of Williams & Wilkins Company.

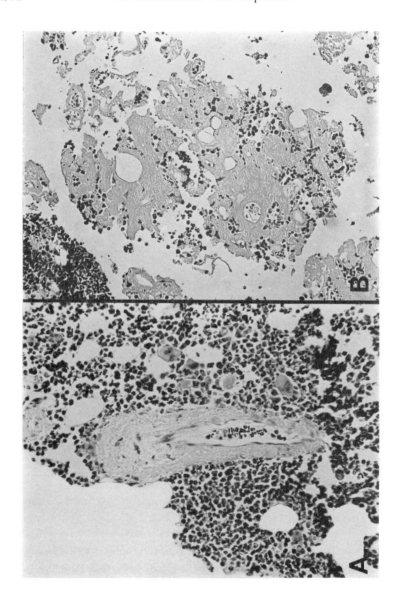

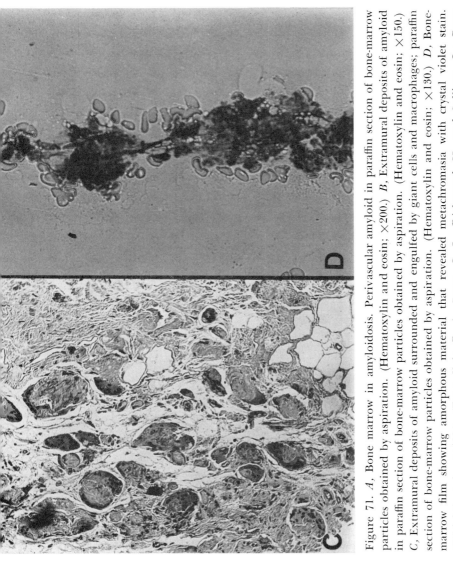

Figure 71. *A*, Bone marrow in amyloidosis. Perivascular amyloid in paraffin section of bone-marrow particles obtained by aspiration. (Hematoxylin and eosin; ×200.) *B*, Extramural deposits of amyloid in paraffin section of bone-marrow particles obtained by aspiration. (Hematoxylin and eosin; ×150.) *C*, Extramural deposits of amyloid surrounded and engulfed by giant cells and macrophages; paraffin section of bone-marrow particles obtained by aspiration. (Hematoxylin and eosin; ×130.) *D*, Bone-marrow film showing amorphous material that revealed metachromasia with crystal violet stain. (Wright's stain: ×400.) (From Kyle, R. A., Pease, G. L., Richmond, H., and Sullivan, L.: Bone marrow aspiration in the antemortem diagnosis of primary systemic amyloidosis. *Am J Clin Pathol, 45:252-257,* 1966. By permission of Williams & Wilkins Company.)

may be useful, especially if suspicious intraoral lesions are biopsied (Schwartz and Olson, 1975). Endomyocardial biopsy has been positive in amyloidosis (Schroeder et al., 1975).

In a previous study of 66 cases of systemic amyloidosis, amyloid was found in antemortem bone marrow preparations from 28 (42%) (Table 71). Paraffin sections made from the aspirated bone marrow showed amyloid in the small-vessel walls in 20 cases, which often produced marked thickening of the vessel wall and partially occluded the lumen (Fig. 71*A*). In 19 cases extramural amyloid occurred as large accumulations dispersed throughout the marrow substance or as isolated masses (Fig. 71*B*). A number of these extramural deposits contained bone-marrow cells, whereas others seemed to replace hematopoietic tissue. In five instances the extramural deposits were surrounded by macrophages and giant cells (Fig. 71*C*); this was regarded as a giant-cell reaction. Rather unexpectedly, in 16 instances amyloid was found in smears of bone marrow aspirates stained by Wright's method; all but 1 of these had extramural deposits of amyloid in the paraffin sections. The amyloid appeared as structureless, pink to purple, irregularly shaped masses of various sizes (Fig. 71*D*). These masses were waxy to transparent, unlike precipitated protein, damaged marrow cells, or megakaryocytic cytoplasm. There were no false-positive reports of amyloid in the bone marrow: all patients with this finding had biopsy or autopsy confirmation of amyloidosis (Kyle et al., 1966b).

In many cases *prostatic biopsy* reveals amyloid. Besides the use of transrectal needle biopsy and open biopsy techniques, tissue for examination may be obtained at transurethral resection or at autopsy. Use of prostatic tissue for diagnosis has been advised (Wilson et al., 1973). Diagnosis of secondary amyloidosis by fine-needle *biopsy of subcutaneous fat* has been reported (Westermark and Stenkvist, 1973).

Dye Tests: The Congo red (Paunz) test is no longer used because it is imprecise and anaphylactic reactions may occur. Testing with Evans blue dye, which is removed at an accelerated rate from the serum of patients with amyloidosis, is insensitive (Cathcart and Cohen, 1963). Larsen and Jarnum (1965), however, obtained positive results with the Evans blue dye test in two-thirds of patients with amyloid, and they reported no false-positive results. Resistance to heparin, manifested by a prolonged clot time 1 hour after the injection of heparin, has been reported as possibly suggesting amyloidosis (Christiansen and Lindqvist, 1967); but this is not of practical value.

Electron Microscopy: We have seen several cases in which staining of renal tissue with Congo red and thioflavine T provided no evidence of amyloid, yet subsequent electron microscopic examination revealed the typical amyloid fibrils. Hobbs (1973) also noted that electron microscopy may be necessary for ultimate diagnosis in some cases. Goodman and associates (1972) have reported a case of primary amyloidosis in which amyloid was demonstrated only by electron microscopy after the usual histochemical staining was inconclusive. A spicular arrangement of amyloid on the basement membrane of the glomerulus, as seen by light microscopy, is ordinarily associated with membranous glomerulonephritis but has been found in 8 of 38 renal biopsies of patients with amyloidosis (Ansell and Joekes, 1972).

TREATMENT AND CLINICAL COURSE

Treatment: The treatment of patients with amyloidosis is not satisfactory. Recent advances in the understanding of the pathogenesis of this disease have included the demonstration that the protein moiety of the amyloid fibril consists of at least a portion of the variable part of the immunoglobulin light chain. Thus, because these polypeptide chains are synthesized by plasma cells, it has seemed reasonable to treat amyloidosis with alkylating agents that are effective against diseases characterized by proliferation of neoplastic plasma cells.

Indeed, two patients with primary amyloidosis have benefited from such therapy (Jones et al., 1972; Lessin et al., 1972). The latter patient, with widespread primary amyloidosis was treated with melphalan and prednisone for 4 days and D-penicillamine, 500 mg 4 times daily, for 17 days. After that, administration of melphalan and prednisone was continued intermittently for more than 4 years. The patient's nephrotic syndrome abated, renal function improved, and the amount of amyloid in the bone marrow decreased (Cohen et al., 1975). It is not possible to determine which agent was responsible for the improvement. We have observed improvement in some patients with primary amyloidosis treated with melphalan; however, a rapidly fatal acute leukemia developed in 2 of them after 4 years of therapy (Kyle et al., 1974b). We believe that melphalan was a factor in this leukemia; and it is therefore always necessary to assess the risks and the benefits, if any, from use of this kind of agent. We hope that a recently instituted prospective, randomized, double-blind study designed to permit a comparison of the therapeutic effects of melphalan and prednisone with those of a placebo in patients with primary amyloidosis will provide an answer; but it is yet too early to report any results.

Mice given casein and thymosin, a thymic hormone, had a lower incidence of amyloid and lesser amounts of it than did mice given casein alone or casein and intraperitoneal injections of splenic extracts (Scheinberg et al., 1975). This may offer therapeutic hope for the future.

Renal transplantation has been performed in 21 patients with amyloidosis, which was primary in 4 cases and secondary in 13. Only one of the transplanted kidneys has shown evidence of amyloid involvement. Five patients have survived for more than 3 years since transplantation (Renal Transplant Registry, 1975).

TABLE 72

AMYLOIDOSIS: FOLLOW-UP OF 193 PATIENTS
(MAYO CLINIC)

Status	Primary (132 Pts.)	With Myeloma (61 Pts.)
Dead	105	59
Alive	27*	2*
Surviving, yr.		
≤ 1	1	0
1.1-2	10	1
2.1-3.0	4	0
3.1-5.0	9	1
> 5	3	0

* Last seen or contacted in 1973 or 1974.

Survival: The mean survival after diagnosis in an earlier Mayo series of 81 patients having primary amyloidosis, with or without myeloma, seen at our institution from 1935 to 1959 was 4.9 months. Daniels and Hewlett (1970) reported that at the Cleveland Clinic the median survival among patients with primary amyloidosis was 5 months, whereas survival among patients with multiple myeloma was 15 months.

In the current Mayo Clinic series, follow-up information was obtained in all 193 cases. Currently, 80% of the patients in group 1 and 97% of those in group 2 have died (Table 72). Duration of the follow-up after diagnosis exceeded 1 year in all but one case, in which the diagnosis had been made less than 1 year before. Three patients of group 1 survived longer than 5 years and were still alive at the time of analysis. One of these three had presented with symptoms of the carpal tunnel syndrome requiring decompression, then manifested macroglossia and fatigue, and was found to have a monoclonal light chain in the urine and was treated with melphalan. Another patient had presented with hepatomegaly and was treated with cyclophosphamide; and the third had presented with peripheral neuropathy that has remained stable. Only two patients of group 2 are living. One of these two presented with carpal tunnel syndrome in 1966. Examination 4 years later revealed overt myeloma with Bence Jones proteinuria (6.5 g/24 h), 55% plasma cells in the bone marrow, and osteoporosis with compression fractures; and subsequently, congestive heart failure has developed. The other patient had presented with renal insufficiency and was surviving at 1 year.

Review of the present series of 193 patients seen since 1960

TABLE 73

AMYLOIDOSIS: SURVIVAL (MAYO CLINIC)

Period, Yr.	Primary: % Survived	With Myeloma: % Survived
1	54	26
3	25	7
5	17	3
(Median survival time, mo.)	(14.7)	(4.0)

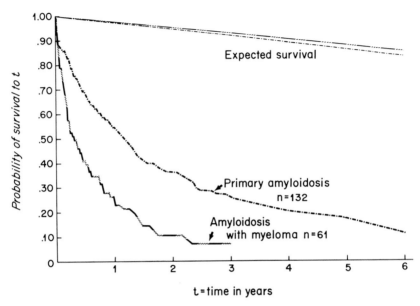

Figure 72. Survival curves of patients with primary amyloidosis and of patients with amyloidosis and myeloma from time of diagnosis to time of last follow-up or death. (From Kyle, R. A., and Bayrd, E. D.: Amyloidosis: review of 236 cases. *Medicine* [Baltimore], *54*:271-299, 1975. By permission of Williams & Wilkins Company.)

TABLE 74

AMYLOIDOSIS: CAUSES OF 164 DEATHS IN 193 CASES
(MAYO CLINIC)

Cause	Primary (132 Pts.): % of 105	With Myeloma (61 Pts.): % of 59	Total, %
"Amyloidosis or myeloma"	18	42	27
Renal failure	16	7	13
Infection	8	5	7
Stroke	5	3	4
Cardiac failure	34	24	30
Other	8	12	9
Unknown	11	7	10
Total	100	100	100

disclosed median survival—after histologic diagnosis of amyloid —as 14.7 months for those with primary amyloidosis and 4 months for those with amyloidosis and myeloma. At 1 year, 54% of group 1 were alive but only 26% of group 2 (Table 73; Fig. 72). In comparison, the 50% survival period from time of diagnosis for 869 cases of multiple myeloma seen in the period from 1960 through 1971 was 20 months and the 1-year survival rate was 66%.

Cause of Death: Among our patients, cardiac failure accounted for 30% of the fatalities and was the most common cause of death (Table 74). Sudden death, presumably from arrhythmia, was frequent. Amyloidosis or myeloma was listed as the cause of death on the death certificates or in letters from the physician or patient's family in 27% of cases. Death certificates were obtained in 63% of this series, and autopsy was done in 56%.

A NOTE ON A NEW CLASSIFICATION OF AMYLOIDOSIS ACCORDING TO CLINICAL PATTERNS

The new classification of amyloidosis by Isobe and Osserman (1974a) is based on three predominant clinical patterns. *Pattern I* comprises principal involvement of the tongue, heart, gastrointestinal tract, skeletal and smooth muscles, carpal ligaments, nerves, and skin. This pattern of distribution was referred to previously as the primary type and is commonly associated with multiple myeloma or occult plasma-cell dyscrasia. *Pattern II* is characterized by principal involvement of the liver, spleen, kidneys, and adrenal glands. This distribution was designated previ-

TABLE 75

AMYLOIDOSIS: CLASSIFICATION OF MAYO CLINIC CASES BY METHOD OF ISOBE AND OSSERMAN (1974a)

| | | *Percentages, by Pattern* | | | |
| | | | | *Mixed* | |
Series	*No. Pts.*	*I*	*II*	*I & II*	*Localized*
Mayo Clinic					
Primary and with myeloma ..	193	57	23	20	0
Total series	236	49	23	19	9
Isobe and Osserman	100	50	17	30	3

ously as the secondary type and is commonly associated with chronic infections, rheumatoid arthritis, familial Mediterranean fever, and Hodgkin's disease. *Mixed pattern I and II* occurs when amyloidosis involves sites of both pattern I and pattern II; it appears to represent an admixture of pathologic processes. The final category is the *localized,* in which amyloid deposits are limited to a single tissue or organ. This classification is based on the clinical features and not on autopsy findings.

To compare this pattern classification with the one we have used (primary amyloidosis, or group 1, and amyloidosis with myeloma, or group 2), we categorized the 193 patients of groups 1 and 2 according to the classification of Isobe and Osserman (1974a, b). If all 236 of our patients (i.e., patients with localized, secondary, or familial forms as well as those of groups 1 and 2) are included, the percentages are very similar to those of

TABLE 76

AMYLOIDOSIS: INITIAL LABORATORY DATA IN MAYO CLINIC CASES, AS CLASSIFIED BY METHOD OF ISOBE AND OSSERMAN (1974a)

Finding	Pattern I Pts., No.	Pattern I Pos., %	Pattern II Pts., No.	Pattern II Pos., %	Mixed I & II Pts., No.	Mixed I & II Pos., %
Hemoglobin, < 12 g/dl	99	39	35	23	38	42
Leukocytes						
< 4,000/mm³	98	4	35	0	38	11
Immature	88	14	32	9	33	18
ESR, > 50 mm in 1 h	93	40	31	74	35	66
Thrombocytes						
< 100,000/mm³	61	13	25	0	23	41
> 300,000/mm³	61	21	25	32	23	43
Proteinuria	99	88	35	100	37	97
Bence Jones protein, positive (heat test)	60	47	30	0	29	14
Creatinine, increased	60	38	26	65	30	57
Uric acid, increased	38	21	7	14	13	46
Calcium, > 10.1 mg/dl	66	21	0	...	34	9
Cholesterol						
Decreased	49	31	27	4	25	4
Increased	49	8	27	58	25	44
Triglycerides						
Decreased	28	11	12	8	16	0
Increased	28	21	12	92	16	37
Plasma cells (bone-marrow), > 15%	83	29	27	0	35	17
Roentgenograms, positive	104	27	38	5	36	17

TABLE 77

AMYLOIDOSIS: CAUSES OF DEATH IN MAYO CLINIC CASES,
AS CLASSIFIED BY METHOD OF ISOBE AND OSSERMAN (1974a)

	Percentages of Deaths		
			Mixed
	Pattern I	Pattern II	I and II
Cause	(N = 90)	(N = 38)	(N = 36)
"Amyloidosis or myeloma"	33	10.5	28
Renal failure	2	39	11
Infection	8	10.5	0
Stroke	7	0	3
Cardiac failure	32	16	42
Other	9	8	11
Unknown	9	16	5

Isobe and Osserman (1974a) except that we categorized more patients as having pattern II and fewer as having mixed pattern I and II (Table 75). This may be explained partially by the large number of patients with the nephrotic syndrome in our series. We also found a larger number with localized amyloidosis, but this most likely reflects the different sources of patients in the two series.

Distributions were made of all pertinent findings in the history and physical examination as well as the results of the laboratory tests, and extensive comparative tables were made of the data; but they revealed no significant differences in clinical correlations. Some of these data are shown in Table 76. Careful comparison with those obtained by use of our classification (primary amyloidosis versus amyloidosis with myeloma fails to show significant clinical advantages in the use of pattern classification.

Course and Survival by Pattern Classification: About 30% of patients with pattern I or the mixed pattern died of myeloma or amyloidosis versus amyloidosis with myeloma) fails to show significant those with pattern II, 2% of those with pattern I, and 11% of those with the mixed pattern. Cardiac causes accounted for a large number of the deaths in patients with pattern I or the mixed pattern (Table 77).

Survival curves relating to patterns I and II and the mixed pat-

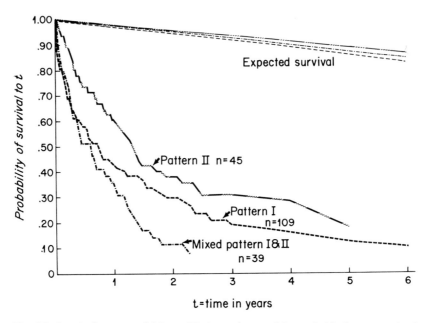

Fig. 73. Survival curves of Mayo Clinic patients with amyloidosis, categorized according to Isobe and Osserman's classification (1974a) from time of diagnosis to time of last follow-up or death. (From Kyle, R. A., and Bayrd, E. D.: Amyloidosis: review of 236 cases. *Medicine* [Baltimore], *54*:271-299, 1975. By permission of Williams & Wilkins Company.)

tern are not significantly different from each other (Fig. 73); median survival times for the three groups were 9.7, 15.6, and 6.0 months, respectively. Classification of amyloidosis on the basis of clinical patterns failed to reveal significant biologic differences. Our classification, which remains open to further pathophysiologic definition, will permit the utilization of knowledge of the biochemistry of the amyloid and amyloid fibrils as it develops. Of added importance is the failure of classification on the basis of "patterns" to reflect survival differences noted between primary amyloidosis and amyloidosis with myeloma when so classified. As a result, we continue to prefer the classification of primary amyloidosis and amyloidosis with myeloma.

SECONDARY AMYLOIDOSIS

Our previous series of amyloidosis from the Mayo Clinic from 1935 through 1959 (Kyle and Bayrd, 1961) comprised 183 cases. Thirty (16%) of these were secondary, with rheumatoid arthritis and tuberculosis the primary disease in two thirds of them. In 72 (39%) of the cases amyloidosis was localized, and involvement of the skin and larynx accounted for more than two-thirds of these.

In the present series, secondary amyloidosis was found in 19 cases (8%). Rheumatoid arthritis was the most common cause; with osteomyelitis, it accounted for two-thirds of the cases. Clinically, the nephrotic syndrome was seen in five instances, sprue (malabsorption) in four, and peripheral neuropathy in two.

Rheumatoid Arthritis: The incidence of amyloidosis in rheumatoid arthritis varies. Among 45 patients with rheumatoid arthritis, 6 (13%) had amyloidosis for which no cause other than rheumatoid arthritis could be found (Missen and Taylor, 1956). In another series of 115 patients with rheumatoid arthritis for more than 3 years, 5% had amyloid as evidenced by rectal biopsy (Arapakis and Tribe, 1963). Reviewing renal biopsies in 32 patients with rheumatoid arthritis, Brun and associates (1965) found amyloid in 4. Calkins and Cohen (1960) reported that amyloidosis was detected in 26% of 42 patients with rheumatoid arthritis who were examined at autopsy.

The organs principally involved are the liver, kidneys, spleen, and adrenals. Usually, rheumatoid arthritis has been present for at least 2 years before the development of amyloidosis. Proteinuria is extremely common; and in a patient with rheumatoid arthritis, this finding should make one consider the possibility of amyloidosis. Pettersson and Wegelius (1972) found malabsorption in 7 of 15 patients with amyloidosis secondary to rheumatoid arthritis and emphasized the value of jejunal biopsy in making the diagnosis of amyloidosis. Massive amyloid deposits in the breasts and abdominal skin appeared in a patient with long-standing rheumatoid arthritis (Sadeghee and Moore, 1974). In an interesting study of 47 patients with rheumatoid arthritis examined at autopsy and compared with a series of 47 controls matched for age and sex, only 1 of the rheumatoid arthritis patients had secondary amyloidosis (Ozdemir et al., 1971). Rheumatoid arthritis, Sjögren's syndrome, and secondary amyloidosis have occurred together (Case Records of the Massachusetts General Hospital, 1968b). Ankylosing spondylitis with amyloidosis has been reported in 13 instances (Benedek and Zawadzki, 1966). The association of amyloidosis and Reiter's disease also has been reported (Caughey and Wakem, 1973).

Infections: Tuberculosis has been a major cause of secondary amyloidosis: Of 468 cases of amyloidosis reported from a tuberculosis hospital, all but 5 were related to tuberculosis (Auerbach and Stemmerman, 1944). Another study disclosed that among 40 cases of renal amyloidosis, tuberculosis was the major preceding disease in 20. However, it was active in only two at the time when amyloidosis was diagnosed (Kennedy et al., 1974); and one might question its etiologic importance in a number of the cases. Tuberculosis no longer is common in this country, and in our experience it is a rare cause of amyloidosis; but that may be different in other parts of the world.

In our experience, osteomyelitis has been a more common cause of amyloidosis. Nephrogenic diabetes insipidus has been attributed to amyloidosis of the basement membrane of the medullary collecting ducts in a patient with a history of osteomyelitis and lung cancer (Carone and Epstein, 1960). Lepromatous leprosy may be associated with amyloidosis. Among patients with lepromatous leprosy at Carville, LA, 31% had secondary amyloidosis; and the incidence among patients with lepromatous leprosy in Mexico was 6% (Williams et al., 1965). A study in South India revealed amyloidosis in only 8% (6 of 79 patients) with lepromatous leprosy (Satyanarayana et al., 1972).

Amyloidosis occurs in up to 25% of patients with paraplegia examined at autopsy and is manifested by proteinuria followed by hepatosplenomegaly and frequently the nephrotic syndrome (Malament et al., 1965); chronic decubitus ulcers, osteomyelitis, and chronic pyelonephritis may contribute to the deposition of amyloid. Amyloid in a patient with syphilitic aortitis, a myocardial gumma, and syphilitic narrowing of the coronary ostia has been reported (Masterton, 1965). Bronchiectasis may also cause amyloidosis; it was a significant factor in the 32 cases of secondary amyloidosis reported by Kuhlbäck and Wegelius (1966). Chronically infected burns reportedly have produced amyloidosis and the nephrotic syndrome (Hoffman et al., 1963).

Neoplasms: Neoplasms other than multiple myeloma may be associated with amyloidosis. It is very difficult, of course, to know exactly how to classify such patients without knowing the biochemical nature of the amyloid substance. One could argue that these are secondary cases (our group 3) or that they are immunoglobulin-related and hence basically instances of plasma-cell disorders (an analogue of our group 2). Without the definitive information, we have chosen to place these patients in our group 3. Amyloidosis in macroglobulinemia has been reported (Forget et al., 1966; Goldberg et al., 1969). A case of macroglobulinemia with nephrotic syndrome from amyloid deposition, peripheral neuropathy, and Charcot joints has been described (Scott et al., 1973). Postnasal obstruction by amyloid deposits in macroglobulinemia has been noted (Elcock and Grimaldi, 1972). Amyloidosis has been seen in μ HCD (Forte et al., 1970).

We have seen two patients with macroglobulinemia of Waldenström, each of whom had severe peripheral neuropathy and documented amyloidosis. Both had severe truncal weakness and were unable to lie back from a sitting position without help. One patient had a significant decrease in the serum concentration of monoclonal protein and subjective improvement of neuropathy while taking chlorambucil daily. The other also experienced subjective neurologic improvement with a decrease in the serum concentration of monoclonal protein while taking chlorambucil intermittently, but death occurred suddenly—presumably from a cardiac arrhythmia (autopsy was not obtained). One other of our patients is of interest: She had presented with a lymphoproliferative infiltrative lesion of the stomach 17 years before and subsequently was found to have a large monoclonal IgM κ protein in the serum and recently developed renal insufficiency. Rectal biopsy revealed amyloidosis.

In a series of 4,033 cases of malignant neoplasm studied at autopsy, Kimball (1961) found amyloidosis in 0.4%. Hodgkin's disease and myeloma were the most common causes; but lymphosarcoma and cancer of the rectum, lung, cervix, esophagus, and kidney were found also. Lender (1974) reported that 5 of 78 patients with secondary amyloidosis had carcinoma of various organs—gallbladder, urinary bladder, stomach, kidney, and rectum.

Falkson and Falkson (1973), who reported a case of Hodgkin's disease and nephrotic syndrome secondary to amyloidosis, reviewed 53 cases of Hodgkin's disease and amyloidosis recorded in the literature. Renal involvement was a major manifestation. Hypernephroma has been associated with amyloidosis in approximately 50 reported cases. Among a series of 59 cases of hypernephroma, Penman and Thomson (1972) found widespread amyloid deposits in the liver, spleen, and kidney in 1 patient and limited amyloid deposits in 2 others. We saw a patient who presented with hypernephroma of the kidney and renal insufficiency. The renal insufficiency increased after operation, and reexamination of the kidney showed obvious amyloidosis.

Other: Amyloidosis was found in 5 of 17 patients with regional enteritis on whom autopsy was performed (Werther et al., 1960). Mir-Madjlessi et al. (1972a) reported 3 cases of amyloidosis and regional enteritis and reviewed 16 others from the literature. Renal failure was the most common cause of death. They could document no regression of amyloidosis after resection of the bowel. In contrast, Fitchen (1975) reported extensive amyloidosis of the liver and kidney in a patient with granulomatous ileocolitis of the terminal ileum and ascending and transverse colon. Resection of involved parts of the gastrointestinal tract resulted in disappearance of the hepatosplenomegaly, striking decrease in amyloid deposits in the liver, and decrease of urinary protein excretion from 18 to 0.3 g/24 h. Amyloidosis associated with chronic ulcerative colitis has been reported in 18 instances (Benedek and Zawadzki, 1966).

Ankylosing spondylitis and amyloidosis in the same patient have been associated with a defect of the proximal renal tubules which was manifested by the nephrotic syndrome, Fanconi's syndrome, hyperchloremic acidosis, and renal failure (Sebastian et al., 1968). A distal tubular defect characterized by renal tubular acidosis and hyperkalemia in chronic osteomyelitis and secondary amyloidosis has been reported (Luke et al., 1969).

Coexistence of primary agammaglobulinemia and amyloidosis in seven cases has been reported, but the influence of recurrent infections must be considered (Conn and Quintiliani, 1966; Mawas et al., 1969).

A patient with chronic neutropenia who subsequently developed vasculitis had extensive amyloidosis at autopsy (Jennings et al., 1973).

Two patients, one with hemophilia and the other with Christmas disease (Factor IX deficiency), received multiple transfusions and developed amyloidosis (Sharma and Geer, 1970; Prentice et al., 1971).

Amyloidosis has been reported in dermatomyositis (Gelderman et al., 1962). We have seen a patient with a monoclonal cryoglobulin in the serum and an undifferentiated connective-tissue process in whom widespread amyloidosis was discovered at autopsy (Maldonado et al., 1973).

Alveolar proteinosis, bronchiectasis, and amyloidosis were noted in one patient (Ganguli et al., 1972); and Whipple's disease (Sander, 1964), acquired epidermolysis bullosa (Muller et al., 1969), Niemann-Pick disease (Case Records of the Massachusetts General Hospital, 1968a), and Behçet's disease (Rosenthal et al., 1975) have been associated with amyloidosis.

Amyloidosis in childhood has been reported in 76 cases. Juvenile rheumatoid arthritis is the most common cause, familial Mediterranean fever and chronic suppurative diseases being significant causes also (Strauss et al., 1969).

The treatment for secondary amyloidosis depends on treatment for the underlying disease. Resorption of amyloid after treatment for osteomyelitis has been reported (Kuhlbäck and Wegelius, 1966). Remission of the nephrotic syndrome with disappearance of proteinuria has occurred in a patient with endocarditis and lung abscess, and in another with pulmonary tuberculosis and suppurative bronchiectasis, when they were treated with appropriate antibiotics (Lowenstein and Gallo, 1970). Two patients with amyloidosis have undergone renal transplantation. One, in whom amyloidosis was associated with familial Mediterranean fever, was doing well at 1 year post transplantation; the other, with osteomyelitis, died of an abscess at 5 months (Cohen et al., 1971).

An instance of almost complete disappearance of amyloid from the liver after nephrectomy for hypernephroma has been reported. Small hepatic foci of amyloid did persist (Paraf et al., 1970). One must make certain that apparent resorption of amyloid from an organ is not merely redistribution of the amyloid. In experimental amyloidosis, deposits in the spleen, liver, intestine, heart, and tongue reportedly may diminish or disappear, whereas renal deposits of amyloid increase (DeLellis et al., 1970).

LOCALIZED AMYLOIDOSIS

Localized amyloidosis was found in 22 cases (9%) in the present series. Involvement of bladder, lung, skin, and larynx accounted for more than half of the cases. Documented systemic amyloidosis never has been demonstrated. One of our patients with amyloid of the bladder was said to have died of amyloidosis, but there was no histologic proof and no autopsy.

Cases in which amyloid is localized to the skin may be classified as lichen amyloidosis (Wong, 1974) or as macular amyloidosis. In these instances, amyloid is not found in any other organ; and such skin lesions are never seen in systemic amyloidosis. Amyloid of the skin may also be tumefactive or nodular and remain localized, but this form sometimes represents the initial phase of systemic amyloidosis (Brownstein and Helwig, 1970a).

Localized amyloidosis of the bladder in 4 cases was reported by Malek et al. (1971) with review of 38 other cases in the literature. Gross hematuria was the most common symptom (85% of cases). Treatment usually consists of transurethral resection and fulguration or partial cystectomy. Strong et al. (1974) reported that a 32-year-old man developed gross hematuria and was found to have amyloid of the bladder. He remained asymptomatic for

16 years and then had painless hematuria from recurrence of amyloid. This case illustrates the indolence of this disease and supports the advisability of a conservative approach. Another patient with amyloid of the bladder had a moderate number of plasma cells surrounding the amyloid nodules (Hofer et al., 1974). This finding raises the possibility that the plasma cells are producing monoclonal light chains that form the amyloid fibrils. Hofer and associates performed pelvic arteriography; and although they could not distinguish between amyloid and carcinoma of the bladder, they found that the extent of the amyloid infiltration was greater than they had seen by cystoscopy. Angiography may be a useful procedure in delineating the extent of amyloidosis of the bladder prior to a surgical procedure.

Amyloidosis of the bladder has caused hemorrhage in several patients with secondary systemic amyloidosis (Montie and Stewart, 1973). Amyloid may also be localized to the renal pelvis (Ullmann, 1973); linear submucosal calcification outlining the pelviocaliceal system of the kidney may be striking and should suggest the diagnosis of amyloidosis (Gardner et al., 1971).

Medullary carcinoma of the thyroid with amyloid stroma may be seen with pheochromocytoma and parathyroid adenomas (Schimke et al., 1968).

In the respiratory tract, amyloidosis may be confined to the larynx (D'Arcy, 1972) or trachea (Keen and Weitzner, 1972). If the trachea and bronchi are involved, submucosal deposits may produce bleeding (Shaheen et al., 1975) or obstruction (Domm et al., 1965); bronchograms often show multiple irregular narrowings of the tracheobronchial tree (Attwood et al., 1972; Cook et al., 1973). Tracheobronchopathia osteoplastica with nodular amyloid deposits in the trachea and bronchi has been reported. Some speculate that tracheobronchopathia osteoplastica is an advanced stage of localized amyloid in the lung (Alroy et al., 1972). Amyloidosis may also be limited to the lung (Prowse, 1958), and focal amyloid tumors of the lower respiratory tract may obstruct the bronchi and lead to pneumonitis (Hayes and Bernhardt, 1969). Systemic amyloidosis does not accompany these problems, and the patients are best managed conservatively with bronchoscopic removal of the obstructive amyloid tumor from the lung (Schmidt et al., 1953).

Solitary or multiple pulmonary nodules consisting of amyloid may be seen without evidence of amyloid elsewhere (Skagseth and Normann, 1970; Moldow et al., 1972; Bonfils-Roberts et al., 1975). Solitary amyloid of the lung has recurred locally 9 years later (Dyke et al., 1974). Nodular amyloid of the lung in Sjögren's syndrome has been reported (Bonner et al., 1973). Acquired epidermolysis bullosa developed in a patient with solitary amyloid tumor of the lung but no systemic amyloidosis (Brauner et al., 1974).

Amyloidosis may be localized to the central nervous system. Involvement of the gasserian ganglion has produced trigeminal neuralgia (Daly et al., 1957), but systemic amyloidosis has not developed in these cases. We have seen a patient with amyloidosis localized to the infraorbital nerve and associated with atypical facial pain; the rectal biopsy, however, was negative for amyloid and there was no evidence of generalized amyloidosis during a 2-year follow-up.

Christensen and Sørensen (1972) reported amyloidosis in the hip-joint capsule of more than one-third of patients with degenerative arthritis.

Amyloid may present as a localized mass in the breast (Fernandez and Hernandez, 1973), in the sella (Barr and Lampert, 1972), and in mesenteric lymph nodes without evidence of amyloid elsewhere in the body (Berardi and Malette, 1973). Bleeding and perforation from heavy amyloid infiltration localized to the small intestine have been reported (Griffel et al., 1975).

We have seen a patient with progressive ptosis of her right eye from localized amyloidosis. Resection of the tarsus (by Dr. Robert R. Waller) reduced the ptosis. No monoclonal protein was detected in the serum or urine and no evidence of systemic amyloidosis was found. Ishwarchandra et al. (1974) described a 17-year-old patient with amyloidosis localized to the lids. She had been treated for leprosy, but the authors did not think that she had systemic amyloidosis.

The presence of small amyloid deposits, particularly in the brain, pancreas, and heart, was emphasized by Schwartz (1965). In his view, these amyloid deposits are factors in the pathogenesis of dementia. The finding of amyloid deposits has been confirmed by Wright and co-workers (1969). At autopsy, they studied 83 general hospital patients (age range: newborn to 97 years). Patients with disease processes known to be associated with amyloidosis were excluded. Amyloid was identified with Congo red staining observed under a polarizing light, and it also gave a positive reaction to one of the fluorochrome dyes. Of those patients over 70 years of age, 63% had cerebral amyloidosis, 37% had cardiac amyloidosis, 50% had aortic amyloidosis, and 30% had pancreatic amyloidosis. This was significantly more than in the patients between the ages of 30 and 70 years. The significance of these findings is unknown, but amyloid may have an important influence in the aging process.

FAMILIAL AMYLOIDOSIS

Our series contained only two patients with familial amyloidosis. This has been reviewed well (Mahloudji et al., 1969; Alexander and Atkins, 1975) and will not be discussed here.

CHAPTER XX

Benign Monoclonal Gammopathy (Monoclonal Gammopathy of Undetermined Significance)

THE TERM "BENIGN MONOCLONAL GAMMOPATHY" denotes the presence of a monoclonal protein in persons without evidence of myeloma, macroglobulinemia, or other related diseases (Hällén, 1966; Zawadzki and Edwards, 1972; Ritzmann et al., 1975). "Monoclonal gammopathy of undetermined significance" is a better term because, in most instances, one cannot tell whether the monoclonal protein will remain unchanged or whether it is an evolving myeloma or macroglobulinemia. Since Waldenström's use of the term "essential hyperglobulinemia" in 1952, many synonyms have been used—including idiopathic, asymptomatic, benign, nonmyelomatous, discrete, cryptogenic, rudimentary, dysimmunoglobulinemia, and lanthanic monoclonal gammopathy; idiopathic paraproteinemias; and asymptomatic paraimmunoglobulinemia. Waldenström (1961) stressed the constancy of the size of the protein peak, contrasting it with the increasing quantity of the monoclonal protein in myeloma.

Staining of bone-marrow plasma cells with monospecific immunofluorescent antisera shows that the plasma cells producing the monoclonal protein are dispersed throughout the bone marrow. The frequency of these plasma cells was the same in marrow preparations taken from different regions, indicating that their distribution in benign monoclonal gammopathy is as widespread as in myeloma (Warner et al., 1974).

Incidence of Monoclonal Proteins: Among 6,995 normal Swedish subjects beyond age 25, the overall occurrence of monoclonal proteins was about 1% (Axelsson et al., 1966). The frequency increased with age, reaching a maximum incidence of 9% in males and 6% in females in the ninth decade. Among the group more than 70 years old, 2.5% had a monoclonal protein in the serum. Hällén (1963, 1966), in a series of subjects more than 70 years old, found monoclonal proteins in 3.1% of 294 who were healthy and in 3.2% of 277 who were infirmary patients because of chronic cardiac, cerebrovascular, or similar diseases.

In a study of the incidence of monoclonal proteins, we collected sera from 1,200 residents of a small Minnesota community who were at least 50 years of age. Cellulose-acetate electrophoresis was applied to all samples, and those with patterns suggesting a monoclonal protein were subjected to immunoelectrophoresis utilizing monospecific antisera. Monoclonal proteins were detected in 15 cases (1.25%) with an incidence of 1.7% in men and 0.9% in women (Table 19). The incidence increased gradually with age. To illustrate: 0.5% of 407 patients 50 to 59 years of age and 4.8% of the 147 persons 80 years of age or older had monoclonal proteins. None of the patients had evidence of multiple myeloma or macroglobulinemia of Waldenström. The monoclonal serum protein peak ranged from 1.3 to 2.6 g/dl, and was less than 2 g/dl in 10 of the 15 cases. The monoclonal proteins were IgG in 11 patients (0.9%), IgA in 1 (0.08%), and IgM in 3 (0.25%); kappa light chains were found in 11 and lambda in 4 (Table 21).

The 15 patients were followed up for a minimum of 3 years. Three, who were more than 80 years of age, died of cardiovascular or cerebrovascular disease during that period without developing evidence of myeloma or macroglobulinemia. When serum samples were obtained from the 12 living patients at 3 years, electrophoresis showed a further increase of monoclonal protein in only 1 patient, and he continued to be asymptomatic. The absence of a further increase in the monoclonal protein in the remaining 11 patients is consistent with benign monoclonal gammopathy (Kyle et al., 1972). After 5 years of follow-up, four more patients had died of cardiovascular or cerebrovascular disease and one from pneumonia without evidence of myeloma or macroglobulinemia. The patient with an increasing IgM monoclonal protein died of macroglobulinemia, and one patient was lost to follow-up. Serum samples from the remaining five patients show no increase in the monoclonal protein; and at present, these cases can be categorized as benign monoclonal gammopathy.

Among 817 unselected residents of a hospital for the aged (mean age 86 years), monoclonal proteins were found in 3% of the men and 1.6% of the women, the overall incidence being 2.1%. One of these patients had probable macroglobulinemia but none had myeloma (Zawadzki and Edwards, 1972).

The incidence of monoclonal proteins is relatively high in certain families, which suggests a genetic predisposition (Axelsson and Hällén, 1965; Williams et al., 1967; Berlin et al., 1968; Grant et al., 1971). However, this appears to account for only a small proportion of the instances occurring in a population.

Differentiation From Myeloma and Macroglobulinemia: At the time when a small concentration of monoclonal protein is discovered, it is impossible in most cases to tell whether the abnormality will remain stable and the patient continue to be asymptomatic or whether he will develop multiple myeloma or macroglobulinemia of Waldenström. Many criteria have been proposed to aid in this differentiation, but none has been completely satisfactory.

The amount of the monoclonal protein is of some help. Bachmann (1965) reported that almost 80% of patients with more than 2 g/dl of IgG monoclonal protein or 1 g/dl of IgA monoclonal protein had myeloma and two thirds of the patients with more than 2 g/dl of IgM monoclonal protein had macroglobulinemia. The presence of anemia suggests a neoplastic process, but a reduction of hemoglobin may occur from lack of iron, vitamin B_{12}, or folic acid or many other causes unrelated to the protein abnormality. The presence of more than 5% plasma cells in the bone marrow suggests myeloma, but patients with greater plasmacytosis have remained stable for long periods; and conversely, patients with overt myeloma may have fewer than 5%

plasma cells in single bone-marrow specimens because the disease is spotty.

Currently we are following a patient with obvious multiple myeloma whose plasma cells never have amounted to as much as 5% in six separate bone-marrow aspirations and biopsies over a 9-month period. During this time the monoclonal protein abnormality has increased progressively (from 2.2 to 4.1 g/dl), anemia has developed (Hb 10.9 g/dl), the patient has had severe pain from collapse of vertebral body T-6 and again from destruction of vertebral body L-5, lytic lesions in the skull have increased and an extradural rib lesion has occurred, and a monoclonal light chain has appeared in the urine (Bence Jones proteinuria).

The morphologic abnormalities of the plasma cells are not always sufficient to differentiate a benign from a malignant process. In one instance a diagnosis of myeloma was made on the basis of 14.5% large, atypical plasma cells in the bone marrow and a sharp gamma peak on serum electrophoresis. No bone lesions, Bence Jones proteinuria, or anemia developed, and the marrow plasma cells and serum protein did not increase. No therapy was given. The patient died 16 years later (Bichel, 1964). This patient had the course of benign monoclonal gammopathy rather than multiple myeloma.

The presence of osteolytic lesions is very suggestive of multiple myeloma, but metastatic carcinoma may be responsible for the roentgenographic changes and plasmacytosis. We have seen a number of patients who had modest amounts of monoclonal protein in their serum, plasmacytosis, and lytic lesions secondary to a metastatic carcinoma.

The association of Bence Jones proteinuria with a monoclonal serum protein usually indicates a neoplastic process. Waldenström (1970) stated that the excretion of demonstrable amounts of Bence Jones protein in the urine of a patient with a monoclonal serum protein is strong evidence of malignancy. Hobbs (1967) said that Bence Jones proteinuria of more than 1.0 mg/dl (10 mg/liter) is of "sinister significance" and suggestive of malignant plasmacytic disease. Seligmann and Basch (1968) have noted that a Bence Jones protein level of 30 mg/100 dl (300 mg/ liter) or more in a patient with pathologic serum immunoglobulins and decreased normal immunoglobulins strongly suggested malignant proliferation. Dammacco and Waldenström (1968), from a study of 42 patients with benign monoclonal gammopathy, reported weakly positive results of a heat test for Bence Jones protein in one patient and small amounts of light chains in 24% of them. None of these patients had more than 60 mg/ liter of Bence Jones protein.

However, Bence Jones proteinuria with apparently benign monoclonal gammopathy has been reported. In these cases the amount of Bence Jones protein has been negligible, the absence of myeloma has not been assured, or the follow-up has been too short to establish that the condition is benign (Rádl and Masopust, 1964; Brittinger and König, 1965; Danon et al., 1967; Migliore and Alexanian, 1968; Kjeldsen et al., 1969; Sleeper and Cawley, 1969; Clauvel et al., 1971). The presence of a monoclonal light chain in the urine is very suggestive of a neoplastic process and such a case must be followed closely for development of multiple myeloma.

Other tests and criteria—including the presence or absence of chromosomal abnormalities, ABO blood group profiles, phytohemagglutinin (PHA) stimulation of lymphocytes, mixed lymphocyte culture reactions, and delayed skin hypersensitivity studies —have not proved to be adequate for distinguishing between benign monoclonal gammopathy and multiple myeloma (Ritzmann et al., 1975). They noted an increased incidence of lambda light chains in patients with benign monoclonal gammopathy, but the number of cases was small. The various immunoglobulin heavy-chain classes occur in approximately the same frequency as in myeloma.

Concentrations of immunoglobulins of classes not associated with the monoclonal protein (normal immunoglobulins) are frequently decreased in multiple myeloma; but this may be true also in benign monoclonal gammopathy, so it is not always a satisfactory differentiating feature. The proportion of B lymphocytes in the blood of patients with myeloma is reported as 10%, whereas the proportion of B lymphocytes in normal persons and those with benign monoclonal gammopathy are 22.9% and 21.4%, respectively (Lindstrom et al., 1973). This may prove helpful in distinguishing benign from malignant plasmacytic processes, but more experience is needed.

At present, periodic reexamination of patients with monoclonal gammopathy is the only way of determining whether the disorder is incipient myeloma or macroglobulinemia or a benign monoclonal gammopathy. In one study, 52 of the 62 patients who had had monoclonal gammopathy without evident neoplastic disease were reexamined after $2\frac{1}{2}$ years (Axelsson and Hällén, 1968) and 39 were again examined after $5\frac{1}{2}$ years (Axelsson and Hällén, 1972), and none of them had developed myeloma or macroglobulinemia. Whether such patients would develop these diseases in a still longer period cannot be answered, and whether some of the patients not available for follow-up actually died of multiple myeloma or macroglobulinemia cannot be ascertained. Patients have developed multiple myeloma and died of it at intervals ranging from 15 to 24 years after the initial demonstration of a monoclonal protein (Nørgaard, 1971). We have seen one patient who developed classic multiple myeloma 16 years after the demonstration of a monoclonal hyperglobulinemia (Kyle and Bayrd, 1966).

We have found the following features likely to be associated with nonprogressive or benign monoclonal gammopathy (Table 78): serum monoclonal protein concentration less than 2.0 g/dl; proportion of plasma cells in the bone-marrow aspirate less than 5%; no anemia; no osteolytic lesions; normal serum albumin; and

TABLE 78

BENIGN MONOCLONAL GAMMOPATHY: CRITERIA

Monoclonal serum protein peak of < 2 g/dl
Normal serum albumin
Marrow plasma cells $< 5\%$
No bone lesions
No anemia
No monoclonal urine protein
Observation without change for > 3 years

absence of monoclonal protein in the urine (Bence Jones proteinuria). Continued observation of the patient is essential: 3 years without deterioration or progression is the minimal period. An increase in the amount of the monoclonal serum protein or appearance of a monoclonal protein in the urine is strong evidence that the patient has a neoplastic process.

Animal Models: Rádl and Hollander (1974) found benign monoclonal gammopathy in mice, which thus provide an animal model for further study of the phenomenon. In their C57BL mice, the incidence of monoclonal serum proteins was 3% at 3 months of age and 50% at 24 months. Usually these proteins were single, but occasional biclonal and triclonal homogeneous proteins were detected. Of the monoclonal proteins, 78% were IgG, 17% IgM, and 5% IgA. The monoclonal protein maintained its same electrophoretic mobility, and the concentration did not increase to high levels as it does in mice with transplantable plasma-cell tumors. None of the mice with a monoclonal protein developed a visible or palpable tumor. Three of the seven autopsied mice with a monoclonal protein were found to have a reticulum-cell sarcoma, but two of five mice without a monoclonal protein also had a reticulum-cell sarcoma.

Association With Other Diseases: Although benign monoclonal gammopathy frequently exists without any other abnormalities, often certain diseases occur in association with it—as would be expected in an older population. It is therefore essential to have a control group when considering the validity of such associations, to show whether it is merely ordinary coincidence.

Carcinoma: Monoclonal gammopathy frequently has been reported as increased with carcinoma of various organs, particularly the colon. In their series of 128 patients with non-reticular neoplasms and a monoclonal protein, Isobe and Osserman (1971) found the rectosigmoid colon most frequently involved (adenocarcinoma 20% and adenomatous polyps 19%). Carcinoma of the prostate (18%) and breast (11%) were the other major categories. Surprisingly, only three cases (4%) of bronchogenic carcinoma were seen in these 128 cases.

In two large studies, the incidence of monoclonal proteins

among patients with non-reticuloendothelial neoplasm was no greater than one would expect in a population of similar age. Migliore and Alexanian (1968) found a monoclonal protein in 0.65% of 5,066 patients referred for evaluation of a known or suspected neoplasm. Of the 33 monoclonal proteins, 31 were IgG and 2 IgM. The median concentration of monoclonal protein was 1.0 g/dl. Talerman and Haije (1973) found no greater frequency of monoclonal components in the sera of patients with solid malignant neoplasms than in sera from a normal adult population. However, they noted an increased frequency of monoclonal proteins in patients with carcinoma of the lung—though Isobe and Osserman (1971) emphasized the infrequency of monoclonal proteins with cancer of the lung.

Surgical removal of tumors has no effect on the concentration of the monoclonal protein, and in no instance has removal of a malignant solid tumor caused the monoclonal protein to disappear. In many cases plasma cells actually infiltrate the tumor, but no reaction between tumor cells and the monoclonal protein has been discovered (Williams et al., 1969). The preponderant findings suggest that the association of monoclonal proteins and neoplasia is fortuitous, or perhaps that both arise through a failure of the patient's immunosurveillance system.

Lymphoma: An increased incidence of monoclonal IgM proteins has been noted with lymphocytic malignancies. In many cases the differentiation from macroglobulinemia is not clear, and a number of them could be classified as Waldenström's macroglobulinemia (Krauss and Sokal, 1966). In a series of 1,150 patients with lymphoma, Alexanian (1975) found monoclonal proteins in 49 (29 IgM, 15 IgG, and 5 not typed). Of 400 patients with chronic lymphocytic leukemia and lymphocytic lymphoma, 2.3% had an IgG monoclonal protein, which is not significantly more than the incidence in a normal population of the same age. However, the incidence of IgM monoclonal proteins in patients with a diffuse histologic infiltration of lymph nodes (chronic lymphocytic leukemia, lymphocytic lymphoma, and reticulum-cell sarcoma) was 100 times greater than in a normal population. No patient with nodular lymphoma or Hodgkin's disease had a monoclonal IgM protein. This study is an extension of a previous one from the same institution (Moore et al., 1970) and confirms the earlier findings.

One would presume that the monoclonal protein in malignant lymphoma was produced by the lymphocytes, but Palutke and McDonald (1973) were unable to detect the production of a monoclonal protein in lymphomatous tissue from two patients with poorly differentiated lymphocytic lymphosarcoma. One of these patients had an IgG κ monoclonal protein, which the malignant lymphocytes might not be expected to produce; but the other patient had an IgM monoclonal protein.

Leukemia: Monoclonal proteins have been found in the serum of children with acute leukemia. A child with acute leukemia in relapse developed a monoclonal IgG λ protein and lambda Bence Jones proteinuria after a Herpes simplex skin infection followed by two other viral infections. No antibody activity against any of the viruses was demonstrated (Stoop et al., 1968). A 4-year-old boy in remission from acute lymphoblastic leukemia had an IgG κ monoclonal protein, but no Bence Jones proteinuria or other evidence of myeloma was noted (Lindqvist et al., 1970). A 12-year-old child with acute leukemia had a modest concentration of IgM κ protein in the serum and Bence Jones proteinuria (Čejka et al., 1974). A monoclonal IgG κ protein appeared in another patient with an acute myeloblastic leukemia (Castoldi et al., 1971). An adult with monocytic leukemia excreted 8 to 10 g of kappa Bence Jones protein in his urine each day and also had an IgG κ monoclonal protein in his serum, but no evidence of myeloma in the bone marrow or on roentgenograms (Poulik et al., 1969). Chronic granulocytic leukemia also has been associated with a monoclonal protein in the serum (Ritzmann et al., 1966). Patients with lymphoma or chronic lymphocytic leukemia and a monoclonal IgM protein do not differ significantly from those without a monoclonal protein (Stein et al., 1975).

We do not yet have the data to determine whether the incidence of a monoclonal protein in leukemia is greater than in a normal population.

Lichen Myxedematosus: Lichen myxedematosus (papular mucinosis, scleromyxedema) is a rare dermatologic condition which is frequently associated with a monoclonal IgG λ protein. It is characterized by dermal papules, macules, and plaques and has a predilection for the upper extremities and upper portion of the trunk, but may involve all of the body. The skin gradually becomes sufficiently infiltrated so that movement becomes difficult, and the condition is easily confused with scleroderma. Biopsy of the skin reveals an increase in fibroblasts and an increased deposition of acid mucopolysaccharides. McCarthy et al. (1964) called attention to the presence of a small monoclonal IgG λ basic protein with cathodal mobility in the serum and skin of one patient. In a review of eight cases of lichen myxedematosus, James et al. (1967) emphasized the frequent appearance of a monoclonal IgG λ protein. This protein often precipitates at low ionic strength (euglobulin). One patient with lichen myxedematosus was thought to have a coincidental myeloma (Perry et al., 1960). A small concentration of monoclonal IgG κ protein rather than λ was found in one case, and in this instance the monoclonal protein was synthesized by cells from the bone marrow and perhaps by the skin as well. The authors could demonstrate no antibody activity against connective-tissue ground substance (Lai A Fat et al., 1973).

Survival is variable. Some patients with lichen myxedematosus live for years, while others have a course of only a few months. Treatment is generally unsatisfactory. We have one unusual patient who presented in 1966 with advanced lichen myxedematosus that thickened her skin so much as to reduce markedly her ability to open her mouth. Objective improvement of the skin and disappearance of the IgG λ monoclonal protein coincided with daily melphalan therapy. When the chemotherapy was discontinued 6 years later, the skin manifestations and the IgG λ monoclonal protein recurred. Intermittent courses of melphalan then were ineffective, but daily oral administration again induced marked improvement of the skin and disappearance of the IgG λ protein. Unquestionably the monoclonal protein figures prominently in lichen myxedematosus, but the pathogenesis has not been elucidated.

Other Hematologic Diseases: Monoclonal gammopathies have been associated with pernicious anemia (Larson, 1962; Selroos and von Knorring, 1973). A patient with acquired sideroblastic anemia developed a monoclonal IgG κ protein and Bence Jones proteinuria, and was found at autopsy to have a malignant lymphoma (Tranchida et al., 1973). Two of seven reported patients with acquired von Willebrand's disease had an IgG monoclonal protein in their serum (Ingram et al., 1971; Mant et al., 1973). Pratt et al. (1968) reported that 4 of 16 patients with Gaucher's disease had a monoclonal IgG κ protein in their serum while 6 others had a diffuse increase of IgG. We have seen apparently benign monoclonal gammopathies in four patients with agnogenic myeloid metaplasia and one with thrombocythemia.

Liver Disease: Although polyclonal increases in immunoglobulins are most common in liver disease, monoclonal proteins have been reported. Zawadzki and Edwards (1970a) found small monoclonal proteins in 12 cases of chronic liver or biliary-tract disease even though the serum electrophoretic pattern suggested a polyclonal hypergammaglobulinemia. They also noted the transformation of a polyclonal increase of immunoglobulins to a monoclonal protein in two patients with alcoholic cirrhosis. One of these patients died of multiple myeloma. On the other hand, Ellman et al. (1969) found monoclonal proteins in only 3 of 387 cases of chronic liver disease, which is no more than the normal incidence.

Connective-Tissue Diseases: Rheumatoid arthritis (Zawadzki and Benedek, 1969), lupus erythematosus, and other connective-tissue diseases have been associated with monoclonal proteins (Michaux and Heremans, 1969). However, in a series of 279 consecutive patients with rheumatoid arthritis in our institution, we found no significant increase in the incidence of either benign monoclonal gammopathy or multiple myeloma.

Neurologic Diseases: Myasthenia gravis (Rowland et al., 1969) and ataxia-telangiectasia (Cawley and Schenken, 1970) are among the neurologic diseases reported with monoclonal proteins. A patient with peripheral neuropathy and a small amount of monoclonal IgM protein (1.1 to 1.3 g/dl) in his serum was found to have infiltration of IgM-producing lymphocytes in a saphenous nerve. Improvement was noted with chlorambucil therapy (Forssman et al., 1973).

Miscellaneous: Monoclonal IgG proteins may be associated with hyperparathyroidism (Dexter et al., 1972). We also have seen several examples of this. Consequently a monoclonal protein associated with hypercalcemia does not always signify myeloma, and hyperparathyroidism must be considered. A gamma peak in the electrophoretic pattern in one case was reported to disappear following removal of a parathyroid adenoma for hyperparathyroidism (Clubb et al., 1964).

Monoclonal proteins have been associated with idiopathic pulmonary fibrosis (Bonanni et al., 1965) and pulmonary alveolar proteinosis (Mork et al., 1968). They have been found with thymoma (Anderson and Vye, 1967), with psoriatic arthritis (Lergier and Gowans, 1975), and with glomerulopathy (Jensen and Wiik, 1975). Monoclonal proteins in pyoderma gangrenosum have been reported—mostly IgA, but some IgG and IgM (Cream, 1971).

"Pseudomyeloma" has been coined as a term for severe osteoporosis and a monoclonal serum protein without evidence of multiple myeloma (Buonocore et al., 1970; Maldonado et al., 1975a). However, in our practice we have seen several dozen patients with osteoporosis, a moderate amount of monoclonal protein in the serum, and minimal plasmacytosis but no evidence of multiple myeloma on follow-up examination. It is likely that postmenopausal or idiopathic osteoporosis is the basis of most of these instances.

Benign Monoclonal Light-Chain Gammopathy: The possibility of a benign monoclonal gammopathy of the light-chain type (Bence Jones proteinuria) must be considered, despite the fact that it is a recognized feature of multiple myeloma, Waldenström's macroglobulinemia, primary amyloidosis, and occasional-

TABLE 79

BENIGN MONOCLONAL LIGHT-CHAIN GAMMOPATHY
(DATA FROM TWO MAYO CLINIC CASES)

	Case 1	Case 2
Clinical data		
Age (yr.) at onset and sex	50, F	49, M
Proteinuria		
Date of onset	2/65	12/55
Date of latest follow-up	7/75	1/74
Duration, yr.	10+	18+
Laboratory data		
Serum		
Hemoglobin, g/dl	13.6	15.9
Albumin, g/dl	3.28	3.77
Globulin peak, g/dl		
Initial	2.59	2.27
Final	2.16	2.40
Monoclonal protein	IgG κ	IgG κ
Immunoglobulin, mg/ml		
IgG	19.5	29.5
IgA	0.45	0.50
IgM	0.55	0.17
Urine		
Protein	3+	2+
Bence Jones protein	3+	± eq
Protein, 24 h		
Initial	1.7	1.0
Final	0.9	1.4
Monoclonal protein	Kappa	Kappa

Modified from Kyle, R. A., Maldonado, J. E., and Bayrd, E. D.: Idiopathic Bence Jones proteinuria: a distinct entity? *Am J Med, 55*:222-226, 1973. By permission of Dun · Donnelley Publishing Corporation.

ly, lymphoma. We have seen periodically two patients who have maintained a stable amount of monoclonal serum protein and excreted 0.8 g or more of Bence Jones protein daily for more than 10 years without evidence of the development of myeloma, amyloidosis, or similar malignant diseases (Table 79; Fig. 74), although the possibility of such future development cannot be excluded (Kyle et al., 1973b). Currently we are following two additional cases in which patients who have excreted more than 1 g/24 h of a monoclonal light chain for 2 and 5 years have no monoclonal protein in the serum, no anemia, no lytic bone lesions, and no

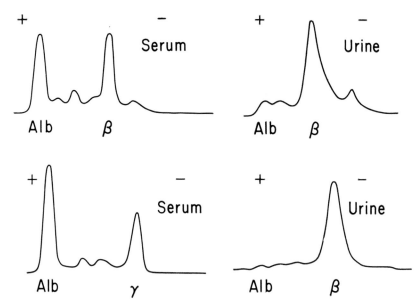

Figure 74. Electrophoretic patterns of serum and urinary proteins. Case 1 *(Upper):* narrow-based beta peaks. Case 2 *(Lower):* narrow-based gamma peak from serum, narrow-based beta peak from urine. (From Kyle, R. A., Maldonado, J. E., and Bayrd, E. D.: Idiopathic Bence Jones proteinuria: a distinct entity? *Am J Med,* 55:222-226, 1973. By permission of Dun · Donnelly Publishing Corporation.)

evidence of multiple myeloma. Cronstedt et al. (1974) reported a case in which decreased IgG and IgA protein had persisted for 5 years and then Bence Jones proteinuria had appeared (175 mg/liter), still without myeloma. Thus, appreciable Bence Jones proteinuria may be benign or idiopathic, and not always an ominous finding.

Management: Treatment for benign monoclonal gammopathy is not required, but frequent reexamination is necessary to be certain that the concentration of the monoclonal protein is stable and that myeloma or macroglobulinemia has not developed.

References

Abdou, N. I., and Abdou, N. L.: Idiotypic immunoglobulin (ID-IG) on monoclonal lymphocytes (Ly) of human multiple myeloma (MM): effects of therapy (abstract). *Clin Res, 23*:408A, 1975.

Abdou, N. L., and Abdou, N. I.: Discoid lupus erythematosus with macroglobulinemia: correlations between autoimmunity and B cell malignancy with hyperimmunoglobulinemia. *Am J Med, 57*:630-637, 1974.

Abrahams, C., Pirani, C. L., and Pollack, V. E.: Ultrastructure of the kidney in a patient with multiple myeloma. *J Pathol, 92*:220-224, 1966.

Abramson, N., and Schur, P. H.: The IgG subclasses of red cell antibodies and relationship to monocyte binding. *Blood, 40*:500-508, 1972.

Abt, A. B., and Deppisch, L. M.: Multiple myeloma involving the extrahepatic biliary system. *Mt Sinai J Med* (NY), *36*:48-54, 1969.

Adams, W. (for Dowse, T. S.) : Mollities ossium. *Trans Pathol Soc Lond, 23*: 186-187, 1872.

Adams, W. S., Alling, E. L., and Lawrence, J. S.: Multiple myeloma: its clinical and laboratory diagnosis with emphasis on electrophoretic abnormalities. *Am J Med, 6*:141-161, 1949.

Adams, W. S., Blahd, W. H., and Bassett, S. H.: A method of human plasmapheresis. *Proc Soc Exp Biol Med, 80*:377-379, 1952.

Adner, P. L., Wallenius, G., and Werner, I.: Macroglobulinemia and myelomatosis. *Acta Med Scand, 168*:431-437, 1960.

Afifi, A. M.: Myeloma cells in the cerebrospinal fluid in plasma cell neoplasia. *J Neurol Neurosurg Psychiatry, 37*:1162-1165, 1974.

Afifi, A. M., and Tawfeek, S.: Deafness due to Waldenström macroglobulinaemia. *J Laryngol Otol, 85*:275-280, 1971.

Akbarian, M., and Fenton, J.: Perforation of small bowel in amyloidosis: includes review of the literature. *Arch Intern Med, 114*:815-821, 1964.

Alarcón-Segovia, D., Fishbein, E., Abruzzo, J. L., and Heimer, R.: Serum hyperviscosity in Sjögren's syndrome: interaction between serum IgG and IgG rheumatoid factor. *Ann Intern Med, 80*:35-43, 1974.

Alberts, D. S., and Golde, D. W.: DNA synthesis in multiple myeloma cells following cell cycle-nonspecific chemotherapy. *Cancer Res, 34*:2911-2914, 1974.

Alberts, D. S., and Salmon, S. E.: Adriamycin (NSC0123127) in the treatment of alkylator-resistant multiple myeloma: a pilot study. *Cancer Chemother Rep, 59*:345-350, 1975.

Alexander, F., and Atkins, E. L.: Familial renal amyloidosis: case reports, literature review and classification. *Am J Med, 59:*121-128, 1975.

Alexanian, R.: Monoclonal gammopathy in lymphoma. *Arch Intern Med, 135:*62-66, 1975.

Alexanian, R., Bergsagel, D. E., Migliore, P. J., Vaughn, W. K., and Howe, C. D.: Melphalan therapy for plasma cell myeloma. *Blood, 31:*1-10, 1968.

Alexanian, R., Bonnet, J., Gehan, E., Haut, A., Hewlett, J., Lane, M., Monto, R., and Wilson, H.: Combination chemotherapy for multiple myeloma. *Cancer, 30:*382-389, 1972.

Alexanian, R., Haut, A., Khan, A. U., Lane, M., McKelvey, E. M., Migliore, P. J., Stuckey, W. J., Jr., and Wilson, H. E.: Treatment for multiple myeloma: combination chemotherapy with different melphalan dose regimens. *JAMA, 208:*1680-1685, 1969.

Alexanian, R., and Migliore, P. J.: Normal immunoglobulins in multiple myeloma: effect of melphalan chemotherapy. *J Lab Clin Med, 75:*225-233, 1970.

Ali, M. A. M., and Blajchman, M. A.: Studies of the antibody on the platelet surface in patients with Factor-VIII inhibitors. *Br J Haematol, 22:*365-368, 1972.

Allan, T. M.: ABO blood groups and myelomatosis (letter to the editor). *Br Med J, 4:*178, 1970a.

Allan, W. S. A.: Acute myeloid leukaemia after treatment with cytostatic agents (letter to the editor). *Lancet, 2:*775, 1970b.

Allen, E. L., Metz, E. N., and Balcerzak, S. P.: Acute myelomonocytic leukemia with macroglobulinemia, Bence Jones proteinuria, and hypercalcemia. *Cancer, 32:*121-124, 1973.

Alroy, G. G., Lichtig, C., and Kaftori, J. K.: Tracheobronchopathia osteoplastica: end stage of primary lung amyloidosis? *Chest, 61:*465-468, 1972.

Alwall, N.: Urethane and stilbamidine in multiple myeloma: report on two cases. *Lancet, 2:*388-389, 1947.

Aly, F. W., Braun, H. J., and Missmahl, H. P.: Amyloid involvement and monoclonal immunoglobins. In Westphal, O., Bock, H.-E., and Grundmann, E. (Eds.): *Current Problems in Immunology* (Bayer-Symposium I). New York, Springer-Verlag, 1969, pp. 295-301.

Andaloro, V. A., Jr., and Babott, D.: Testicular involvement in plasma-cell leukemia. *Urology, 3:*636-638, 1974.

Anday, G. J., Fishkin, B., and Gabor, E. P.: Cytogenetic studies in multiple myeloma. *J Natl Cancer Inst, 52:*1069-1079, 1974.

Andersen, B. R., and Terry, W. D.: Gamma G4-globulin antibody causing inhibition of clotting Factor VIII (letter to the editor). *Nature, 217:*174-175, 1968.

Andersen, E., and Videbaek, A.: Stem cell leukaemia in myelomatosis. *Scand J Haematol, 7:*201-207, 1970.

Anderson, E. T., and Vye, M. V.: Dysproteinemia of the myeloma type associated with a thymoma. *Ann Intern Med, 66:*141-149, 1967.

Anderson, R. E.: Disseminated amyloidosis in germfree mice: spontaneous prevalence, relationship to ionizing radiation and pathogenetic implications. *Am J Pathol, 65*:43-49, 1971.

Anderson, R. E., and Ishida, K.: Malignant lymphoma in survivors of the atomic bomb in Hiroshima. *Ann Intern Med, 61*:853-862, 1964.

Ansell, I. D., and Joekes, A. M.: Spicular arrangement of amyloid in renal biopsy. *J Clin Pathol, 25*:1056-1062, 1972.

Arapakis, G., and Tribe, C. R.: Amyloidosis in rheumatoid arthritis investigated by means of rectal biopsy. *Ann Rheum Dis, 22*:256-262, 1963.

Arend, W. P., and Adamson, J. W.: Nonsecretory myeloma: immunofluorescent demonstration of paraprotein within bone marrow plasma cells. *Cancer, 33*:721-728, 1974.

Argani, I., and Kipkie, G. F.: Macroglobulinemic nephropathy: acute renal failure in macroglobulinemia of Waldenström. *Am J Med, 36*:151-157, 1964.

Arinkin, M. I.: Die intravitale Untersuchungsmethodik des Knochenmarks. *Folia Haematol* (Leipz), *38*:233-240, 1929.

Askanazy-Königsberg, M.: Ueber knötchenförmige lokale Amyloidbildung in der Darmmuskulatur. *Verh Dtsch Ges Pathol, 7*:32-34, 1904.

Atkinson, K., McElwain, T. J., and Mackay, A. M.: Myeloma of the heart. *Br Heart J, 36*:309-312, 1974.

Attwood, H. D., Price, C. G., and Riddell, R. J.: Primary diffuse tracheobronchial amyloidosis. *Thorax, 27*:620-624, 1972.

Auerbach, O., and Stemmerman, M. G.: Renal amyloidosis. *Arch Intern Med, 74*:244-253, 1944.

Axelsson, U., Bachmann, R., and Hällén, J.: Frequency of pathological proteins (M-components) in 6,995 sera from an adult population. *Acta Med Scand, 179*:235-247, 1966.

Axelsson, U., Hällén, A., and Rausing, A.: Amyloidosis of bone: report of two cases. *J Bone Joint Surg* [Br], *52*:717-723, 1970.

Axelsson, U., and Hällén, J.: Familial occurrence of pathological serum-proteins of different γ-globulin groups. *Lancet, 2*:369-370, 1965.

Axelsson, U., and Hällén, J.: Review of fifty-four subjects with monoclonal gammopathy. *Br J Haematol, 15*:417-420, 1968.

Axelsson, U., and Hällén, J.: A population study on monoclonal gammopathy: follow-up after 5½ years on 64 subjects detected by electrophoresis of 6,995 sera. *Acta Med Scand, 191*:111-113, 1972.

Azam, L., and Delamore, I. W.: Combination therapy for myelomatosis. *Br Med J, 4*:560-564, 1974.

Azar, H. A.: Experimental plasmacytomas in relation to human multiple myeloma. *Ann Clin Lab Sci, 4*:157-163, 1974.

Azar, H. A., and Potter, M.: *Multiple Myeloma and Related Disorders.* Vol 1. Hagerstown, Maryland, Harper & Row, Publishers, 1973.

Azar, H. A., Zaino, E. C., Pham, T. D., and Yannopoulos, K.: "Nonsecretory" plasma cell myeloma: observations on seven cases with electron microscopic studies. *Am J Clin Pathol, 58*:618-629, 1972.

Bachmann, R.: The diagnostic significance of the serum concentration of pathological proteins (M-components). *Acta Med Scand, 178*:801-808, 1965.

Badrinas, F., Rodriguez-Roisin, R., Rives, A., and Picado, C.: Multiple myeloma with pleural involvement. *Am Rev Respir Dis, 110*:82-87, 1974.

Baitz, T., and Kyle, R. A.: Solitary myeloma in chronic osteomyelitis: report of case. *Arch Intern Med, 113*:872-876, 1964.

Baker, T. R., and Spencer, W. H.: Ocular findings in multiple myeloma: a report of two cases. *Arch Ophthalmol, 91*:110-113, 1974.

Ballard, H. S., Hamilton, L. M., Marcus, A. J., and Illes, C. H.: A new variant of heavy-chain disease (μ-chain disease). *N Engl J Med, 282*:1060-1062, 1970.

Bannick, E. G., and Greene, C. H.: Renal insufficiency associated with Bence-Jones proteinuria: report of thirteen cases with a note on the changes in the serum proteins. *Arch Intern Med, 44*:486-501, 1929.

Barclay, G. P. T., Cameron, H. M., and Loughridge, L. W.: Amyloid disease of the kidney and renal vein thrombosis. *Q J Med, ns, 29*:137-151, 1960.

Bark, C. J., and Feinberg, S.: Solitary plasmacytoma and obstructive jaundice (letter to the editor). *JAMA, 201*:491, 1967.

Barr, R., and Lampert, P.: Intrasellar amyloid tumor. *Acta Neuropathol* (Berl), *21*:83-86, 1972.

Bartels, E. D., Brun, G. C., Gammeltoft, A., and Gjørup, P. A.: Acute anuria following intravenous pyelography in a patient with myelomatosis. *Acta Med Scand, 150*:297-302, 1954.

Barth, R. F., Willerson, J. T., Buja, L. M., Decker, J. L., and Roberts, W. C.: Amyloid coronary artery disease, primary systemic amyloidosis and paraproteinemia. *Arch Intern Med, 126*:627-630, 1970.

Barth, W. F., Glenner, G. G., Waldmann, T. A., and Zelis, R. F.: Primary amyloidosis. *Ann Intern Med, 69*:787-805, 1968a.

Barth, W. F., Gordon, J. K., and Willerson, J. T.: Amyloidosis induced in mice by *Escherichia coli* endotoxin. *Science, 162*:694-695, 1968b.

Barth, W. F., Willerson, J. T., Waldmann, T. A., and Decker, J. L.: Primary amyloidosis: clinical, immunochemical and immunoglobulin metabolism studies in fifteen patients. *Am J Med, 47*:259-273, 1969.

Baumal, R., Birshtein, B. K., Coffino, P., and Scharff, M. D.: Mutations in immunoglobulin-producing mouse myeloma cells. *Science, 182*:164-166, 1973.

Bayrd, E. D.: The bone marrow on sternal aspiration in multiple myeloma. *Blood, 3*:987-1018, 1948.

Bayrd, E. D.: Continuous chlorambucil therapy in primary macroglobulinemia of Waldenström: report of four cases. *Proc Staff Meet Mayo Clin, 36*:135-147, 1961.

Bazin, H., Querinjean, P., Beckers, A., Heremans, J. F., and Dessy, F.: Transplantable immunoglobulin-secreting tumours in rats. IV. Sixty-three IgE-secreting immunocytoma tumours. *Immunology*, 26:713-723, 1974.

Bedine, M. S., Yardley, J. H., Elliott, H. L., Banwell, J. G., and Hendrix, T. R.: Intestinal involvement in Waldenström's macroglobulinemia. *Gastroenterology*, 65:308-315, 1973.

Beker, S. G., Grases, P. J., Merino, F., Arends, T., and Guevara, J.: Intestinal malabsorption in macroglobulinemia. *Am J Dig Dis*, ns, 16:648-656, 1971.

Bell, E. T.: Renal lesions associated with multiple myeloma. *Am J Pathol, 9:* 393-420, 1933.

Bence Jones, H.: On a new substance occurring in the urine of a patient with mollities ossium. *Proc R Soc* (Lond), 5:673, 1847a.

Bence Jones, H.: Papers on chemical pathology: Lecture III. *Lancet*, 2:88-92, 1847b.

Bence Jones, H.: On a new substance occurring in the urine of a patient with mollities ossium. *Philos Trans R Soc* (Lond), 1848, pp. 55-62.

Benditt, E. P., and Eriksen, N.: Chemical classes of amyloid substance. *Am J Pathol*, 65:231-249, 1971.

Benedek, T. G., and Zawadzki, Z. A.: Ankylosing spondylitis with ulcerative colitis and amyloidosis: report of a case and review of the literature. *Am J Med, 40:*431-439, 1966.

Benedict, K. T., Jr.: Destructive lesion of the proximal radius. *JAMA, 212:* 464-465, 1970.

Benjamin, I., Taylor, H., and Spindler, J.: Orbital and conjunctival involvement in multiple myeloma: report of a case. *Am J Clin Pathol*, 63:811-817, 1975.

Benson, M. D., Aldo-Benson, M. A., Shirahama, T., Borel, Y., and Cohen, A. S.: Suppression of in vitro antibody response by a serum factor (SAA) in experimentally induced amyloidosis. *J Exp Med*, 142:236-241, 1975a.

Benson, M. D., Cohen, A. S., Brandt, K. D., and Cathcart, E. S.: Neuropathy, M components, and amyloid. *Lancet, 1:*10-12, 1975b.

Benson, M. D., Skinner, M., and Cohen, A. S.: Antigenicity and cross-reactivity of denatured fibril proteins of primary, secondary, and myeloma associated amyloids. *J Lab Clin Med, 85:*650-659, 1975c.

Bentwich, Z., Rosenmann, E., and Eliakim, M.: Prevalence of hypertension in renal amyloidosis: correlation with clinical and histological parameters; a study of 56 patients and review of the literature. *Am J Med Sci, 262:*93-100, 1971.

Benvenisti, D. S., and DeBellis, R. H.: Carcinoma of the breast, chronic lymphocytic leukemia, macroglobulinemia, eosinophilic chloroma and myelosclerosis—a unique association. *Cancer, 23:*1204-1209, 1969.

Berardi, R. S., and Malette, W. G.: Focal amyloidosis of small bowel mesentery. *Int Surg, 58:*491-494, 1973.

Berg, J. W.: The incidence of multiple primary cancers. I. Development of further cancers in patients with lymphomas, leukemias, and myeloma. *J Natl Cancer Inst, 38:*741-752, 1967.

Bergsagel, D. E.: Total body irradiation for myelomatosis. *Br Med J, 2*:325, 1971.

Bergsagel, D. E., Cowan, D. H., and Hasselback, R.: Plasma cell myeloma: response of melphalan-resistant patients to high-dose intermittent cyclophosphamide. *Can Med Assoc J, 107*:851-855, 1972.

Bergsagel, D. E., Migliore, P. J., and Griffith, K. M.: Myeloma proteins and the clinical response to melphalan therapy. *Science, 148*:376-377, 1965.

Bergsagel, D. E., and Pruzanski, W.: Treatment of plasma cell myeloma with cytotoxic agents. *Arch Intern Med, 135*:172-176, 1975.

Bergsagel, D. E., Sprague, C. C., Austin, C., and Griffith, K. M.: Evaluation of new chemotherapeutic agents in the treatment of multiple myeloma. IV. L-Phenylalanine mustard (NSC-8806). *Cancer Chemother Rep, 21*:87-99, 1962.

Berlin, S.-O., Odeberg, H., and Weingart, L.: Familial occurrence of M-components. *Acta Med Scand, 183*:347-350, 1968.

Berman, H. H.: Waldenström's macroglobulinemia with lytic osseous lesions and plasma-cell morphology: report of a case. *Am J Clin Pathol, 63*:397-402, 1975.

Bernard, D. B., Lynch, S. R., Bothwell, T. H., Bezwoda, W. R., Stevens, K., and Shulman, G.: Multiple myeloma. II. The value of melphalan. *S Afr Med J, 48*:1026-1028, 1974.

Bernhardt, B., Valletta, M., Brook J., and Lejnieks, I.: Amyloidosis with Factor X deficiency. *Am J Med Sci, 264*:411-414, 1972.

Bertrams, J., Kuwert, E., Böhme, U., Reis, H. E., Gallameier, W. M., Wetter, O., and Schmidt, C. G.: HL-A antigens in Hodgkin's disease and multiple myeloma: increased frequency of W18 in both diseases. *Tissue Antigens, 2*:41-46, 1972.

Bevan, M. J., Parkhouse, R. M. E., Williamson, A. R., and Askonas, B. A.: Biosynthesis of immunoglobulins. *Prog Biophys Mol Biol, 25*:133-162, 1972.

Bhan, A. K., Baez-Giangreco, A., and Vawter, G. F.: Lymphoreticular malignancy in immunodeficiency with lymphocytotoxic antibody. *Cancer, 34*:1612-1619, 1974.

Bichel, J.: Megaloblastic anaemia and myxoedema in a patient suffering from myeloma, observed for a period of 16 years. *Acta Med Scand, 176*:165-168, 1964.

Bichel, J., Bing, J., and Harboe, N.: Another case of hyperglobulinemia and affection of the central nervous system. *Acta Med Scand, 138*:1-14, 1950.

Bichel, J., Effersøe, P., Gormsen, H., and Harboe, N.: Leukemic myelomatosis (plasma cell leukemia): a review with report of four cases. *Acta Radiol, 37*:196-207, 1952.

Bigner, D. D., Olson, W. H., and McFarlin, D. E.: Peripheral polyneuropathy, high and low molecular weight IgM, and amyloidosis. *Arch Neurol, 24*:365-373, 1971.

Bihrer, R., Flury, R., and Morell, A.: Biklonale Paraproteinämie. *Schweiz Med Wochenschr, 104:*39-45, 1974.

Bing, J., and Neel, A. V.: Two cases of hyperglobulinaemia with affection of the central nervous system on a toxi-infectious basis. *Acta Med Scand, 88:* 492-506, 1936.

Biserte, G., Lebreton, J. P., Ropartz, C., Tijou, G., Mouty, B., Rodat, G., Maillet, J. Y., Letournou, A., Guimbretiere, J., Bray, B., and Boudart, D.: Un cas de maladie des chaînes lourdes μ (letter to the editor). *Nouv Presse Med, 2:*1997, 1973.

Bjerrum, O. J., and Weeke, B.: Two M components (γGK and γML) in different cells of the same patient. *Scand J Haematol, 5:*215-234, 1968.

Bjørneboe, M., and Jensen, K. B.: Plasma volume, colloid-osmotic pressure and gamma globulin in multiple myeloma. *Acta Med Scand, 186:*475-478, 1969.

Bjørn-Hansen, R.: Primary plasmocytoma of the spleen. *Am J Roentgenol Radium Ther Nucl Med, 117:*81-83, 1973.

Bladen, H. A., Nylen, M. U., and Glenner, G. G.: The ultrastructure of human amyloid as revealed by the negative staining technique. *J Ultrastruc Res, 14:*449-459, 1966.

Blaylock, W. M., Waller, M., and Normansell, D. E.: Sjögren's syndrome: hyperviscosity and intermediate complexes. *Ann Intern Med, 80:*27-34, 1974.

Bloch, K. J., Lee, L., Mills, J. A., and Haber, E.: Gamma heavy chain disease: an expanding clinical and laboratory spectrum. *Am J Med, 55:*61-70, 1973.

Bloch, K. J., and Maki, D. G.: Hyperviscosity syndrome associated with immunoglobulin abnormalities. *Semin Hematol, 10:*113-124, 1973.

Blokhin, N., Larionov, L., Perevodchikova, N., Chebotareva, L., and Merkulova, N.: Clinical experiences with sarcolysin in neoplastic diseases. *Ann NY Acad Sci, 68:*1128-1132, 1958.

Blom, J.: The ultrastructure of contact zones between plasma cells and dendritic macrophages from patients with multiple myeloma. *Acta Pathol Microbiol Scand* [A], *81:*734-736, 1973.

Bloth, B., and Svehag, S.-E.: Further studies on the ultrastructure of dimeric IgA of human origin. *J Exp Med, 133:*1035-1042, 1971.

Bohrod, M. G., and Bottcher, E. J.: Multiple myeloma, hemolytic anemia, and protein phagocytosis. *Arch Pathol, 76:*700-707, 1963.

Bonanni, P. P., Frymoyer, J. W., and Jacox, R. F.: A family study of idiopathic pulmonary fibrosis: a possible dysproteinemic and genetically determined disease. *Am J Med, 39:*411-421, 1965.

Bonfils-Roberts, E., Marx, A. J., and Nealon, T. F., Jr.: Primary amyloidosis of the respiratory tract. *Ann Thorac Surg, 19:*313-318, 1975.

Bonhomme, J., Seligmann, M., Mihaesco, C., Clauvel, J. P., Danon, F., Brouet, J. C., Bouvry, P., Martine, J., and Clerc, M.: Mu-chain disease in an African patient. *Blood, 43:*485-492, 1974.

Bonner, H., Jr., Ennis, R. S., Geelhoed, G. W., and Tarpley, T. M., Jr.: Lymphoid infiltration and amyloidosis of lung in Sjögren's syndrome. *Arch Pathol, 95*:42-44, 1973.

Booth, J. B., Cheesman, A. D., and Vincenti, N. H.: Extramedullary plasmacytomata of the upper respiratory tract. *Ann Otol Rhinol Laryngol, 82*: 709-715, 1973.

Booth, L. J., Minielly, J. A., and Smith, E. K. M.: Acute renal failure in multiple myeloma. *Can Med Assoc J, 111*:334-335, 1974.

Bottomley, J. P., Bradley, J., and Whitehouse, G. H.: Waldenström's macroglobulinaemia and amyloidosis with subcutaneous calcification and lymphographic appearances. *Br J Radiol, 47*:232-235, 1974.

Bouroncle, B. A., Datta, P., and Frajola, W. J.: Waldenström's macroglobulinemia: report of three patients treated with cyclophosphamide. *JAMA, 189*:729-732, 1964.

Bowie, E. J. W., Maldonado, J. E., Brown, A. L., Jr., Didisheim, P., and Owen, C. A., Jr.: Intravascular coagulation in systemic amyloidosis. *Thromb Diath Haemorrh* Suppl, *36*:305-312, 1969.

Bradley, J., Hawkins, C. F., Rowe, D. S., and Stanworth, D. R.: Macroglobulinaemia and steatorrhoea. *Gut, 9*:564-568, 1968.

Brambell, F. W. R.: The transmission of immunity from mother to young and the catabolism of immunoglobulins. *Lancet, 2*:1087-1093, 1966.

Brandt, K., Cathcart, E. S., and Cohen, A. S.: A clinical analysis of the course and prognosis of forty-two patients with amyloidosis. *Am J Med, 44*:955-969, 1968.

Braun, D. G., Eichmann, K., and Krause, R. M.: Rabbit antibodies to streptococcal carbohydrates: influence of primary and secondary immunization and of possible genetic factors on the antibody response. *J Exp Med, 129*: 809-830, 1969.

Brauner, G. J., Al Bazzaz, F., and Mihm, M. C., Jr.: Acquired bullous disease of the skin and solitary amyloidoma of the lung. *Am J Med, 57*:978-986, 1974.

Brecher, G., Tanaka, Y., Malmgren, R. A., and Fahey, J. L.: Morphology and protein synthesis in multiple myeloma and macroglobulinemia. *Ann NY Acad Sci, 113*:642-653, 1964.

Briccetti, A. B., Cathcart, E. S., and Cohen, A. S.: Lymphocyte transformation and amyloidosis: an immunologic study of 14 patients with biopsy-proved disease. *Int Arch Allergy Appl Immunol, 44*:349-357, 1973.

Brittin, G. M., Tanaka, Y., and Brecher, G.: Intranuclear inclusions in multiple myeloma and macroglobulinemia. *Blood, 21*:335-351, 1963.

Brittinger, G., and König, E.: Zur Klinik der Paraproteinämien. *Schweiz Med Wochenschr, 95*:1584-1588, 1965.

Brody, I. A., Wertlake, P. T., and Laster, L.: Causes of intestinal symptoms in primary amyloidosis. *Arch Intern Med, 113*:512-518, 1964a.

Brody, J. I., Beizer, L. H., and Schwartz, S.: Multiple myeloma and the myeloproliferative syndromes. *Am J Med, 36*:315-319, 1964b.

Brody, J. I., and Samitz, M. H.: Cutaneous signs of cryoparaproteinemia: control with burst Alkeran and prednisone. *Am J Med, 55*:211-214, 1973.

Brook, J., Bateman, J. R., Gocka, E. F., Nakamura, E., and Steinfeld, J. L.: Long-term low dose melphalan treatment of multiple myeloma. *Arch Intern Med, 131*:545-548, 1973.

Brook, J., Bateman, J. R., and Steinfeld, J. L.: Evaluation of melphalan (NSC-8806) in treatment of multiple myeloma. *Cancer Chemother Rep, 36*:25-34, 1964.

Brouet, J.-C., Clauvel, J.-P., Danon, F., Klein, M., and Seligmann, M.: Biologic and clinical significance of cryoglobulins: a report of 86 cases. *Am J Med, 57*:775-788, 1974.

Brown, A. K., Elves, M. W., Gunson, H. H., and Pell-Ilderton, R.: Waldenström's macroglobulinaemia: a family study. *Acta Haematol* (Basel), *38*:184-192, 1967.

Brown, M., and Battle, J. D., Jr.: The effect of urography on renal function in patients with multiple myeloma. *Can Med Assoc J, 91*:786-790, 1964.

Brown, T. S., and Paterson, C. R.: Osteosclerosis in myeloma. *J Bone Joint Surg* [Br], *55*:621-623, 1973.

Brownstein, M. H., and Helwig, E. B.: The cutaneous amyloidoses. I. Localized forms. *Arch Dermatol, 102*:8-19, 1970a.

Brownstein, M. H., and Helwig, E. B.: The cutaneous amyloidoses. II. Systemic forms. *Arch Dermatol, 102*:20-28, 1970b.

Brun, C., Olsen, T. S., Raaschou, F., and Sørensen, A. W. S.: Renal biopsy in rheumatoid arthritis. *Nephron, 2*:65-81, 1965.

Bryan, C. W., and Healy, J. K.: Acute renal failure in multiple myeloma. *Am J Med, 44*:128-133, 1968.

Bryan, C. W., and McIntire, K. R.: Effect of sustained diuresis on the renal lesions of mice with Bence Jones protein-producing tumors. *J Lab Clin Med, 83*:409-416, 1974.

Buckley, C. E., III, and Dorsey, F. C.: The effect of aging on human serum immunoglobulin concentrations. *J Immunol, 105*:964-972, 1970.

Buckley, R. H., and Fiscus, S. A.: Serum IgD and IgE concentrations in immunodeficiency diseases. *J Clin Invest, 55*:157-165, 1975.

Buja, L. M., Khoi, N. B., and Roberts, W. C.: Clinically significant cardiac amyloidosis: clinicopathologic findings in 15 patients. *Am J Cardiol, 26*:394-405, 1970.

Buonocore, E., Solomon, A., and Kerley, H. E.: Pseudomyeloma. *Radiology, 95*:41-46, 1970.

Bush, S. T., Swedlund, H. A., and Gleich, G. J.: Low molecular weight IgM in human sera. *J Lab Clin Med, 73*:194-201, 1969.

Buxbaum, J., and Scharff, M. D.: The synthesis, assembly, and secretion of gamma globulin by mouse myeloma cells. VI. Assembly of IgM proteins. *J Exp Med, 138*:278-288, 1973.

Buxbaum, J., Zolla, S., Scharff, M. D., and Franklin, E. C.: Synthesis and assembly of immunoglobulins by malignant human plasmacytes and lymphocytes. II. Heterogeneity of assembly in cells producing IgM proteins. *J Exp Med, 133:*1118-1130, 1971.

Buxbaum, J. N.: The biosynthesis, assembly, and secretion of immunoglobulins. *Semin Hematol, 10:*33-52, 1973.

Buxbaum, J. N., and Preud'homme, J.-L.: Alpha and gamma heavy chain diseases in man: intracellular origin of the aberrant polypeptides. *J Immunol, 109:*1131-1137, 1972.

Buxbaum, J. N., Zolla, S., Scharff, M. D., and Franklin, E. C.: The synthesis and assembly of immunoglobulins by malignant human plasmacytes. III. Heterogeneity in IgA polymer assembly. *Eur J Immunol, 4:*367-369, 1974.

Cabrera, A., de la Pava, S., and Pickren, J. W.: Intestinal localization of Waldenström's disease. *Arch Intern Med, 114:*399-407, 1964.

Calkins, E., and Cohen, A. S.: Diagnosis of amyloidosis. *Bull Rheum Dis, 10:* 215-218, 1960.

Callerame, M. L., and Nadel, M.: *Pneumocystis carinii* pneumonia in two adults with multiple myeloma. *Am J Clin Pathol, 45:*258-263, 1966.

Callis, M. N., and Sheets, R. F.: Multiple myeloma in Iowa, *J Iowa Med Soc, 64:*429-433, 1974.

Campbell, A. E., De Vine, J., Azam, L., Hamid, J., Delamore, I. W., and McFarlane, H.: Lymphocyte transformation in patients with paraproteinaemia. *Br J Haematol, 29:*179-188, 1975.

Canale, D. D., Jr., and Collins, R. D.: Use of bone marrow particle sections in the diagnosis of multiple myeloma. *Am J Clin Pathol, 61:*382-392, 1974.

Capra, J. D., and Kehoe, J. M.: Hypervariable regions, idiotypy, and the antibody-combining site. *Adv Immunol, 20:*1-40, 1975.

Capra, J. D., and Kunkel, H. G.: Aggregation of γG3 proteins: relevance to the hyperviscosity syndrome. *J Clin Invest, 49:*610-621, 1970.

Carbone, P. P., Frei, E., III, Owens, A. H., Jr., Olson, K. B., and Miller, S. P.: 6-Thioguanine (NSC-752) therapy in patients with multiple myeloma. *Cancer Chemother Rep, 36:*59-62, 1964.

Carbone, P. P., Kellerhouse, L. E., and Gehan, E. A.: Plasmacytic myeloma: a study of the relationship of survival to various clinical manifestations and anomalous protein type in 112 patients. *Am J Med, 42:*937-948, 1967.

Carbone, P. P., Zipkin, I., Sokoloff, L., Frazier, P., Cook, P., and Mullins, F.: Fluoride effect on bone in plasma cell myeloma. *Arch Intern Med, 121:* 130-140, 1968.

Cardamone, J. M., Kimmerle, R. I., and Marshall, E. Y.: Development of acute erythroleukemia in B-cell immunoproliferative disorders after prolonged therapy with alkylating drugs. *Am J Med, 57:*836-842, 1974.

Carone, F. A., and Epstein, F. H.: Nephrogenic diabetes insipidus caused by amyloid disease: evidence in man of the role of the collecting ducts in concentrating urine. *Am J Med, 29:*539-544, 1960.

Carter, J. B.: Macroglobulin-producing histiocytic lymphoma: of hepatic origin. *Minn Med, 57*:22-24, 1974.

Carter, P. M., and Hobbs, J. R.: Clinical significance of 7s IgM in monoclonal IgM diseases. *Br Med J, 2*:260-261, 1971.

Carter, P. M., and Rushman, R. W.: Solitary plasmacytoma of the clavicle. *Proc R Soc Med, 67*:1097-1098, 1974.

Casad, D. E., and Bocian, J. J.: Primary systemic amyloidosis simulating acute idiopathic ulcerative colitis: report of a case. *Am J Dig Dis*, ns, *10*:63-74, 1965.

Case Records of the Massachusetts General Hospital (Case 23-1968). *N Engl J Med, 278*:1276-1286, 1968a.

Case Records of the Massachusetts General Hospital (Case 42-1968). *N Engl J Med, 279*:876-883, 1968b.

Case Records of the Massachusetts General Hospital (Case 31-1972). *N Engl J Med, 287*:243-248, 1972.

Case Records of the Massachusetts General Hospital (Case 3-1973). *N Engl J Med, 288*:150-156, 1973.

Castaldi, P. A., and Penny, R.: A macroglobulin with inhibitory activity against coagulation Factor VIII. *Blood, 35*:370-376, 1970.

Castoldi, G. L., Grusovin, G. D., Scapoli, G. L., and Spanedda, R.: Association of multiple haematological disorders (acute myeloblastic leukaemia, paraproteinaemia, and thalassaemia) in a 46,XX/46,XXqi female. *Acta Haematol* (Basel), *46*:294-306, 1971.

Castro, E. B., Lewis, J. S., and Strong, E. W.: Plasmacytoma of paranasal sinuses and nasal cavity. *Arch Otolaryngol, 97*:326-329, 1973a.

Castro, G. A. M., Church, A., Pechet, L., and Snyder, L. M.: Leukemia after chemotherapy of Hodgkin's disease (letter to the editor). *N Engl J Med, 289*:103-104, 1973b.

Catalona, W. J., and Biles, J. D., III: Therapeutic considerations in renal plasmacytoma. *J Urol, 111*:582-583, 1974.

Cathcart, E. S., and Cohen, A. S.: Evans blue as a diagnostic test for amyloidosis. *Arch Intern Med, 112*:875-881, 1963.

Cathcart, E. S., Mullarkey, M., and Cohen, A. S.: Amyloidosis: an expression of immunological tolerance? *Lancet, 2*:639-640, 1970.

Cathcart, E. S., Ritchie, R. F., Cohen, A. S., and Brandt, K.: Immunoglobulins and amyloidosis. *Am J Med, 52*:93-101, 1972a.

Cathcart, E. S., Rodgers, O. G., and Cohen, A. S.: Amyloid-inducing factor and immunological unresponsiveness. *Ann Rheum Dis, 31*:303-307, 1972b.

Catovsky, D., and Galton, D. A. G.: Myelomonocytic leukaemia supervening on chronic lymphocytic leukaemia. *Lancet, 1*:478-479, 1971.

Catovsky, D., Holt, P. J. L., and Galton, D. A. G.: Binucleated blast-cells in lymphocyte cultures from myelomatosis. *Immunology, 22*:1103-1109, 1972a.

Catovsky, D., Holt, P. J. L., and Galton, D. A. G.: Lymphocyte transformation in immunoproliferative disorders. *Br J Cancer, 26*:154-163, 1972b.

Catovsky, D., Ikoku, N. B., Pitney, W. R., and Galton, D. A. G.: Thromboembolic complications in myelomatosis. *Br Med J, 3:*438-439, 1970.

Catovsky, D., Shaw, M. T., Hoffbrand, A. V., and Dacie, J. V.: Sideroblastic anaemia and its association with leukaemia and myelomatosis: a report of five cases. *Br J Haematol, 20:*385-393, 1971.

Caughey, D. E., and Wakem, C. J.: A fatal case of Reiter's disease complicated by amyloidosis. *Arthritis Rheum, 16:*695-700, 1973.

Cawley, J. C., Goldstone, A. H., Arno, J., Rees, J. H. K., and Grant, A.: Myeloma in a case of Hodgkin's disease. *Acta Haematol* (Basel), *52:*349-355, 1974.

Cawley, L. P., and Schenken, J. R.: Monoclonal hypergammaglobulinemia of the γM type in a nine-year-old girl with ataxia-telangiectasia. *Am J Clin Pathol, 54:*790-801, 1970.

Čejka, J., Bollinger, R. O., Schuit, H. R. E., Lusher, J. M., Chang, C.-H., and Zuelzer, W. W.: Macroglobulinemia in a child with acute leukemia. *Blood, 43:*191-199, 1974.

Chambers, R. A., Medd, W. E., and Spencer, H.: Primary amyloidosis: with special reference to involvement of the nervous system. *Q J Med,* ns, *27:* 207-226, 1958.

Chantar, C., Escartín, P., Plaza, A. G., Corugedo, A. F., Arenas, J. I., Sanz, E., Anaya, A., Bootello, A., and Segovia, J. M.: Diffuse plasma cell infiltration of the small intestine with malabsorption associated to IgA monoclonal gammapathy. *Cancer, 34:*1620-1630, 1974.

Chapman, R. S., Neville, E. A., and Lawson, J. W.: Xanthoma-like skin lesions as a presenting feature in primary systemic amyloidosis. *Br J Clin Pract, 27:*271-273, 1973.

Chen, Y., Yakulis, V., and Heller, P.: Passive immunity to murine plasmacytoma by anti-idiotypic antibody to myeloma protein (abstract). *Clin Res, 23:*446A, 1975.

Chernenkoff, R. M., Costopoulos, L. B., and Bain, G. O.: Gastrointestinal manifestations of primary amyloidosis. *Can Med Assoc J, 106:*567-569, 1972.

Chesebro, B., Bloth, B., and Svehag, S.-E.: The ultrastructure of normal and pathological IgM immunoglobulins. *J Exp Med, 127:*399-410, 1968.

Christensen, H. E., and Rask-Nielsen, R.: Comparative morphologic, histochemical, and serologic studies on the pathogenesis of casein-induced and reticulosarcoma-induced amyloidosis in mice. *J Natl Cancer Inst, 28:*1-33, 1962.

Christensen, H. E., and Sørensen, K. H.: Local amyloid formation of capsula fibrosa in arthrosis coxae. *Acta Pathol Microbiol Scand* [A] Suppl, *233:*128-131, 1972.

Christiansen, J., and Lindqvist, B.: Heparin-resistance in amyloidosis. *Acta Med Scand, 181:*723-724, 1967.

Christine, B., Flannery, J. T., and Sullivan, P. D.: *Cancer in Connecticut, 1966-1968.* Connecticut Tumor Registry, 1971.

Christopherson, W. M., and Miller, A. J.: A re-evaluation of solitary plasma-cell myeloma of bone. *Cancer, 3*:240-252, 1950.

Clamp, J. R.: Some aspects of the first recorded case of multiple myeloma. *Lancet, 2*:1354-1356, 1967.

Clatanoff, D. V., and Meyer, O. O.: Response to chlorambucil in macroglobu-linemia. *JAMA, 183*:40-44, 1963.

Clauvel, J. P., Danon, F., and Seligmann, M.: Immunoglobulines mono-clonales décelées en l'absence de myélome ou de macroglobulinémie de Waldenström: evolution dans 54 observations. *Nouv Rev Fr Hematol, 11*: 677-687, 1971.

Cline, M. J., and Berlin, N. I.: Studies of the anemia of multiple myeloma. *Am J Med, 33*:510-525, 1962.

Cline, M. J., Solomon, A., Berlin, N. I., and Fahey, J. L.: Anemia in macro-globulinemia. *Am J Med, 34*:213-220, 1963.

Clinicopathologic Conference: Multiple malignancies: chronic lymphocytic leukemia, malignant melanoma, multiple myeloma and acute myelomono-cytic leukemia. *Am J Med, 58*:408-416, 1975.

Clinicopathological Conference: A case of Waldenström's macroglobulinae-mia with slow progression. *Br Med J, 3*:237-242, 1968.

Clubb, J. S., Posen, S., and Neale, F. C.: Disappearance of a serum parapro-tein after parathyroidectomy. *Arch Intern Med, 114*:616-620, 1964.

Clyne, D. H., Brendstrup, L., First, M. R., Pesce, A. J., Finkel, P. N., Pollak, V. E., and Pirani, C. L.: Renal effects of intraperitoneal kappa chain in-jection: introduction of crystals in renal tubular cells. *Lab Invest, 31*: 131-142, 1974.

Codling, B. W., and Chakera, T. M. H.: Pulmonary fibrosis following thera-py with melphalan for multiple myeloma. *J Clin Pathol, 25*:668-673, 1972.

Cohen, A. S.: Amyloidosis. *N Engl J Med, 277*:522-530; 574-583; 628-638, 1967.

Cohen, A. S., Bricetti, A. B., Harrington, J. T., and Mannick, J. A.: Renal transplantation in two cases of amyloidosis. *Lancet, 2*:513-516, 1971.

Cohen, A. S., and Calkins, E.: Electron microscopic observations on a fibrous component in amyloid of diverse origins (letter to the editor). *Nature, 183*:1202-1203, 1959.

Cohen, A. S., and Cathcart, E. S.: Amyloidosis and immunoglobulins. *Adv Intern Med, 19*:41-55, 1974.

Cohen, A. S., and Shirahama, T.: Electron microscopic analysis of isolated amyloid fibrils from patients with primary, secondary and myeloma-asso-ciated disease: a study utilizing shadowing and negative staining tech-niques. *Isr J Med Sci, 9*:849-856, 1973.

Cohen, D. M., Svien, H. J., and Dahlin, D. C.: Long-term survival of patients with myeloma of the vertebral column. *JAMA, 187*:914-917, 1964.

Cohen, H. J., and Lefer, L. G.: Intranuclear inclusions in Bence Jones lambda plasma cell myeloma. *Blood, 45*:131-139, 1975.

Cohen, H. J., Lessin, L. S., Hallal, J., and Burkholder, P.: Resolution of primary amyloidosis during chemotherapy: studies in a patient with nephrotic syndrome. *Ann Intern Med, 82*:466-473, 1975.

Cohen, H. J., and Rundles, R. W.: Managing the complications of plasma cell myeloma. *Arch Intern Med, 135*:177-184, 1975.

Cohen, I., Amir, J., Ben-Shaul, Y., Pick, A., and De Vries, A.: Plasma cell myeloma associated with an unusual myeloma protein causing impairment of fibrin aggregation and platelet function in a patient with multiple malignancy. *Am J Med, 48*:766-776, 1970.

Cohen, P., and Gardner, F. H.: Induction of subacute skeletal fluorosis in a case of multiple myeloma. *N Engl J Med, 271*:1129-1133, 1964.

Cohen, P., Nichols, G. L., Jr., and Banks, H. H.: Fluoride treatment of bone rarefaction in multiple myeloma and osteoporosis: a review. *Clin Orthop, 64*:221-249, 1969.

Cohen, R. J., Bohannon, R. A., and Wallerstein, R. O.: Waldenström's macroglobulinemia: a study of ten cases. *Am J Med, 41*:274-284, 1966.

Coleman, M., Vigliano, E. M., Weksler, M. E., and Nachman, R. L.: Inhibition of fibrin monomer polymerization by lambda myeloma globulins. *Blood, 39*:210-223, 1972.

Collins-Williams, C., Tkachyk, S. J., Toft, B., and Moscarello, M.: Quantitative immunoglobulin levels (IgG, IgA and IgM) in children. *Int Arch Allergy Appl Immunol, 31*:94-103, 1967.

Committee of the Chronic Leukemia-Myeloma Task Force, National Cancer Institute: Proposed guidelines for protocol studies. II. Plasma cell myeloma. *Cancer Chemother Rep, 4*:145-158, 1973.

Cone, L., and Uhr, J. W.: Immunological deficiency disorders associated with chronic lymphocytic leukemia and multiple myeloma. *J Clin Invest, 43*: 2241-2248, 1964.

Conklin, R., and Alexanian, R.: Clinical classification of plasma cell myeloma. *Arch Intern Med, 135*:139-143, 1975.

Conn, H. O., and Quintiliani, R.: Severe diarrhea controlled by gamma globulin in a patient with agammaglobulinemia, amyloidosis, and thymoma. *Ann Intern Med, 65*:528-541, 1966.

Cook, A. J., Weinstein, M., and Powell, R. D.: Diffuse amyloidosis of the tracheobronchial tree: bronchographic manifestations. *Radiology, 107*: 303-304, 1973.

Cooper, M. R., Cohen, H. J., Huntley, C. C., Waite, B. M., Spees, L., and Spurr, C. L.: A monoclonal IgM with antibodylike specificity for phospholipids in a patient with lymphoma. *Blood, 43*:493-504, 1974.

Cooperative Study by Acute Leukemia Group B: Correlation of abnormal immunoglobulin with clinical features of myeloma. *Arch Intern Med,* *135*:46-52, 1975.

Cornelius, C. E.: Animal models: a neglected medical resource. *N Engl J Med,* *281*:934-944, 1969.

Cornes, J. S., Jones, T. G., and Fisher, G. B.: The incidence of carcinoma in patients dying from leukaemia, malignant disorders of plasma cells, and malignant lymphoma. *Br J Cancer, 15*:200-205, 1961.

Corwin, N. D.: Multiple myeloma with myeloid metaplasia. *J Med Soc NJ,* *69*:847-849, 1972.

Costa, G., Engle, R. L., and Taliente, P.: Criteria for defining risk groups and response to chemotherapy in multiple myeloma (abstract). *Proc Am Assoc Cancer Res, 10*:15, 1969.

Costa, G., Engle, R. L., Jr., Schilling, A., Carbone, P., Kochwa, S., Nachman, R. L., and Glidewell, O.: Melphalan and prednisone: an effective combination for the treatment of multiple myeloma. *Am J Med, 54*:589-599, 1973.

Costea, N., Yakulis, V. J., Libnoch, J. A., Pilz, C. G., and Heller, P.: Two myeloma globulins (IgG and IgA) in one subject and one cell line. *Am J Med, 42*:630-635, 1967.

Cream, J. J.: Pyoderma gangrenosum with a monoclonal IgM red cell agglomerating factor. *Br J Dermatol, 84*:223-226, 1971.

Crockett, L. K., Thompson, M., and Dekker, A.: A review of cardiac amyloidosis: report of a case presenting as constrictive pericarditis. *Am J Med Sci, 264*:149-156, 1972.

Cronstedt, J., Carling, L., and Östberg, H.: Idiopathic light chain dyscrasia— a new distinct entity? *Acta Med Scand, 196*:445-447, 1974.

Crosbie, W. A., Lewis, M. L., Ramsay, I. D., and Doyle, D.: Pulmonary amyloidosis with impaired gas transfer. *Thorax, 27*:625-630, 1972.

Cunningham, A. J.: Antibody formation studied at the single-cell level. *Prog Allergy, 17*:5-50, 1973.

Cunningham-Rundles, C., Lamm, M. E., and Franklin, E. C.: Primary structure of human secretory component (abstract). *Fed Proc, 33*:747, 1974.

Cutler, S. J., Myers, M. H., and Green, S. B.: Trends in survival rates of patients with cancer. *N Engl J Med, 293*:122-124, 1975.

Dahlin, D. C.: Primary amyloidosis, with report of six cases. *Am J Pathol, 25:* 105-123, 1949.

Dalrymple, J.: On the microscopical character of mollities ossium. *Dublin Q J Med Sci, 2*:85-95, 1846.

Dalton, A. J., Potter, M., and Merwin, R. M.: Some ultrastructural characteristics of a series of primary and transplanted plasma-cell tumors of the mouse. *J Natl Cancer Inst, 26*:1221-1267, 1961.

Daly, D. D., Love, J. G., and Dockerty, M. B.: Amyloid tumor of the gasserian ganglion: report of case. *J Neurosurg, 14*:347-352, 1957.

Dammacco, F., and Clausen, J.: Antibody deficiency in paraproteinemia. *Acta Med Scand, 179*:755-768, 1966.

Dammacco, F., and Waldenström, J.: Bence Jones proteinuria in benign monoclonal gammopathies: incidence and characteristics. *Acta Med Scand, 184*:403-409, 1968.

Daniels, J. D., and Hewlett, J. S.: Renal manifestations in multiple myeloma and in primary amyloidosis. *Cleve Clin Q, 37*:181-187, 1970.

Danon, F., Clauvel, J. P., and Seligmann, M.: Les "Paraprotéines" de type IgG et IgA en dehors de la maladie de Kahler. *Rev Fr Etud Clin Biol, 12*:681-701, 1967.

Danon, F., and Seligmann, M.: Transient human monoclonal immunoglobulins. *Scand J Immunol, 1*:323-328, 1972.

Daoud, F. S., Nieman, R. E., and Vilter, R. W.: Amyloid goiter in a case of generalized primary amyloidosis. *Am J Med, 43*:604-608, 1967.

Darbari, B. S., Bansal, N. C., Phadke, S. N., and Arora, M. M.: Bilateral orbit plasmacytoma. *Indian J Ophthalmol, 20*:28-30, 1972.

D'Arcy, F.: Localized amyloidosis of the larynx. *J Laryngol Otol, 86*:929-931, 1972.

Darnley, J. D.: Polyneuropathy in Waldenström's macroglobulinemia: case report and discussion. *Neurology* (Minneap), *12*:617-623, 1962.

Dartnall, J. A., Mundy, G. R., and Baikie, A. G.: Cytogenetic studies in myeloma. *Blood, 42*:229-239, 1973.

Davidson, S.: Solitary myeloma with peripheral polyneuropathy—recovery after treatment. *Calif Med, 116*:68-71, Jan. 1972.

Davies-Jones, G. A. B., and Esiri, M. M.: Neuropathy due to amyloid in myelomatosis. *Br Med J, 2*:444, 1971.

Davis, H, L., Jr., Prout, M. N., McKenna, P. J., Cole, D. R., and Korbitz, B. C.: Acute leukemia complicating metastatic breast cancer. *Cancer, 31*: 543-546, 1973.

Davis, L. E., and Drachman, D. B.: Myeloma neuropathy: successful treatment of two patients and review of cases. *Arch Neurol, 27*:507-511, 1972.

Dawson, A. A., and Ogston, D.: Factors influencing the prognosis in myelomatosis. *Postgrad Med J, 47*:635-638, 1971.

Dawson, A. A., and Ogston, D.: High incidence of myelomatosis in northeast Scotland. *Scott Med J, 18*:75-77, 1973.

Dayan, A. D., and Lewis, P. D.: Demyelinating neuropathy in macrocryoglobulinemia. *Neurology* (Minneap), *16*:1141-1144, 1966.

Dayan, A. D., Urich, H., and Gardner-Thorpe, C.: Peripheral neuropathy and myeloma. *J Neurol Sci, 14*:21-35, 1971.

DeCoteau, W. E.: The role of secretory IgA in defense of the distal lung. *Ann NY Acad Sci, 221*:214-219, 1974.

DeFronzo, R. A., Cooke, C. R., Wright, J. R., and Humphrey, R. L.: Bence

Jones proteinuria and renal failure in multiple myeloma (abstract). *Clin Res, 22:*486A, 1974.

DeFronzo, R. A., Humphrey, R. L., Wright, J. R., and Cooke, C. R.: Acute renal failure in multiple myeloma. *Medicine* (Baltimore), *54:*209-223, 1975.

Deftos, L. J., and Neer, R.: Medical management of the hypercalcemia of malignancy. *Annu Rev Med, 25:*323-331, 1974.

DelDuca, V., Jr., and Morningstar, W. A.: Multiple myeloma associated with progressive multifocal leukoencephalopathy. *JAMA, 199:*671-673, 1967.

DeLellis, R. A., Ram, J. S., and Glenner, G. G.: Amyloid. IX. Further kinetic studies on experimental murine amyloidosis. *Int Arch Allergy Appl Immunol, 37:*175-183, 1970.

Derechin, M. M., Goldberg, L. S., and Herron, L.: Extraosseous plasmacytomas causing extrahepatic cholestasis and cardiac tamponade: a unique case of multiple myeloma. *Scand J Haematol, 7:*318-321, 1970.

Despont, J.-P. J., Abel, C. A., Grey, H. M., and Penn, G. M.: Structural studies on a human IgA1 myeloma protein with a carboxy-terminal deletion. *J Immunol, 112:*1517-1525, 1974.

Devey, M., Carter, D., Sanderson, C. J., and Coombs, R. R. A.: IgD antibody to insulin. *Lancet, 2:*1280-1283, 1970.

Dexter, R. N., Mullinax, F., Estep, H. L., and Williams, R. C., Jr.: Monoclonal IgG gammopathy and hyperparathyroidism. *Ann Intern Med, 77:* 759-764, 1972.

Diaz-Buxo, J. A., Hermans, P. E., and Elveback, L. R.: Prevalence of cholelithiasis in idiopathic late-onset immunoglobulin deficiency. *Ann Intern Med, 82:*213-214, 1975.

Dillman, C. E., Jr., and Silverstein, M. N.: Alkaline phosphatase in multiple myeloma. *Am J Med Sci, 249:*445-447, 1965.

Dine, M. E., Guay, A. T., and Snyder, L. M.: Hyperviscosity syndrome with IgA myeloma. *Am J Med Sci, 264:*111-115, 1972.

Dittmar, K., Kochwa, S., Zucker-Franklin, D., and Wasserman, L. R.: Coexistence of polycythemia vera and biclonal gammopathy (γGK and γAL) with two Bence Jones proteins (BJK and BJL). *Blood, 31:*81-92, 1968.

Doe, W. F.: Alpha chain disease: clinicopathological features and relationship to so-called Mediterranean lymphoma. *Br J Cancer 31* Suppl, *2:*350-355, 1975.

Dolin, S., and Dewar, J. P.: Extramedullary plasmacytoma. *Am J Pathol, 32:* 83-103, 1956.

Domm, B. M., Vassallo, C. L., and Adams, C. L.: Amyloid deposition localized to the lower respiratory tract. *Am J Med, 38:*151-155, 1965.

Douglass, H. O., Jr., Sika, J. V., and LeVeen, H. H.: Plasmacytoma: a not so rare tumor of the small intestine. *Cancer, 28:*456-460, 1971.

Drapiewski, J. F., Sternlieb, S. B., and Jones, R.: Primary amyloidosis with spontaneous rupture of the spleen and sudden death. *Ann Intern Med, 43*:406-412, 1955.

Drewinko, B., Brown, B. W., Humphrey, R., and Alexanian, R.: Effect of chemotherapy on the labelling index of myeloma cells. *Cancer, 34*:526-531, 1974.

Drivsholm, A., and Clausen, J.: The relationship between the cytology and the immuno-electrophoretic pattern in 105 cases of myelomatosis. *Acta Med Scand, 175*:609-620, 1964.

Drusin, L. M., Litwin, S. D., Armstrong, D., and Webster, B. P.: Waldenström's macroglobulinemia in a patient with a chronic biologic false-positive serologic test for syphilis. *Am J Med, 56*:429-432, 1974.

Duarte-Amaya, A., and Mansour, N. J., Jr.: Acute renal failure in multiple myeloma. *Ariz Med, 29*:483-486, 1972.

Dudley, F. J., and Blackburn, C. R. B.: Extraskeletal calcification complicating oral neutral phosphate therapy. *Lancet, 2*:628-630, 1970.

Durant, J. R., Barry, W. E., and Learner, N.: The changing face of myeloma. *Lancet, 1*:119-124, 1966.

Durie, B. G. M., and Salmon, S. E.: High-speed scintillation autoradiography (HSARG) for clinical and research hematology (abstract). *Blood, 44*:914, 1974.

Dutcher, T. F., and Fahey, J. L.: The histopathology of the macroglobulinemia of Waldenström. *J Natl Cancer Inst, 22*:887-917, 1959.

Dyke, P. C., Demaray, M. J., Delavan, J. W., and Rasmussen, R. A.: Pulmonary amyloidoma. *Am J Clin Pathol, 61*:301-305, 1974.

Edelman, G. M.: Antibody structure and molecular immunology. *Science, 180*:830-840, 1973.

Edelman, G. M., and Gally, J. A.: The nature of Bence-Jones proteins: chemical similarities to polypeptide chains of myeloma globulins and normal γ-globulins. *J Exp Med, 116*:207-227, 1962.

Edwards, G. A., and Zawadzki, Z. A.: Extraosseous lesions in plasma cell myeloma: a report of six cases. *Am J Med, 43*:194-205, 1967.

Ein, D., and Fahey, J. L.: Two types of lambda polypeptide chains in human immunoglobulins. *Science, 156*:947-948, 1967.

Eisen, H. N.: Primary systemic amyloidosis. *Am J Med, 1*:144-160, 1946.

Eisen, H. N., Little, J. R., Osterland, C. K., and Simms, E. S.: A myeloma protein with antibody activity. *Cold Spring Harbor Symp Quant Biol, 32*:75-81, 1967.

Eisenberg, H.: *Cancer in Connecticut, Incidence and Rates 1935-1962.* Chronic Disease Control Section, Connecticut State Department of Health, Hartford, Connecticut, 1966.

Eisenberg, P., Aster, R. H., and Abramson, N.: Post-transfusion purpura: new aspects of diagnosis and therapy (abstract). *Blood, 42*:1024, 1973.

Ekelund, L., and Lindholm, T.: Angiography in renal amyloidosis. *Acta Radiol [Diagn]* (Stockh), *15*:393-400, 1974.

Elcock, H. W., and Grimaldi, P. M. G. B.: Post-nasal obstruction by amyloid, secondary to Waldenström's macroglobulinaemia. *J Laryngol Otol, 86:* 1075-1079, 1972.

Elias, E. G., Gailani, S., Jones, R., Jr., and Mittelman, A.: Extraosseous multiple myeloma: a cause of intestinal obstruction. *Ann Surg, 170*:857-861, 1969.

Elias, E. G., Holyoke, E. D., and Mittelman, A.: Obstructive jaundice in macroglobulinemia. *J Surg Oncol, 4*:380-384, 1972.

Ellman, L. L., and Bloch, K. J.: Heavy-chain disease: report of a seventh case. *N Engl J Med, 278*:1195-1201, 1968.

Ellman, L. L., Pachas, W. N., Pinals, R. S., and Bloch, K. J.: M-components in patients with chronic liver disease. *Gastroenterology, 57*:138-142, 1969.

Elveback, L.: Estimation of survivorship in chronic disease: the actuarial method. *J Am Stat Assoc, 53*:420-440, 1958.

Elves, M. W., and Brown, A. K.: Cytogenetic studies in a family with Waldenström's macroglobulinaemia. *J Med Genet, 5*:118-122, 1968.

Elves, M. W., and Israëls, M. C. G.: Chromosomes and serum proteins: a linked abnormality. *Br Med J, 2*:1024-1026, 1963.

Emori, H. W., Bluestone, R., and Goldberg, L. S.: Pseudo-leukocytosis associated with cryoglobulinemia. *Am J Clin Pathol, 60*:202-204, 1973.

Engle, R. L., Jr., and Wallis, L. A.: Multiple myeloma and the adult Fanconi syndrome. I. Report of a case with crystal-like deposits in the tumor cells and in the epithelial cells of the kidney. *Am J Med, 22*:5-12, 1957.

Engle, R. L., Jr., and Wallis, L. A.: Amyloidosis. In Tice, F. (Ed.) : *Practice of Medicine*, Vol 1. Hagerstown, Maryland, W. F. Prior, 1966, pp. 365-394.

Engle, R. L., Jr., and Wallis, L. A.: *Immunoglobulinopathies: Immunoglobulins, Immune Deficiency Syndromes, Multiple Myeloma and Related Disorders.* Springfield, Illinois, Charles C Thomas, Publisher, 1969, 270 pp.

Epp, O., Colman, P., Fehlhammer, H., Bode, W., Schiffer, M., and Huber, R.: Crystal and molecular structure of a dimer composed of the variable portions of the Bence-Jones protein REI. *Eur J Biochem, 45*:513-524, 1974.

Epstein, L. B., and Salmon, S. E.: The production of interferon by malignant plasma cells from patients with multiple myeloma. *J Immunol, 112:* 1131-1138, 1974.

Epstein, W. V., Tan, M., and Wood, I. S.: Formation of "amyloid" fibrils in vitro by action of human kidney lysosomal enzymes on Bence Jones proteins. *J Lab Clin Med, 84*:107-110, 1974.

Estrada, P. C., and Scardino, P. L.: Myeloma of the prostate: a case report. *J Urol, 106*:586-587, 1971.

Evison, G., and Evans, K. T.: Bone sclerosis in multiple myeloma. *Br J Radiol*, ns, *40*:81-89, 1967.

Fadem, R. S.: Differentiation of plasmocytic responses from myelomatous diseases on the basis of bone-marrow findings. *Cancer, 5:*128-137, 1952.

Fahey, J. L., Barth, W. F., and Solomon, A.: Serum hyperviscosity syndrome. *JAMA, 192:*464-467, 1965.

Fahey, J. L., Carbone, P. P., Rowe, D. S., and Bachmann, R.: Plasma cell myeloma with D-myeloma protein (^{I}gD myeloma). *Am J Med, 45:*373-380, 1968.

Fahey, J. L., and McKelvey, E. M.: Quantitative determination of serum immunoglobulins in antibody-agar plates. *J Immunol, 94:*84-90, 1965.

Fahey, J. L., Scoggins, R., Utz, J. P., and Szwed, C. F.: Infection, antibody response and gamma globulin components in multiple myeloma and macroglobulinemia. *Am J Med, 35:*698-707, 1963.

Fair, D. S., Krueger, R. G., Gleich, G. J., and Kyle, R. A.: Studies on IgA and IgG monoclonal proteins derived from a single patient. I. Evidence for shared individually specific antigenic determinants. *J Immunol, 112:*201-209, 1974.

Fairley, K. F., Barrie, J. U., and Johnson, W.: Sterility and testicular atrophy related to cyclophosphamide therapy. *Lancet, 1:*568-569, 1972.

Falkson, G., and Falkson, H. C.: Amyloidosis in Hodgkin's disease. *S Afr Med J, 47:*62-64, 1973.

Farhangi, M., and Osserman, E. F.: The treatment of multiple myeloma. *Semin Hematol, 10:*149-161, 1973.

Farmer, R. G., Cooper, T., and Pascuzzi, C. A.: Cryoglobulinemia: report of twelve cases with bone marrow findings. *Arch Intern Med, 106:*483-495, 1960.

Farrow, G. M., Harrison, E. G., Jr., and Utz, D. C.: Sarcomas and sarcomatoid and mixed malignant tumors of the kidney in adults. *Cancer, 22:*551-555, 1968.

Fayemi, A. O., and Wisniewski, M.: Pulmonary calcification in a patient with multiple myeloma. *Chest, 64:*765-769, 1973.

Feinberg, D. H., and Harlan, W. K.: Amyloidosis of the pituitary gland linked with multiple myeloma. *Pa Med J, 64:*761-764, 1961.

Feingold, M. L., Goldstein, M. J., and Lieberman, P. H.: Multiple myeloma involving the stomach: report of a case with gastroscopic observations. *Gastrointest Endosc, 16:*107-110, 1969.

Feinleib, M., and MacMahon, B.: Duration of survival in multiple myeloma. *J Natl Cancer Inst, 24:*1259-1269, 1960.

Feinstein, D., and Franklin, E. C.: Two antigenically distinguishable subclasses of human A myeloma proteins differing in their heavy chains (letter to the editor). *Nature, 212:*1496-1498, 1966.

Fermin, E. A., Johnson, C. A., Eckel, R. E., and Bernier, G. M.: Renal removal of low molecular weight proteins in myeloma and renal transplant patients. *J Lab Clin Med, 83:*681-694, 1974.

Fernandez, B. B., and Hernandez, F. J.: Amyloid tumor of the breast. *Arch Pathol, 95:*102-105, 1973.

Fine, J. D., Luke, R. G., and Rees, E. D.: Multiple myeloma and renal involvement (letter to the editor). *Lancet, 2:*1205-1206, 1973a.

Fine, J. D., and Rees, E. D.: Bence-Jones protein: detection and implications (letter to the editor). *N Engl J Med, 290:*106-107, 1974.

Fine, J. M.: Study of the frequency of kappa and lambda light chains in 347 sera containing a monoclonal IgG, IgA, IgD, or Bence-Jones protein. *Rev Eur Etud Clin Biol, 40:*199-202, 1970.

Fine, J. M., Lambin, P., and Frommel, D.: Size heterogeneity of human IgA myeloma proteins: relationships between polymers and "J" chain. *Biomedicine, 18:*145-151, 1973b.

Fine, J. M., Lambin, P., Valentin, L., and Blatrix, C.: IgG monoclonal gammapathy in the sister of a patient with Waldenström's macroglobulinaemia. *Biomedicine* [Express], *19:*117-121, 1973c.

Fine, J. M., Rivat, C., Lambin, P., and Ropartz, C.: Monoclonal IgD: a comparative study of 60 sera with IgD "M" component. *Biomedicine* [Express], *21:*119-125, 1974.

Finkel, P. N., Kronenberg, K., Pesce, A. J., Pollak, V. E., and Pirani, C. L.: Adult Fanconi syndrome, amyloidosis and marked κ-light chain proteinuria. *Nephron, 10:*1-24, 1973.

Finkle, H. I., Brownlow, K., and Elevitch, F. R.: Monoclonal IgG-lysozyme (muramidase) complex in acute myelomonocytic leukemia: an unusual finding. *Am J Clin Pathol, 60:*936-940, 1973.

Fisher, E. R., and Zawadzki, Z. A.: Ultrastructural features of plasma cells in patients with paraproteinemias. *Am J Clin Pathol, 54:*779-789, 1970.

Fishkin, B. G., Orloff, N., Scaduto, L. E., Borucki, D. T., and Spiegelberg, H. L.: IgE multiple myeloma: a report of the third case. *Blood, 39:*361-367, 1972.

Fitchen, J. H.: Amyloidosis and granulomatous ileocolitis: regression after surgical removal of the involved bowel. *N Engl J Med, 292:*352-353, 1975.

Fitzgerald, P. H., Rastrick, J. M., and Hamer, J. W.: Acute plasma cell leukaemia following chronic lymphatic leukaemia: transformation or two separate diseases? *Br J Haematol, 25:*171-177, 1973.

Florin-Christensen, A., Doniach, D., and Newcomb, P. B.: Alpha-chain disease with pulmonary manifestations. *Br Med J, 2:*413-415, 1974.

Font, R. L., and Zimmerman, L. E.: Macroglobulinemia complicated by pneumocystis pneumonia and cytomegalic inclusion disease including postmortem examination of the eyes: report of a case. *Med Ann DC, 39:*428-432, 1970.

Forbes, I. J.: Development of acute leukaemia in Waldenström's macroglobulinaemia after prolonged treatment with chlorambucil. *Med J Aust, 1:*918-919, 1972.

Forget, B. G., Squires, J. W., and Sheldon, H.: Waldenström's macroglobu-linemia with generalized amyloidosis. *Arch Intern Med, 118*:363-375, 1966.

Forssman, O., Björkman, G., Hollender, A., and Englund, N.-E.: IgM-produc-ing lymphocytes in peripheral nerve in a patient with benign monoclonal gammopathy. *Scand J Haematol, 11*:332-335, 1973.

Forte, F. A., Prelli, F., Yount, W. J., Jerry, L. M., Kochwa, S., Franklin, E. C., and Kunkel, H. G.: Heavy chain disease of the μ (γM) type: report of the first case. *Blood, 36*:137-144, 1970.

Frangione, B., and Franklin, E. C.: Heavy chain diseases: clinical features and molecular significance of the disordered immunoglobulin structure. *Semin Hematol, 10*:53-64, 1973.

Frangione, B., Milstein, C., and Franklin, E. C.: Chemical typing of immuno-globulins. *Nature, 221*:149-151, 1969a.

Frangione, B., Milstein, C., and Pink, J. R. L.: Structural studies of immuno-globulin G. *Nature, 221*:145-148, 1969b.

Franklin, E. C.: μ-Chain disease. *Arch Intern Med, 135*:71-72, 1975.

Franklin, E. C., and Frangione, B.: Structural differences between macro-globulins belonging to two serologically distinguishable subclasses. *Bio-chemistry, 7*:4203-4211, 1968.

Franklin, E. C., Lowenstein, J., Bigelow, B., and Meltzer, M.: Heavy chain disease—a new disorder of serum γ-globulins: report of the first case. *Am J Med, 37*:332-350, 1964.

Franklin, E. C., and Zucker-Franklin, D.: Current concepts of amyloid. *Adv Immunol, 15*:249-304, 1972.

Frantzen, E., Hertz, H., Matzke, J., and Videbaek, A.: Protein studies on cerebrospinal fluid and neurological symptoms in myelomatosis: with some remarks on EEG and EMG findings. *Acta Neurol Scand, 45*:1-17, 1969.

Franzén, S., Johansson, B., and Kaigas, M.: Primary polycythemia associated with multiple myeloma. *Acta Med Scand 179* Suppl, *445*:336-343, 1966.

Fraser, J. G., and Kaye, M.: Renal amyloidosis: a review of 12 cases. *Can Med Assoc J, 85*:967-973, 1961.

Fraser, K. J.: Multiple myeloma and pernicious anaemia. *Med J Aust, 1*:298-299, 1969.

Freel, R. J., Maldonado, J. E., and Gleich, G. J.: Hyperviscosity syndrome associated with immunoglobulin A myeloma. *Am J Med Sci, 264*:117-122, 1972.

French, J. D.: Plasmacytoma of the hypothalamus: clinical-pathological re-port of a case. *J Neuropathol Exp Neurol, 6*:265-270, 1947.

French, J. M., Hall, G., Parish, D. J., and Smith, W. T.: Peripheral and auto-nomic nerve involvement in primary amyloidosis associated with uncon-trollable diarrhoea and steatorrhoea. *Am J Med, 39*:277-284, 1965.

Frenkel, E. P., and Tourtellotte, C. D.: Elevated serum acid phosphatase associated with multiple myeloma: case report with tissue enzyme assay. *Arch Intern Med, 110*:345-349, 1962.

Frick, P. G., Schmid, J. R., Kistler, H. J., and Hitzig, W. H.: Hyponatremia associated with hyperproteinemia in multiple myeloma. *Helv Med Acta, 33*:317-329, 1967.

Fulmer, D. H., Dimich, A. B., Rothschild, E. O., and Myers, W. P. L.: Treatment of hypercalcemia: comparison of intravenously administered phosphate, sulfate, and hydrocortisone. *Arch Intern Med, 129*:923-930, 1972.

Furgerson, W. B., Jr., Bachman, L. B., and O'Toole, W. F.: Waldenström's macroglobulinemia with diffuse pulmonary infiltration: lung biopsy and response to chlorambucil therapy. *Am Rev Respir Dis, 88*:689-697, 1963.

Gaan, D., Mahoney, M. P., Rowlands, D. J., and Jones, A. W.: Postural hypotension in amyloid disease. *Am Heart J, 84*:395-400, 1972.

Gabriel, S.: Multiple myeloma presenting as pulmonary infiltration: report of a case. *Dis Chest, 47*:123-126, 1965.

Gach, J., Simar, L., and Salmon, J.: Multiple myeloma without M-type proteinemia: report of a case with immunologic and ultrastructure studies. *Am J Med, 50*:835-844, 1971.

Galbraith, P. A., Sharma, N., Parker, W. L., and Kilgour, J. M.: Acquired Factor X deficiency: Altered plasma antithrombin activity and association with amyloidosis. *JAMA, 230*:1658-1660, 1974.

Ganguli, P. C., Lynne-Davies, P., and Sproule, B. J.: Pulmonary alveolar proteinosis, bronchiectasis and secondary amyloidosis: a case report. *Can Med Assoc J, 106*:569-573, 1972.

Garcia, R., and Saeed, S. M.: Amyloidosis: cardiovascular manifestations in five illustrative cases. *Arch Intern Med, 121*:259-266, 1968.

Gardner, K. D., Jr., Castellino, R. A., Kempson, R., Young, B. W., and Stamey, T. A.: Primary amyloidosis of the renal pelvis. *N Engl J Med, 284*: 1196-1198, 1971.

Garfield, D. H.: Acute erythromegakaryocytic leukaemia after treatment with cytostatic agents (letter to the editor). *Lancet, 2*:1037, 1970.

Garrett, M. J.: Spinal myeloma and cord compression: diagnosis and management. *Clin Radiol, 21*:42-46, 1970.

Garrett, T. J., McCans, J. L., and Parker, J. O.: Fatal involvement of the heart with multiple myeloma. *Can Med Assoc J, 107*:979-980, 1972.

Gaudin, D., and Yielding, K. L.: Response of a "resistant" plasmacytoma to alkylating agents and x-ray in combination with the "excision repair inhibitors caffeine and chloroquine." *Proc Soc Exp Biol Med, 131*:1413-1416, 1969.

Gelderman, A. H., Levine, R. A., and Arndt, K. A.: Dermatomyositis complicated by generalized amyloidosis: report of a case. *N Engl J Med, 267*: 858-861, 1962.

George, R. P., Poth, J. L., Gordon, D., and Schrier, S. L.: Multiple myeloma—

intermittent, combination chemotherapy compared to continuous therapy. *Cancer, 29:*1665-1670, 1972.

Gerber, M. A.: Asbestosis and neoplastic disorders of the hematopoietic system. *Am J Clin Pathol, 53:*204-208, 1970.

Getaz, P., Handler, L., Jacobs, P., and Tunley, I.: Osteosclerotic myeloma with peripheral neuropathy. *S Afr Med J, 48:*1246-1250, 1974.

Ghosh, M. L., and Sayeed, A.: Unusual cases of myelomatosis. *Scand J Haematol, 12:*147-154, 1974.

Gilat, T., Revach, M., and Sohar, E.: Deposition of amyloid in the gastrointestinal tract. *Gut, 10:*98-104, 1969.

Gilat, T., and Spiro, H. M.: Amyloidosis and the gut. *Am J Dig Dis,* ns, *13:* 619-633, 1968.

Gilbert, E. F., Harley, J. B., Anido, V., Mengoli, H. F., and Hughes, J. T.: Thymoma, plasma cell myeloma, red cell aplasia and malabsorption syndrome. *Am J Med, 44:*820-829, 1968.

Ginsberg, D. M.: Elevated alkaline phosphatase levels in multiple myeloma: fact or fiction. *J Ky Med Assoc, 65:*36-38, 1967.

Gleich, G. J., Bieger, R. C., and Stankievic, R.: Antigen combining activity associated with immunoglobulin D. *Science, 165:*606, 1969.

Glenner, G. G., Eanes, E. D., Bladen, H. A., Linke, R. P., and Termine, J. D.: β-Pleated sheet fibrils: a comparison of native amyloid with synthetic protein fibrils. *J Histochem Cytochem, 22:*1141-1158, 1974.

Glenner, G. G., Ein, D., Eanes, E. D., Bladen, H. A., Terry, W., and Page, D. L.: Creation of "amyloid" fibrils from Bence Jones proteins in vitro. *Science, 174:*712-714, 1971a.

Glenner, G. G., Terry, W., Harada, M., Isersky, C., and Page, D.: Amyloid fibril proteins: proof of homology with immunoglobulin light chains by sequence analyses. *Science, 172:*1150-1151, 1971b.

Glenner, G. G., and Terry, W. D.: Characterization of amyloid. *Annu Rev Med, 25:*131-135, 1974.

Glenner, G. G., Terry, W. D., and Isersky, C.: Amyloidosis: its nature and pathogenesis. *Semin Hematol, 12:*65-86, 1973.

Gloor, B.: Diffuse Hornhautdegeneration bei einem Fall von Makroglobulinämie Waldenström. *Ophthalmologica, 155:*449-463, 1968.

Godard, J. E., Fox, J. E., and Levinson, M. J.: Primary gastric plasmacytoma: case report and review of the literature. *Am J Dig Dis,* ns, *18:*508-512, 1973.

Godeau, P., Sicard, D., Herreman, G., and Slama, G.: Macroglobulinémie de Waldenström de localisation pleuropulmonaire, orbitaire et sous-cutanée: effet favorable du chlorambucil. *Sem Hop Paris, 48:*3111-3116, 1972.

Goebel, H. H., and Friedman, A. H.: Extraocular muscle involvement in idiopathic primary amyloidosis. *Am J Ophthalmol, 71:*1121-1127, 1971.

Götze, O., and Müller-Eberhard, H. J.: The C3-activator system: an alternate pathway of complement activation. *J Exp Med, 134*:90S-108S, 1971.

Goh, K. O., and Swisher, S. N.: Macroglobulinemia of Waldenström and the chromosomal morphology. *Am J Med Sci, 260*:237-244, 1970.

Goldberg, A., Brodsky, I., and McCarty, D.: Multiple myeloma with paramyloidosis presenting as rheumatoid disease. *Am J Med, 37*:653-658, 1964.

Goldberg, E., and Mori, K.: Multiple myeloma with isolated visceral (epicardial) involvement and cardiac tamponade. *Chest, 57*:584-587, 1970.

Goldberg, L. S., Fisher, R., Castronova, E. A., and Calabro, J. J.: Amyloid arthritis associated with Waldenström's macroglobulinemia. *N Engl J Med, 281*:256-257, 1969.

Goldenberg, G. J., Paraskevas, F., and Israels, L. G.: The association of rheumatoid arthritis with plasma cell and lymphocytic neoplasms. *Arthritis Rheum, 12*:569-579, 1969.

Goldsmith, R. S., Bartos, H., Hulley, S. B., Ingbar, S. H., and Moloney, W. C.: Phosphate supplementation as an adjunct in the therapy of multiple myeloma. *Arch Intern Med, 122*:128-133, 1968.

Gomez, A. R., and Harley, J. B.: Multiple myeloma and pernicious anemia. *W Va Med J, 66*:38-41, 1970.

Gompels, B. M., Votaw, M. L., and Martel, W.: Correlation of radiological manifestations of multiple myeloma with immunoglobulin abnormalities and prognosis. *Radiology, 104*:509-514, 1972.

Goodman, S. I., Rodgerson, D. O., and Kauffman, J.: Hypercupremia in a patient with multiple myeloma. *J Lab Clin Med, 70*:57-62, 1967.

Goodman, T. F., Jr., Abele, D. C., and West, C. S., Jr.: Electron microscopy in the diagnosis of amyloidosis. *Arch Dermatol, 106*:393-397, 1972.

Gordon, D. A., Pruzanski, W., Ogryzlo, M. A., and Little, H. A.: Amyloid arthritis simulating rheumatoid disease in five patients with multiple myeloma. *Am J Med, 55*:142-154, 1973.

Gordon, H., Bandmann, M., and Sandbank, U.: Multiple myeloma associated with progressive multifocal leukoencephalopathy and *Pneumocystis carinii* pneumonia. *Isr J Med Sci, 7*:581-588, 1971.

Gordon-Smith, E. C., Harrison, R. J., and Hobbs, J. R.: Multiple myeloma presenting as cryoglobulinaemia. *Proc R Soc Med, 61*:1112-1115, 1968.

Gothoni, G., Wasastjerna, C., and Jeglinsky, B.: Macroglobulinaemia: primary (Waldenström) and symptomatic in rheumatoid arthritis. *Acta Med Scand, 177*:263-273, 1965.

Goyert, S. M., and Spiegelberg, H. L.: IgD: partial amino acid sequence of the Fc fragment resembles IgE and IgG (abstract). *Fed Proc, 34*:971, 1975.

Grabar, P., and Williams, C. A.: Méthode permettant l'étude conjuguée des propriétés électrophorétiques et immunochimiques d'un mélange de protéines: application au sérum sanguin. *Biochim Biophys Acta, 10:*193-194, 1953.

Grader, J., and Moynihan, J. W.: Multiple myeloma and osteogenic sarcoma in a patient with Paget's disease. *JAMA, 176:*685-687, 1961.

Graham, R. C., Jr., and Bernier, G. M.: The bone marrow in multiple myeloma: correlation of plasma cell ultrastructure and clinical state. *Medicine* (Baltimore), *54:*225-243, 1975.

Grant, J. A., Blumenschein, G. R., and Buckley, C. E., III: Familial paraproteinemia. *Arch Intern Med, 128:*427-431, 1971.

Greenspan, E. M., and Tung, B. G.: Acute myeloblastic leukemia after cure of ovarian cancer. *JAMA, 230:*418-420, 1974.

Gregg, J. A., Herskovic, T., and Bartholomew, L. G.: Ascites in systemic amyloidosis. *Arch Intern Med, 116:*605-610, 1965.

Grey, H. M., Abel, C. A., Yount, W. J., and Kunkel, H. G.: A subclass of human γA-globulins (γA2) which lacks disulfide bonds linking heavy and light chains. *J Exp Med, 128:*1223-1236, 1968a.

Grey, H. M., and Kohler, P. F.: Cryoimmunoglobulins. *Semin Hematol, 10:* 87-112, 1973.

Grey, H. M., Kohler, P. F., Terry, W. D., and Franklin, E. C.: Human monoclonal γG-cryoglobulins with anti-γ-globulin activity. *J Clin Invest, 47:* 1875-1884, 1968b.

Grey, H. M., and Kunkel, H. G.: H chain subgroups of myeloma proteins and normal 7S γ-globulin. *J Exp Med, 120:*253-266, 1964.

Griffel, B., Man, B., and Kraus, L.: Selective massive amyloidosis of small intestine. *Arch Surg, 110:*215-217, 1975.

Griffiths, C., and Brown, G.: Extramedullary plasmacytoma. *Can J Otolaryngol, 3:*81-85, 1974.

Groch, G. S., Perillie, P. E., and Finch, S. C.: Reticuloendothelial phagocytic function in patients with leukemia, lymphoma and multiple myeloma. *Blood, 26:*489-499, 1965.

Grossman, J., Abraham, G. N., Leddy, J. P., and Condemi, J. L.: Crystalglobulinemia. *Ann Intern Med, 77:*395-400, 1972.

Grubb, R.: Agglutination of erythrocytes coated with "incomplete" anti-Rh by certain rheumatoid arthritic sera and some other sera: the existence of human serum groups. *Acta Pathol Microbiol Scand, 39:*195-197, 1956.

Grundbacher, F. J.: Human X chromosome carries quantitative genes for immunoglobulin M. *Science, 176:*311-312, 1972.

Gudas, P. P., Jr.: Optic nerve myeloma. *Am J Ophthalmol, 71:*1085-1089, 1971.

Gupta, R. M., Roy, D. C., Gupta, I. M., and Khanna, S.: Extramedullary plasmacytoma IgG type I presenting as mediastinal syndrome. *Br J Dis Chest, 68:*65-70, 1974.

Habeshaw, J. A., Hayward, M. J., and McVie, J. G.: Extramedullary plasmacytoma of stomach. *Scand J Haematol, 14:*57-64, 1975.

Hällén, J.: Frequency of "abnormal" serum globulins (M-components) in the aged. *Acta Med Scand, 173:*737-744, 1963.

Hällén, J.: Discrete gammaglobulin (M-)components in serum: clinical study of 150 subjects without myelomatosis. *Acta Med Scand* [Suppl], *462:*1-127, 1966.

Hall, A. J., and Mackay, N. N. S.: The results of laminectomy for compression of the cord or cauda equina by extradural malignant tumour. *J Bone Joint Surg* [Br] *55:*497-505, 1973.

Halpern, M. S., and Koshland, M. E.: Novel subunit in secretory IgA. *Nature, 228:*1276-1278, 1970.

Handley, G. J., and Arney, G. K.: Plasma cell myeloma and associated amino acid disorder: case with crystalline deposition in the cornea and lens. *Arch Intern Med, 120:*353-355, 1967.

Hanicki, Z., Hirszel, P., Magdoń, M., Pajdak, W., Szczepkowska, W., and Żebro, T.: Nephropathy in the course of myeloma. *Pol Med J, 11:*1446-1458, 1972.

Hansen, O. P., Jessen, B., and Videbaek, A.: Prognosis of myelomatosis on treatment with prednisone and cytostatics. *Scand J Haematol, 10:*282-290, 1973.

Harbaugh, M. E., Hill, E. M., and Conn, R. B.: Antithrombin and antithromboplastin activity accompanying IgG myeloma: report of a case with a severe bleeding tendency. *Am J Clin Pathol, 63:*57-67, 1975.

Harboe, M., Deverill, J., and Godal, H. C.: Antigenic heterogeneity of Waldenström type γM-globulins. *Scand J Haematol, 2:*137-147, 1965.

Harboe, M., Hannestad, K., and Sletten, K.: Oligoclonal macroglobulinaemia. *Scand J Immunol, 1:*13-26, 1972.

Hardt, F.: Acceleration of casein induced amyloidosis in mice by immunosuppressive agents. *Acta Pathol Microbiol Scand* [A], *79:*61-64, 1971.

Hardt, F., and Claësson, M. H.: Casein-induced amyloidosis in the nude mouse. I. Acceleration of amyloidosis in recipients of spleen grafts from casein-sensitized donor mice. II. Transfer of amyloidosis by spleen cells. *Acta Pathol Microbiol Scand* [B], *82:*403-408, 1974.

Harley, J. B., Ramanan, S. V., Kim, I., Thiagarajan, P. V., Chen, J. H., Gomez, R., Koppel, D., Hyde, F., Gustke, S., and Krall, J.: The cyclic use of multiple alkylating agents in multiple myeloma. *W Va Med J, 68:*1-3, 1972a.

Harley, J. B., Schilling, A., and Glidewell, O.: Ineffectiveness of fluoride therapy in multiple myeloma. *N Engl J Med, 286:*1283-1288, 1972b.

Harris, J., Alexanian, R., Hersh, E., and Migliore, P.: Immune function in multiple myeloma: impaired responsiveness to keyhole limpet hemocyanin. *Can Med Assoc J, 104:*389-392, 1971.

Harris, J., and Copeland, D.: Impaired immunoresponsiveness in tumor patients. *Ann NY Acad Sci, 230*:56-85, 1974.

Harris, R. I., and Kohn, J.: A urinary cryo-Bence Jones protein gelling at room temperature. *Clin Chim Acta, 53*:233-237, 1974.

Harrison, C. V.: The morphology of the lymph node in the macroglobulinaemia of Waldenström. *J Clin Pathol, 25*:12-16, 1972.

Hauptman, S., and Tomasi, T. B., Jr.: A monoclonal IgM protein with antibody-like activity for human albumin. *J Clin Invest, 53*:932-940, 1974.

Hayes, D. M., Costa, J., Moon, J. H., Hoogstraten, B., and Harley, J. B.: Combination therapy with thioguanine (NSC-752) and azaserine (NSC-742) for multiple myeloma. *Cancer Chemother Rep, 51*:235-238, 1967.

Hayes, D. W., Bennett, W. A., and Heck, F. J.: Extramedullary lesions in multiple myeloma: review of literature and pathologic studies. *Arch Pathol, 53*:262-272, 1952.

Hayes, W. T., and Bernhardt, H.: Solitary amyloid mass of the lung: report of a case with 6-year follow-up. *Cancer, 24*:820-825, 1969.

Heading, R. C., Girdwood, R. H., and Eastwood, M. A.: Macroglobulinaemia treated with prednisone, azathioprine, and folic acid. *Br Med J, 3*:750, 1970.

Heffernan, A. G. A.: Unusual presentation of multiple myeloma. *Postgrad Med J, 48*:238-240, 1972.

Heinle, E. W., Jr., Sarasti, H. O., Garcia, D., Kenny, J. J., and Westerman, M. P.: Polycythemia vera associated with lymphomatous diseases and myeloma. *Arch Intern Med, 118*:351-355, 1966.

Heitzman, E. J., Heitzman, G. C., and Elliott, C. F.: Primary esophageal amyloidosis: report of a case with bleeding, perforation, and survival following resection. *Arch Intern Med, 109*:595-600, 1962.

Hellwig, C. A.: Extramedullary plasma cell tumors as observed in various locations. *Arch Pathol, 36*:95-111, 1943.

Henderson, J. W.: *Orbital Tumors*. Philadelphia, W. B. Saunders Company, 1973, pp. 382-408.

Henson, P. M., and Spiegelberg, H. L.: Release of serotonin from human platelets induced by aggregated immunoglobulins of different classes and subclasses. *J Clin Invest, 52*:1282-1288, 1973.

Heremans, J. F.: Immunochemical studies on protein pathology: the immunoglobulin concept. *Clin Chim Acta, 4*:639-646, 1959.

Heremans, J. F., Heremans, M.-T., and Schultze, H. E.: Isolation and description of a few properties of the β_{2A}-globulin of human serum. *Clin Chim Acta, 4*:96-102, 1959.

Herskovic, T., Andersen, H. A., and Bayrd, E. D.: Intrathoracic plasmacytomas: presentation of 21 cases and review of literature. *Dis Chest, 47*:1-6, 1965.

Herskovic, T., Bartholomew, L. G., and Green, P. A.: Amyloidosis and malabsorption syndrome. *Arch Intern Med, 114*:629-633, 1964.

Hicks, K. A., and Dickie, W. R.: Amyloidosis: report of a case presenting with macroglossia. *Br J Plast Surg, 26*:274-276, 1973.

Higgins, W. H., and Higgins, W. H., Jr.: Primary amyloidosis: a clinical and pathological study. *Am J Med Sci, 220*:610-615, 1950.

Himmelfarb, E., Sebes, J., and Rabinowitz, J.: Unusual roentgenographic presentations of multiple myeloma: report of three cases. *J Bone Joint Surg* [Am], *56*:1723-1728, 1974.

Hippe, E., Paaske Hansen, O., and Drivsholm, A.: Decreased serum cobalamin in multiple myeloma without signs of vitamin B_{12} deficiency: a preliminary report. *Scand J Gastroenterol 9* Suppl *29*:85-87, 1974.

Hiramoto, R., Ghanta, V., and Durant, J. R.: Evaluation of a cooperative group human myeloma protocol using the MOPC 104E myeloma model. *Cancer Res, 35*:1309-1313, 1975.

Hobbs, J. R.: Paraproteins, benign or malignant? *Br Med J, 3*:699-704, 1967.

Hobbs, J. R.: Immunochemical classes of myelomatosis: including data from a therapeutic trial conducted by a medical research council working party. *Br J Haematol, 16*:599-606, 1969a.

Hobbs, J. R.: Growth rates and responses to treatment in human myelomatosis. *Br J Haematol, 16*:607-617, 1969b.

Hobbs, J. R.: Immunocytoma o' mice an' men. *Br Med J, 2*:67-72, 1971.

Hobbs, J. R.: The emergence of new tumour lines during therapy (abstract). *J Clin Pathol, 25*:556, 1972.

Hobbs, J. R.: An ABC of amyloid. *Proc R Soc Med, 66*:705-710, 1973.

Hobbs, J. R.: Monitoring myelomatosis. *Arch Intern Med, 135*:125-130, 1975.

Hobbs, J. R., and Corbett, A. A.: Younger age of presentation and extraosseous tumour in IgD myelomatosis. *Br Med J, 1*:412-414, 1969.

Hobbs, J. R., Slot, G. M. J., Campbell, C. H., Clein, G. P., Scott, J. T., Crowther, D., and Swan, H. T.: Six cases of gamma-D myelomatosis. *Lancet, 2*: 614-618, 1966.

Hofer, P.-Å., Winblad, B., Andersson, L., Schönebeck, J., Lingårdh, G., and Hietala, S.-O.: Primary localized amyloidosis of the bladder. *Scand J Urol Nephrol, 8*:193-197, 1974.

Hoffbrand, A. V., Hobbs, J. R., Kremenchuzky, S., and Mollin, D. L.: Incidence and pathogenesis of megaloblastic erythropoiesis in multiple myeloma. *J Clin Pathol, 20*:699-705, 1967.

Hoffman, S., Simon, B. E., Fischel, R. A., and Gribetz, D.: Renal amyloidosis resulting from a chronically infected burn. *Pediatrics, 32*:888-894, 1963.

Holland, J. F., Hosley, H., Scharlau, C., Carbone, P. P., Frei, E., III, Brindley, C. O., Hall, T. C., Shnider, B. I., Gold, G. L., Lasagna, L., Owens, A. H., Jr., and Miller, S. P.: A controlled trial of urethane treatment in multiple myeloma. *Blood, 27*:328-342, 1966.

Hollander, V. P., Takakura, K., and Yamada, H.: Endocrine factors in the pathogenesis of plasma cell tumors. *Recent Prog Horm Res, 24*:81-137, 1968.

Holt, J. M., and Robb-Smith, A. H. T.: Multiple myeloma: development of plasma cell sarcoma during apparently successful chemotherapy. *J Clin Pathol, 26:*649-659, 1973.

Hood, L., and Talmage, D. W.: Mechanism of antibody diversity: germ line basis for variability. *Science, 168:*325-334, 1970.

Hoogstraten, B.: Steroid therapy of multiple myeloma and macroglobulinemia. *Med Clin North Am, 57:*1321-1330, 1973.

Hoogstraten, B., Costa, J., Cuttner, J., Forcier, R. J., Leone, L. A., Harley, J. B., and Glidewell, O. J.: Intermittent melphalan therapy in multiple myeloma. *JAMA, 209:*251-253, 1969.

Hoogstraten, B., Cuttner, J., and Wasserman, L. R.: Prognostic indicators in multiple myeloma (abstract). *Proc Am Assoc Cancer Res, 8:*31, 1967a.

Hoogstraten, B., Sheehe, P. R., Cuttner, J., Cooper, T., Kyle, R. A., Oberfield, R. A., Townsend, S. R., Harley, J. B., Hayes, D. M., Costa, G., and Holland, J. F.: Melphalan in multiple myeloma. *Blood, 30:*74-83, 1967b.

Hopper, J. E., and Nisonoff, A.: Individual antigenic specificity of immunoglobulins. *Adv Immunol, 13:*58-99, 1971.

Horn, M. E., Knapp, M. S., Page, F. T., and Walker, W. H. C.: Adult Fanconi syndrome and multiple myelomatosis. *J Clin Pathol, 22:*414-416, 1969.

Horvath, W. L., Montana, G. S., and Palmer, J. G.: Comparison of total body irradiation and L-phenylalanine mustard in myeloma (abstract). *Clin Res, 22:*395A, 1974.

Houston, E. W., Ritzmann, S. E., and Levin, W. C.: Chromosomal aberrations common to three types of monoclonal gammopathies. *Blood, 29:*214-232, 1967.

Hurez, D., Preud'homme, J.-L., and Seligmann, M.: Intracellular "monoclonal" immunoglobulin in nonsecretory human myeloma. *J Immunol, 104:* 263-264, 1970.

Hurvitz, A. I., Haskins, S. C., and Fischer, C. A.: Macroglobulinemia with hyperviscosity syndrome in a dog. *J Am Vet Med Assoc, 157:*455-460, 1970.

Husby, G., and Natvig, J. B.: A serum component related to nonimmunoglobulin amyloid protein AS, a possible precursor of the fibrils. *J Clin Invest, 53:*1054-1061, 1974.

Husby, G., Natvig, J. B., and Harboe, M.: The occurrence in sera with M-components of different proteins related to amyloid fibrils. *Scand J Immunol, 3:*391-396, 1974.

Husby, G., Natvig, J. B., Michaelsen, T. E., Sletten, K., and Höst, H.: Unique amyloid protein subunit common to different types of amyloid fibril (letter to the editor). *Nature, 244:*362-364, 1973.

Imahori, S., and Moore, G. E.: Multiple myeloma and prolonged stimulation of reticuloendothelial system. *NY State J Med, 72:*1625-1628, 1972.

Indiveri, F., Barabino, A., Santolini, M. E., and Santolini, B.: "Nonsecretory" multiple myeloma: report of a case. *Acta Haematol* (Basel), *51:*302-309, 1974.

Ingram, G. I. C., Kingston, P. J., Leslie, J., and Bowie, E. J. W.: Four cases of acquired von Willebrand's syndrome. *Br J Haematol, 21:*189-199, 1971.

Invernizzi, F., Cattaneo, R., Rosso di San Secondo, V., Balestrieri, G., and Zanussi, C.: Pyroglobulinemia: a report of eight patients with associated paraproteinemia. *Acta Haematol* (Basel), *50:*65-74, 1973.

Ironside, P.: Clinical value of immunoelectrophoresis in multiple myeloma. *Pathology, 2:*53-60, 1970.

Ishizaka, K., Ishizaka, T., and Hornbrook, M. M.: Physicochemical properties of reaginic antibody. V. Correlation of reaginic activity with γE-globulin antibody. *J Immunol, 97:*840-853, 1966.

Íshwarchandra, Deshmukh, P. C., and Hardas, U.: Amyloid tumour of the lids. *Indian J Ophthalmol, 22:*30-32, 1974.

Isobe, T., and Osserman, E. F.: Pathologic conditions associated with plasma cell dyscrasias: a study of 806 cases. *Ann NY Acad Sci, 190:*507-518, 1971.

Isobe, T., and Osserman, E. F.: Patterns of amyloidosis and their association with plasma-cell dyscrasia, monoclonal immunoglobulins and Bence-Jones proteins. *N Engl J Med, 290:*473-477, 1974a.

Isobe, T., and Osserman, E. F.: Plasma cell dyscrasia associated with the production of incomplete (? deleted) IgG λ molecules, gamma heavy chains, and free lambda chains containing carbohydrate: description of the first case. *Blood, 43:*505-526, 1974b.

Iwashita, H., Argyrakis, A., Lowitzsch, K., and Spaar, F.-W.: Polyneuropathy in Waldenström's macroglobulinaemia. *J Neurol Sci, 21:*341-354, 1974.

Jabłońska, S., and Stachow, A.: Scleroderma-like lesions in multiple myeloma. *Dermatologica, 144:*257-269, 1972.

Jacobson, R. J., Sandler, S. G., and Rath, C. E.: Systemic amyloidosis associated with micro-angiopathic haemolytic anaemia and Factor X (Stuart factor) deficiency. *S Afr Med J, 46:*1634-1637, 1972.

James, K., Fudenberg, H., Epstein, W. L., and Shuster, J.: Studies on a unique diagnostic serum globulin in papular mucinosis (lichen myxedematosus). *Clin Exp Immunol, 2:*153-166, 1967.

James, T. N.: Pathology of the cardiac conduction system in amyloidosis. *Ann Intern Med, 65:*28-36, 1966.

Jamshidi, K., and Swaim, W. R.: Bone marrow biopsy with unaltered architecture: a new biopsy device. *J Lab Clin Med, 77:*335-342, 1971.

Jancelewicz, Z., Takatsuki, K., Sugai, S., and Pruzanski, W.: IgD multiple myeloma: review of 133 cases. *Arch Intern Med, 135:*87-93, 1975.

Jao, W., and Pirani, C. L.: Renal amyloidosis: electron microscopic observations. *Acta Pathol Microbiol Scand* [A] Suppl, *233:*217-227, 1972.

Jean, G., Lambertenghi-Deliliers, G., Ranzi, T., and Polli, E.: Ultrastructural aspects of bone marrow and peripheral blood cells in a case of plasma cell leukemia. *Acta Haematol* (Basel) *45:*36-49, 1971.

Jennings, G. H., Levi, A. J., and Reeve, J.: A case of chronic granulocytopenia associated with vasculitis and amyloidosis. *J Clin Pathol, 26*:592-595, 1973.

Jensen, H., and Wiik, A.: Monoclonal immunoglobulinaemia associated with glomerulopathy. *Acta Med Scand, 197*:265-269, 1975.

Johansson, S. G. O.: Raised levels of a new immunoglobulin class (IgND) in asthma. *Lancet, 2*:951-953, 1967.

Johansson, S. G. O., and Bennich, H.: Immunological studies of an atypical (myeloma) immunoglobulin. *Immunology, 13*:381-394, 1967.

Johner, C. H., Widen, A. H., and Sahgal, S.: Amyloidosis of the head and neck. *Trans Am Acad Ophthalmol Otolaryngol, 76*:1354-1355, 1972.

Johnson, W. W., and Meadows, D. C.: Urinary-bladder fibrosis and telangiectasia associated with long-term cyclophosphamide therapy. *N Engl J Med, 284*:290-294, 1971.

Jones, N. F., Hilton, P. J., Tighe, J. R., and Hobbs, J. R.: Treatment of "primary" renal amyloidosis with melphalan. *Lancet, 2*:616-619, 1972.

Jowsey, J., Riggs, B. L., Kelly, P. J., and Hoffman, D. L.: Effect of combined therapy with sodium fluoride, vitamin D and calcium in osteoporosis. *Am J Med, 53*:43-49, 1972.

Kahler, O.: Zur Symptomatologie des multiplen Myeloms: Beobachtung von Albumosurie. *Prag Med Wochenschr, 14*:33; 45, 1889.

Kahn, T., and Levitt, M. F.: Salt wasting in myeloma. *Arch Intern Med, 126*: 664-667, 1970.

Kaji, H., and Parkhouse, R. M. E.: Control of J chain biosynthesis in relation to heavy and light chain synthesis, polymerization and secretion. *J Immunol, 114*:1218-1220, 1975.

Kalff, M. W., and Hijmans, W.: Immunoglobulin analysis in families of macroglobulinaemia patients. *Clin Exp Immunol, 5*:479-498, 1969.

Kaplan, G. A., and Bennett, J.: Solitary myeloma of the lumbar spine successfully treated with radiation: report of case. *Radiology, 91*:1017-1018; 1032, 1968.

Kapp, J. P.: Hepatic amyloidosis with portal hypertension. *JAMA, 191*:497-499, 1965.

Karakousis, C. P., and Elias, E. G.: Spontaneous (pathologic) rupture of spleen in malignancies. *Surgery, 76*:674-677, 1974.

Karchmer, R. K., Amare, M., Larsen, W. E., Mallouk, A. G., and Caldwell, G. G.: Alkylating agents as leukemogens in multiple myeloma. *Cancer, 33*:1103-1107, 1974.

Kaslow, R. A., Wisch, N., and Glass, J. L.: Acute leukemia following cytotoxic chemotherapy. *JAMA, 219*:75-76, 1972.

Katz, G. A., Peter, J. B., Pearson, C. M., and Adams, W. S.: The shoulder-pad sign: a diagnostic feature of amyloid arthropathy. *N Engl J Med, 288*: 354-355, 1973.

Kaye, R. L., Martin, W. J., Campbell, D. C., and Lipscomb, P. R.: Long survival in disseminated myeloma with onset as solitary lesion: two cases. *Ann Intern Med, 54*:535-544, 1961.

Kedar, I., Sohar, E., and Gafni, J.: Demonstration of amyloid-degrading activity in normal human serum. *Proc Soc Exp Biol Med, 145*:343-345, 1974.

Keen, P. E., and Weitzner, S.: Primary localized amyloidosis of trachea. *Arch Otolaryngol, 96*:142-145, 1972.

Keith, D. A.: Oral features of primary amyloidosis. *Br J Oral Surg, 10*:107-115, 1972.

Keizman, I., Rimon, A., Sohar, E., and Gafni, J.: Amyloid accelerating factor: purification of a substance from human amyloidotic spleen that accelerates the formation of casein-induced murine amyloid. *Acta Pathol Microbiol Scand* [A] Suppl, *233*:172-177, 1972.

Keller, H., Spengler, G. A., Skvaril, F., Flury, W., Noseda, G., and Riva, G.: Zur Frage der Heavy chain disease: Ein Fall von IgG-heavy-chain-Fragment- und IgM-Typ K-Paraproteinämie mit Plasmazellenleukämie. *Schweiz Med Wochenschr, 100*:1012-1022, 1970.

Kennedy, A. C., Burton, J. A., and Allison, M. E. M.: Tuberculosis as a continuing cause of renal amyloidosis. *Br Med J, 3*:795-797, 1974.

Kennerdell, J. S., Jannetta, P. J., and Johnson, B. L.: A steroid-sensitive solitary intracranial plasmacytoma. *Arch Ophthalmol, 92*:393-398, 1974.

Kenny, J. J., and Moloney, W. C.: Long-term survival in multiple myeloma: report of three cases. *Ann Intern Med, 45*:950-957, 1956.

Kenyon, A. J., Williams, R. C., Jr., and Howard, E. B.: Monoclonal gamma-globulins in ferrets with lymphoproliferative lesions. *Proc Soc Exp Biol Med, 123*:510-513, 1966.

Khaleeli, M., Keane, W. M., and Lee, G. R.: Sideroblastic anemia in multiple myeloma: a preleukemic change. *Blood, 41*:17-25, 1973.

Khilnani, M. T., Keller, R. J., and Cuttner, J.: Macroglobulinemia and steatorrhea: roentgen and pathologic findings in the intestinal tract. *Radiol Clin North Am, 7*:43-55, 1969.

Kiang, D. T., Sundberg, R. D., Fortuny, I. E., Brunning, R. D., Theologides, A., Goldman, A., and Kennedy, B. J.: Multiple myeloma: clinical evolution. *Minn Med, 57*:542-548, 1974.

Kiely, J. M., and Perry, H. O.: Sturge-Weber syndrome associated with multiple myeloma. *Arch Dermatol, 100*:63-65, 1969.

Kim, I., Harley, J. B., and Weksler, B.: Multiple myeloma without initial paraproteins. *Am J Med Sci, 264*:267-275, 1972.

Kimball, K. G.: Amyloidosis in association with neoplastic disease: report of an unusual case and clinicopathological experience at Memorial Center for Cancer and Allied Diseases during eleven years (1948-1958). *Ann Intern Med, 55*:958-974, 1961.

King, F. H., and Oppenheimer, G. D.: Rupture of amyloid spleen. *Ann Intern Med, 29*:374-378, 1948.

Kjeldsberg, C. R., and Holman, R. E.: Acute renal failure in multiple myeloma. *J Urol, 105*:21-23, 1971.

Kjeldsen, K., Clausen, J., and Frøland, A.: Pernicious anaemia, paraproteinaemia with unusual features, and chromosome aberrations. *Acta Med Scand, 186*:209-215, 1969.

Kochwa, S., Makuku, E., and Frangione, B.: Chemical typing of immunoglobulins and their subtypes. *Arch Intern Med, 135*:37-39, 1975.

Kohn, J.: A cellulose acetate supporting medium for zone electrophoresis. *Clin Chim Acta, 2*:297-303, 1957.

Koletsky, S., and Stecher, R. M.: Primary systemic amyloidosis: involvement of cardiac valves, joints and bones, with pathologic fracture of the femur. *Arch Pathol, 27*:267-288, 1939.

Kopéc, M., Świerczyńska, Z., Pazdur, J., Luft, S., Płachecka, M., Dabska, M., Glińska, D., and Woźniczko-Orłowska, G.: Diffuse lymphoma of the intestines with a monoclonal gammopathy of IgG$_3$ kappa type. *Am J Med, 56*: 381-385, 1974.

Kopp, W. L., MacKinney, A. A., Jr., and Wasson, G.: Blood volume and hematocrit value in macroglobulinemia and myeloma. *Arch Intern Med 123*:394-396, 1969.

Korst, D. R., Clifford, G. O., Fowler, W. M., Louis, J., Will, J., and Wilson, H. E.: Multiple myeloma. II. Analysis of cyclophosphamide therapy in 165 patients. *JAMA, 189*:758-762, 1964.

Korst, D. R., and Kratochvil, C. H.: "Cryofibrinogen" in a case of lung neoplasm associated with thrombophlebitis migrans. *Blood, 10*:945-953, 1955.

Koshland, M. E.: Structure and function of the J chain. *Adv Immunol, 20*: 41-69, 1975.

Kosova, L. A., and Schwartz, S. O.: Multiple myeloma in normal pregnancy: report of a case. *Blood, 28*:102-111, 1966.

Kotner, L. M., and Wang, C. C.: Plasmacytoma of the upper air and food passages. *Cancer, 30*:414-418, 1972.

Kramer, W.: Plasmocytoma of the brain in Kahler's disease (multiple myeloma). *Acta Neuropathol* (Berl), *2*:438-450, 1963.

Krause, R. M.: The search for antibodies with molecular uniformity. *Adv Immunol, 12*:1-56, 1970.

Krauss, S., and Sokal, J. E.: Paraproteinemia in the lymphomas. *Am J Med, 40*:400-413, 1966.

Kretschmer, R. R., Pizzuto, J., González, J., and López-Osuna, M.: Heavy chain disease, rheumatoid arthritis and cryoglobulinemia. *Clin Immunol Immunopathol, 2*:195-215, 1974.

Krogh Jensen, M., Eriksen, J., and Djernes, B. W.: Cytogenetic studies in myelomatosis. *Scand J Haematol, 14*:201-209, 1975.

Kuczynski, A., Evans, R. J. C., and Mitchinson, M. J.: Sicca syndrome due to primary amyloidosis. *Br Med J, 2*:506, 1971.

Kuhlbäck, B., and Wegelius, O.: Secondary amyloidosis: a study of clinical and pathological findings. *Acta Med Scand, 180*:737-745, 1966.

Kunkel, H. G.: Myeloma proteins and antibodies. *Harvey Lect, 59*:219-242, 1965.

Kunkel, H. G.: The "abnormality" of myeloma proteins. *Cancer Res, 28*: 1351-1353, 1968.

Kunkel, H. G., Joslin, F. G., Penn, G. M., and Natvig, J. B.: Genetic variants of γG4 globulin: a unique relationship to other classes of γG globulin. *J Exp Med, 132*:508-520, 1970.

Kunkel, H. G., and Prendergast, R. A.: Subgroups of γA immune globulins. *Proc Soc Exp Biol Med, 122*:910-913, 1966.

Kunwar, K. B., and Kumar, S.: Multiple myeloma with myeloma cells in the urine: case report. *Indian J Med Sci, 20*:641-643, 1966.

Kutcher, R., Ghatak, N. R., and Leeds, N. E.: Plasmacytoma of the calvaria. *Radiology, 113*:111-115, 1974.

Kyle, R. A.: Solitary myeloma (solitary plasmacytoma) of bone. *Minn Med, 50*:1651-1653, 1967.

Kyle, R. A.; Multiple Myeloma (plasmacytic myeloma). In Conn, H. F. (Ed.) : *Current Therapy*. Philadelphia, W. B. Saunders Company, 1973, pp. 288-290.

Kyle, R. A.: Multiple myeloma: review of 869 cases. *Mayo Clin Proc, 50*:29-40, 1975.

Kyle, R. A., and Bayrd, E. D.: "Primary" systemic amyloidosis and myeloma: discussion of relationship and review of 81 cases. *Arch Intern Med, 107*: 344-353, 1961.

Kyle, R. A., and Bayrd, E. D.: "Benign" monoclonal gammopathy: a potentially malignant condition? *Am J Med, 40*:426-430, 1966.

Kyle, R. A., and Bayrd, E. D.: Amyloidosis: review of 236 cases. *Medicine* (Baltimore), *54*:271-299, 1975.

Kyle, R. A., Bieger, R. C., and Gleich, G. J.: Diagnosis of syndromes associated with hyperglobulinemia. *Med Clin North Am, 54*:917-938, 1970a.

Kyle, R. A., Carbone, P. P., Lynch, J. J., Owens, A. H., Jr., Costa, G., Silver, R. T., Cuttner, J., Harley, J. B., Leone, L. A., Shnider, B. I., and Holland, J. F.: Evaluation of tryptophan mustard (NSC-62403) in patients with plasmacytic myeloma. *Cancer Res, 27*:510-515, 1967.

Kyle, R. A., Costa, G., Cooper, M. R., Ogawa, M., Silver, R. T., Glidewell, O., and Holland, J. F.: Evaluation of aniline mustard in patients with multiple myeloma. *Cancer Res, 33*:956-960, 1973a.

Kyle, R. A., Finkelstein, S., Elveback, L. R., and Kurland, L. T.: Incidence of monoclonal proteins in a Minnesota community with a cluster of multiple myeloma. *Blood, 40*:719-724, 1972.

Kyle, R. A., and Gleich, G. J.: Syndromes associated with hyperglobulinemia. In *Tice's Practice of Medicine*, Vol. 1. Hagerstown, Maryland, Harper & Row, Publishers, 1972, pp. 1-37.

Kyle, R. A., Heath, C. W., Jr., and Carbone, P.: Multiple myeloma in spouses. *Arch Intern Med, 127*:944-946, 1971.

Kyle, R. A., Henderson, E. S., Randolph, V. L., and Budge, W. R.: Multiple myeloma, acute leukemia, and Hodgkin's disease: occurrence in three of four family members. *Cancer, 37*:1496-1499, 1976.

Kyle, R. A., Herber, L., Evatt, B. L., and Heath, C. W., Jr.: Multiple myeloma: a community cluster. *JAMA, 213*:1339-1341, 1970b.

Kyle, R. A.: Jowsey, J., Kelly, P. J., and Taves, D. R.: Multiple-myeloma bone disease: the comparative effect of sodium fluoride and calcium carbonate or placebo. *N Engl J Med, 293*:1334-1338, 1975a.

Kyle, R. A., Kottke, B. A., and Schirger, A.: Orthostatic hypotension as a clue to primary systemic amyloidosis. *Circulation, 34*:883-888, 1966a.

Kyle, R. A., Maldonado, J. E., and Bayrd, E. D.: Idiopathic Bence Jones proteinuria: a distinct entity? *Am J Med, 55*:222-226, 1973b.

Kyle, R. A., Maldonado, J. E., and Bayrd, E. D.: Plasma cell leukemia: report on 17 cases. *Arch Intern Med, 133*:813-818, 1974a.

Kyle, R. A., Nobrega, F. T., and Kurland, L. T.: Multiple myeloma in Olmsted County, Minnesota, 1945-1964. *Blood, 33*:739-745, 1969.

Kyle, R. A., Pease, G. L., Richmond, H., and Sullivan, L.: Bone marrow aspiration in the antemortem diagnosis of primary systemic amyloidosis. *Am J Clin Pathol, 45*:252-257, 1966b.

Kyle, R. A., Pierre, R. V., and Bayrd, E. D.: Multiple myeloma and acute myelomonocytic leukemia: report of four cases possibly related to melphalan. *N Engl J Med, 283*:1121-1125, 1970c.

Kyle, R. A., Pierre, R. V., and Bayrd, E. D.: Primary amyloidosis and acute leukemia associated with melphalan therapy. *Blood, 44*:333-337, 1974b.

Kyle, R. A., Pierre, R. V., and Bayrd, E. D.: Multiple myeloma and acute leukemia associated with alkylating agents. *Arch Intern Med, 135*:185-192, 1975b.

Kyle, R. A., Seligman, B. R., Wallace, H. J., Jr., Silver, R. T., Glidewell, O., and Holland, J. F.: Multiple myeloma resistant to melphalan (NSC-8806) treated with cyclophosphamide (NSC-26271), prednisone (NSC-10023), and chloroquine (NSC-187208). *Cancer Chemother Rep, 59*:557-562, 1975c.

Kyle, R. A., Spencer, R. J., and Dahlin, D. C.: Value of rectal biopsy in the diagnosis of primary systemic amyloidosis. *Am J Med Sci, 251*:501-506, 1966c.

Lackner, H.: Hemostatic abnormalities associated with dysproteinemias. *Semin Hematol, 10*:125-133, 1973.

Ladefoged, A. J., Nielsen, B., and Pedersen, K.: Akut nyreinsufficiens ved myelomatose. *Ugeskr Laeger, 132*:641-646, 1970.

Lai A Fat, R. F. M., Suurmond, D., Rádl, J., and van Furth, R.: Scleromyxoedema (lichen myxoedematosus) associated with a paraprotein, IgG$_1$ of type kappa. *Br J Dermatol, 88*:107-116, 1973.

Lam, C. W. K., and Stevenson, G. T.: Detection in normal plasma of immunoglobulin resembling the protein of γ-chain disease (letter to the editor). *Nature, 246*:419-421, 1973.

Lane, S. L.: Plasmacytoma of the mandible. *Oral Surg, 5*:434-442, 1952.

Langley, G. R., Sabean, H. B., and Sorger, K.: Sclerotic lesions of bone in myeloma. *Can Med Assoc J, 94*:940-946, 1966.

LaPerriere, R. J., Wolf, J. E., and Gellin, G. A.: Primary cutaneous plasmacytoma. *Arch Dermatol, 107*:99-100, 1973.

Larsen, O. A., and Jarnum, S.: The Evans blue test in amyloidosis. *Scand J Clin Lab Invest, 17*:287-294, 1965.

Larson, S. O.: Myeloma and pernicious anaemia. *Acta Med Scand, 172*:195-205, 1962.

Law, I. P.: Kaposi sarcoma and plasma cell dyscrasia. *JAMA, 229*:1329-1331, 1974.

Lawrence, D. A., Weigle, W. O., and Spiegelberg, H. L.: Immunoglobulins cytophilic for human lymphocytes, monocytes, and neutrophils. *J Clin Invest, 55*:368-376, 1975.

Lee, B. J., Korngold, L., and Weiner, M. J.: Melphalan and antigenic type of Bence Jones proteins in myeloma. *Science, 149*:564-565, 1965.

Lee, B. J., Sahakian, G., Clarkson, B. D., and Krakoff, I. H.: Combination chemotherapy of multiple myeloma with Alkeran, Cytoxan, vincristine, prednisone, and BCNU. *Cancer, 33*:533-538, 1974.

Leech, S. H., Polesky, H. F., and Shapiro, F. L.: Chronic hemodialysis in myelomatosis. *Ann Intern Med, 77*:239-242, 1972.

Legge, D. A., Carlson, H. C., and Wollaeger, E. E.: Roentgenologic appearance of systemic amyloidosis involving gastrointestinal tract. *Am J Roentgenol Radium Ther Nucl Med, 110*:406-412, 1970a.

Legge, D. A., Wollaeger, E. E., and Carlson H. C.: Intestinal pseudo-obstruction in systemic amyloidosis. *Gut, 11*:764-767, 1970b.

Lender, M.: Amyloidosis associated with neoplastic diseases. *S Afr Med J, 48*: 1944-1946, 1974.

Lergier, J. E., and Gowans, J. D. C.: Monoclonal IgM immunoglobulinemia in psoriatic arthritis. *JAMA, 231*:171-173, 1975.

Lergier, J. E., Jiménez, E., Maldonado, N., and Veray, F.: Normal pregnancy in multiple myeloma treated with cyclophosphamide. *Cancer, 34*:1018-1022, 1974.

Lerner, A. B., and Watson, C. J.: Studies of cryoglobulins. I. Unusual purpura associated with the presence of a high concentration of cryoglobulin (cold precipitable serum globulin). *Am J Med Sci, 214*:410-415, 1947.

Lessin, L. S., Hallal, J., Burkholder, P., and Cohen, H.: Ultrastructural studies of the role of the reticuloendothelial (RE) cell in clinical resolution of amyloidosis (abstract). *Clin Res, 20*:512, 1972.

Levi, D. F., Williams, R. C., Jr., and Lindström, F. D.: Immunofluorescent studies of the myeloma kidney with special reference to light chain disease. *Am J Med, 44:*922-933, 1968.

Levin, H. S., and Mostofi, F. K.: Symptomatic plasmacytoma of the testis. *Cancer, 25:*1193-1203, 1970.

Levin, M., Franklin, E. C., Frangione, B., and Pras, M.: The amino acid sequence of a major nonimmunoglobulin component of some amyloid fibrils. *J Clin Invest, 51:*2773-2776, 1972.

Levine, R. A.: Amyloid disease of the liver: correlation of clinical, functional and morphologic features in forty-seven patients. *Am J Med, 33:*349-357, 1962.

Lewis, E. B.: Leukemia, multiple myeloma, and aplastic anemia in American radiologists. *Science, 142:*1492-1494, 1963.

Lewis, L. A., and Page, I. H.: Serum proteins and lipoproteins in multiple myelomatosis. *Am J Med, 17:*670-673, 1954.

Lewis, M.: Gastrocamera findings in a patient with gastric amyloidosis and multiple myeloma. *Gastrointest Endosc, 14:*190-193, 1968.

Lindberg, J.: Rupture of the right ventricle of the heart in a case of advanced heart amyloidosis. *Acta Pathol Microbiol Scand* [A], *79:*53-54, 1971.

Lindgärde, F., and Zettervall, O.: Hypercalcemia and normal ionized serum calcium in a case of myelomatosis. *Ann Intern Med, 78:*396-399, 1973.

Lindgärde, F., and Zettervall, O.: Characterization of a calcium-binding IgG myeloma protein. *Scand J Immunol, 3:*277-285, 1974.

Lindh, E.: Increased resistance of immunoglobulin A dimers to proteolytic degradation after binding of secretory component. *J Immunology, 114:*284-286, 1975.

Lindqvist, K. J., Ragab, A. H., and Osterland, C. K.: Paraproteinemia in a child with leukemia. *Blood, 35:*213-221, 1970.

Lindsley, H., Teller, D., Noonan, B., Peterson, M., and Mannik, M.: Hyperviscosity syndrome in multiple myeloma: a reversible, concentration-dependent aggregation of the myeloma protein. *Am J Med, 54:*682-688, 1973.

Lindström, F. D., Hardy, W. R., Eberle, B. J., and Williams, R. C., Jr.: Multiple myeloma and benign monoclonal gammopathy: differentiation by immunofluorescence of lymphocytes. *Ann Intern Med, 78:*837-844, 1973.

Lindström, F. D., Williams, R. C., Jr., and Brunning, R. D.: Thymoma associated with multiple myeloma. *Arch Intern Med, 122:*526-531, 1968.

Linke, R. P., Tischendorf, F. W., Zucker-Franklin, D., and Franklin, E. C.: The formation of amyloid-like fibrils in vitro from Bence Jones proteins of the VλI subclass. *J Immunol, 111:*24-26, 1973a.

Linke, R. P., Zucker-Franklin, D., and Franklin, E. C.: Morphologic, chemical, and immunologic studies of amyloid-like fibrils formed from Bence Jones proteins by proteolysis. *J Immunol, 111:*10-23, 1973b.

Lipman, I. J.: Pyroglobulinemia, an unusual presenting sign in multiple myeloma. *JAMA, 188*:1002-1004, 1964.

Little, J. M.: Waldenström's macroglobulinemia in the lacrimal gland. *Trans Am Acad Ophthalmol Otolaryngol, 71*:875-879, 1967.

Littman, E.: Renal amyloidosis with nephrotic syndrome associated with retroperitoneal fibrosis. *Ann Intern Med, 74*:240-241, 1971.

Liu, C. T., and Dahlke, M. B.: Bone marrow findings of reactive plasmacytosis. *Am J Clin Pathol, 48*:546-551, 1967.

Lock, J. P., Castro, G. A. M., Pechet, L. N., and Snyder, L. M.: Hemodialysis in myelomatosis (letter to the editor). *Ann Intern Med, 78*:454, 1973.

Logothetis, J., Silverstein, P., and Coe, J.: Neurologic aspects of Waldenström's macroglobulinemia: report of a case. *Arch Neurol, 3*:564-573, 1960.

Lohrmann, H.-P., Schneider, G., Merten, K., and Tenbaum, A.: Koinzidenz von familiär gehäuft auftretendem Plasmozytom, chronischer lymphatischer Leukämie und Rektumkarzinom. *Blut, 24*:356-364, 1972.

Longsworth, L. G., Shedlovsky, T., and MacInnes, D. A.: Electrophoretic patterns of normal and pathological human blood serum and plasma. *J Exp Med, 70*:399-413, 1939.

Loughrey, J. R., and Meyer, R. L.: Plasmapheresis in hyperviscosity syndrome—a better way? *JAMA, 229*:1211, 1974.

Lowenstein, J., and Gallo, G.: Remission of the nephrotic syndrome in renal amyloidosis. *N Engl J Med, 282*:128-132, 1970.

Lubarsch, O.: Zur Kenntnis ungewöhnlicher Amyloidablagerungen. *Virchows Arch* [Pathol Anat], *271*:867-889, 1929.

Luke, R. G., Allison, M. E. M., Davidson, J. F., and Duguid, W. P.: Hyperkalemia and renal tubular acidosis due to renal amyloidosis. *Ann Intern Med, 70*:1211-1217, 1969.

Lyon, L. W., McCormick, W. F., and Schochet, S. S., Jr.: Progressive multifocal leukoencephalopathy. *Arch Intern Med, 128*:420-426, 1971.

Lyons, R. M., Chaplin, H., Tillack, T. W., and Majerus, P. W.: Gamma heavy chain disease: rapid, sustained response to cyclophosphamide and prednisone. *Blood, 46*:1-9, 1975.

Macintyre, W.: Case of mollities and fragilitas ossium, accompanied with urine strongly charged with animal matter. *Med Chir Trans* (Lond), *33*: 211-232, 1850.

Mackenzie, D. H.: Amyloidosis presenting as lymphadenopathy. *Br Med J, 2*: 1449-1450, 1963.

MacKenzie, M. R., and Babcock, J.: Studies of the hyperviscosity syndrome. II. Macroglobulinemia. *J Lab Clin Med, 85*:227-234, 1975.

MacKenzie, M. R., Brown, E., Fudenberg, H. H., and Goodenday, L.: Waldenström's macroglobulinemia: correlation between expanded plasma volume and increased serum viscosity. *Blood, 35*:394-408, 1970.

MacKenzie, M. R., and Fudenberg, H. H.: Macroglobulinemia: an analysis for forty patients. *Blood, 39*:874-889, 1972.

MacKenzie, M. R., Warner, N., Linscott, D., and Fudenberg, H. H.: Differentiation of human IgM subclass by the ability or inability to interact with C'1 (abstract). *J Lab Clin Med, 72*:993, 1968.

Maeda, K., Abesamis, C. M., Kuhn, L. M., and Hyun, B. H.: Multiple myeloma in childhood: report of a case with breast tumors as a presenting manifestation. *Am J Clin Pathol, 60*:552-558, 1973.

Mäkelä, O., and Cross, A. M.: The diversity and specialization of immunocytes. *Prog Allergy, 14*:145-207, 1970.

Magnus-Levy, A.: Bence-Jones-Eiweiss und Amyloid. *Z Klin Med, 116*:510-531, 1931.

Magnus-Levy, A.: Amyloidosis in multiple myeloma: progress noted in 50 years of personal observation. *Mt Sinai J Med* (NY), *19*:8-9, 1952.

Mahloudji, M., Teasdall, R. D., Adamkiewicz, J. J., Hartmann, W. H., Lambird, P. A., and McKusick, V. A.: The genetic amyloidoses with particular reference to hereditary neuropathic amyloidosis, type II (Indiana or Rukavina type). *Medicine* (Baltimore), *48*:1-37, 1969.

Maize, J. C., Ahmed, A. R., and Provost, T. T.: Xanthoma disseminatum and multiple myeloma. *Arch Dermatol, 110*:758-761, 1974.

Major, D., Meltzer, M. H., Nedwich, A., Hayes, B., and Oaks, W. W.: Waldenström's macroglobulinemia presenting as a pulmonary mass. *Chest, 64*: 760-762, 1973.

Malament, M., Friedman, M., and Pschibul, F.: Amyloidosis of paraplegia. *Arch Phys Med Rehabil, 46*:406-411, 1965.

Maldonado, J. E., Brown, A. L., Jr., Bayrd, E. D., and Pease, G. L.: Ultrastructure of the myeloma cell. *Cancer, 19*:1613-1627, 1966a.

Maldonado, J. E., and Kyle, R. A.: Familial myeloma: report of eight families and a study of serum proteins in their relatives. *Am J Med, 57*:875-884, 1974.

Maldonado, J. E., Kyle, R. A., Brown, A. L., Jr., and Bayrd, E. D.: "Intermediate" cell types and mixed cell proliferation in multiple myeloma: electron microscopic observations. *Blood, 27*:212-226, 1966b.

Maldonado, J. E., Kyle, R. A., Ludwig, J., and Okazaki, H.: Meningeal myeloma. *Arch Intern Med, 126*:660-663, 1970.

Maldonado, J. E., McNutt, D. R., Kyle, R. A., Baggenstoss, A. H., and Fudenberg, H. H.: IgG cryoglobulinemia associated with amyloidosis. *Blood, 41*:569-576, 1973.

Maldonado, J. E., Riggs, B. L., and Bayrd, E. D.: Pseudomyeloma: is association of severe osteoporosis with serum monoclonal gammopathy an entity or a coincidence? *Arch Intern Med, 135*:267-270, 1975a.

Maldonado, J. E., Velosa, J. A., Kyle, R. A., Wagoner, R. D., Holley, K. E., and Salassa, R. M.: Fanconi syndrome in adults: a manifestation of a latent form of myeloma. *Am J Med, 58*:354-364, 1975b.

Malek, R. S., Greene, L. F., and Farrow, G. M.: Amyloidosis of the urinary bladder. *Br J Urol, 43*:189-200, 1971.

Mancini, G., Carbonara, A. O., and Heremans, J. F.: Immunochemical quantitation of antigens by single radial immunodiffusion. *Immunochemistry, 2*:235-254, 1965.

Mangalik, A., and Veliath, A. J.: Osteosclerotic myeloma and peripheral neuropathy: a case report. *Cancer, 28*:1040-1045, 1971.

Mannik, M.: Blood viscosity in Waldenström's macroglobulinemia. *Blood, 44*:87-98, 1974.

Mant, M. J., Hirsh, J., Gauldie, J., Bienenstock, J., Pineo, G. F., and Luke, K. H.: Von Willebrand's syndrome presenting as an acquired bleeding disorder in association with a monoclonal gammopathy. *Blood, 42*:429-436, 1973.

Marcović, N., Hansson, B.-G., and Hällén, J.: Myelomatosis and acute monocytic leukaemia. *Scand J Haematol, 12*:32-36, 1974.

Marien, K. J., and Smeenk, G.: Generalised planar xanthomata associated with multiple myeloma and hyperlipoproteinemia. *Arch Belg Dermatol Syphiligr, 29*:317-318, 1973.

Markel, S. F., and Janich, S. L.: Complexing of lactate dehydrogenase isoenzymes with immunoglobulin A of the kappa class. *Am J Clin Pathol, 61*:328-332, 1974.

Markowitz, H., and Tschida, A. R.: Automated quantitative immunochemical analysis of human immunoglobulins. *Clin Chem, 18*:1364-1367, 1972.

Martelo, O. J., Schultz, D. R., Pardo, V., and Perez-Stable, E.: Immunologically-mediated renal disease in Waldenström's macroglobulinemia. *Am J Med, 58*:567-575, 1975.

Martin, J. H., Brown, A. L., Jr., and Daugherty, G. W.: Renal amyloidosis: a biopsy study. *Am J Med Sci, 251*:129-132, 1966.

Martin, N. H.: Macroglobulinaemia. *Clin Chim Acta, 22*:15-25, 1968.

Martin, W. E., and Heller, P.: Radiation therapy for paraplegia due to multiple myeloma. *JAMA, 191*:247-249, 1965.

Martin, W. J., and Mathieson, D. R.: Pyroglobulinemia (heat-coagulable globulin in the blood). *Proc Staff Meet Mayo Clin, 28*:545-554, 1953.

Martin, W. J., Mathieson, D. R., and Eigler, J. O. C.: Pyroglobulinemia: further observations and review of 20 cases. *Proc Staff Meet Mayo Clin, 34*: 95-101, 1959.

Martinez-Maldonado, M., Yium, J., Suki, W. N., and Eknoyan, G.: Renal complications in multiple myeloma: pathophysiology and some aspects of clinical management. *J Chronic Dis, 24*:221-237, 1971.

Maruyama, Y., and Thomson, J., Jr.: Radiotherapeutic response of plasma cell tumors associated with monoclonal gammopathy. *Cancer, 26*:110-113, 1970.

Massari, R., Fine, J. M., and Metais, R.: Waldenström's macroglobulinaemia observed in two brothers (letter to the editor) . *Nature, 196*:176-178, 1962.

Masterton, G.: Cardiovascular syphilis with amyloidosis and periods of alternating heart block. *Br J Vener Dis, 41*:181-185, 1965.

Mathews, W. H.: Primary systemic amyloidosis. *Am J Med Sci, 228*:317-333, 1954.

Mathison, D. A., Condemi, J. J., Leddy, J. P., Callerame, M. L., Panner, B. J., and Vaughan, J. H.: Purpura, arthralgia, and IgM-IgG cryoglobulinemia with rheumatoid factor activity: response to cyclophosphamide and splenectomy. *Ann Intern Med, 74*:383-390, 1971.

Mawas, C., Sors, C., and Bernier, J.-J.: Amyloidosis associated with primary agammaglobulinemia, severe diarrhea and familial hypogammaglobulinemia. *Am J Med, 46*:624-634, 1969.

Maxwell, M. H., Adams, D. A., and Goldman, R.: Corticosteroid therapy of amyloid nephrotic syndrome. *Ann Intern Med, 60*:539-555, 1964.

Mazzaferri, E. L., and Penn, G. M.: Kaposi's sarcoma associated with multiple myeloma: report of a patient and review of the literature. *Arch Intern Med, 122*:521-525, 1968.

McArthur, J. R., Athens, J. W., Wintrobe, M. M., and Cartwright, G. E.: Melphalan and myeloma: experience with a low-dose continuous regimen. *Ann Intern Med, 72*:665-670, 1970.

McCaffrey, J., Kingston, C. W., and Hacker, W. E.: Extramedullary plasmacytoma of the gastro-intestinal tract. *Aust NZ J Surg, 41*:351-353, 1972.

McCallister, B. D., Bayrd, E. D., Harrison, E. G., Jr., and McGuckin, W. F.: Primary macroglobulinemia: review with a report of thirty-one cases and notes on the value of continuous chlorambucil therapy. *Am J Med, 43*: 394-434, 1967.

McCarthy, J. T., Osserman, E., Lombardo, P. C., and Takatsuki, K.: An abnormal serum globulin in lichen myxedematosus. *Arch Dermatol, 89*:446-450, 1964.

McDougal, J. S., Hardisdangkul, V., and Christian, C. L.: Naturally-occurring low molecular weight IgM in patients with rheumatoid arthritis, systemic lupus erythematosus, and macroglobulinemia. II. Structural studies and comparison of some physicochemical properties of reduced and alkylated IgM, and low molecular weight IgM. *J Immunol, 115*:223-229, 1975.

McIntire, K. R., Asofsky, R. M., Potter, M., and Kuff, E. L.: Macroglobulin-producing plasma-cell tumor in mice: identification of a new light chain. *Science, 150*:361-363, 1965.

McIntire, K. R., and Princler, G. L.: Plasma cell tumors (PCT) in germfree (GF) mice: effect of subcellular extracts (abstract). *Proc Am Assoc Cancer Res, 12*:65, 1971.

McKelvey, E. M., and Kwaan, H. C.: An IgM circulating anticoagulant with Factor VIII inhibitory activity. *Ann Intern Med, 77*:571-575, 1972.

McLauchlan, J.: Solitary myeloma of the clavicle with long survival after total excision: report of a case. *J Bone Joint Surg* [Br], *55*:357-358, 1973.

McNutt, D. R., and Fudenberg, H. H.: IgG myeloma and Waldenström macroglobulinemia: coexistence and clinical manifestations in one patient. *Arch Intern Med, 131*:731-734, 1973.

McPhedran, P., Finch, S. C., Nemerson, Y. R., and Barnes, M. G.: Alpha-2 globulin "spike" in renal carcinoma. *Ann Intern Med, 76*:439-441, 1972a.

McPhedran, P., and Heath, C. W., Jr.: Acute leukemia occurring during chronic lymphocytic leukemia. *Blood, 35*:7-11, 1970.

McPhedran, P., Heath, C. W., Jr., and Garcia, J.: Multiple myeloma incidence in metropolitan Atlanta, Georgia: racial and seasonal variations. *Blood, 39*:866-873, 1972b.

Medical Research Council's Working Party for Therapeutic Trials in Leukaemia: Myelomatosis: comparison of melphalan and cyclophosphamide therapy. *Br Med J, 1*:640-641, 1971.

Medical Research Council's Working Party for Therapeutic Trials in Leukaemia: Report on the first myelomatosis trial. I. Analysis of presenting features of prognostic importance. *Br J Haematol, 24*:123-139, 1973.

Meinke, G. C.: Antigenic studies of J chain (abstract). *Fed Proc, 32*:968, 1973.

Mellstedt, H., and Holm, G.: *In vitro* studies of lymphocytes from patients with plasma cell myeloma. I. Stimulation by mitogens and cytotoxic activities. *Clin Exp Immunol, 15*:309-320, 1973.

Meltzer, L. E., Palmon, F. P., Jr., Paik, Y. K., and Custer, R. P.: Acute pancreatitis secondary to hypercalcemia of multiple myeloma. *Ann Intern Med, 57*:1008-1012, 1962.

Meltzer, M., and Franklin, E. C.: Cryoglobulinemia: a study of twenty-nine patients. I. IgG and IgM cryoglobulins and factors affecting cryoprecipitability. *Am J Med, 40*:828-836, 1966.

Meltzer, M., Franklin, E. C., Elias, K., McCluskey, R. T., and Cooper, N.: Cryoglobulinemia: a clinical and laboratory study. II. Cryoglobulins with rheumatoid factor activity. *Am J Med, 40*:837-856, 1966.

Mestecky, J., and Lawton, A. R. (Eds.): International Symposium on the Immunoglobulin A System, Volume 45: *Advances in Experimental Medicine and Biology*. New York, Plenum Press, 1974, 555 pp.

Mestecky, J., Schrohenloher, R. E., and Kulhavy, R.: J chain attachment to human IgM (abstract). *Fed Proc, 33*:747, 1974.

Meszaros, W. T.: The many facets of multiple myeloma. *Semin Roentgenol, 9*:219-228, 1974.

Metzger, H.: Structure and function of γM macroglobulins. *Adv Immunol, 12*:57-116, 1970.

Meyer, J. E., and Schulz, M. D.: "Solitary" myeloma of bone: a review of 12 cases. *Cancer, 34*:438-440, 1974.

Meyers, B. R., Hirschman, S. Z., and Axelrod, J. A.: Current patterns of infection in multiple myeloma. *Am J Med, 52:*87-92, 1972.

Meytes, D., and Katz, D. R.: Breast cancer and acute leukemia in a patient with multiple myeloma treated with melphalan. *Isr J Med Sci, 9:*1044-1047, 1973.

Michaux, J.-L., and Heremans, J. F.: Thirty cases of monoclonal immunoglobulin disorders other than myeloma or macroglobulinemia: a classification of diseases associated with the production of monoclonal-type immunoglobulins. *Am J Med, 46:*562-579, 1969.

Michels, N. A.: The plasma cell: a critical review of its morphogenesis, function and developmental capacity under normal and under abnormal conditions. *Arch Pathol, 11:*775-793, 1931.

Midwest Cooperative Chemotherapy Group: Multiple myeloma: general aspects of diagnosis, course, and survival. *JAMA, 188:*741-745, 1964.

Migliore, P. J., and Alexanian, R.: Monoclonal gammopathy in human neoplasia. *Cancer, 21:*1127-1131, 1968.

Milham, S., Jr.: Leukemia and multiple myeloma in farmers. *Am J Epidemiol, 94:*307-310, 1971.

Mill, W. B.: Radiation therapy in multiple myeloma. *Radiology, 115:*175-179, 1975.

Millard, L. G.: Generalized plane xanthomata with macroglobulinaemia. *Proc R Soc Med, 66:*325-326, 1973.

Milstein, C., and Pink, J. R. L.: Structure and evolution of immunoglobulins. *Prog Biophys Mol Biol, 21:*209-263, 1970.

Mir-Madjlessi, S. H., Brown, C. H., and Hawk, W. A.: Amyloidosis associated with Crohn's disease. *Am J Gastroenterol, 58:*563-577, 1972a.

Mir-Madjlessi, S. H., Farmer, R. G., and Hawk, W. A., Jr.: Cholestatic jaundice associated with primary amyloidosis. *Cleve Clin Q, 39:*167-175, 1972b.

Missen, G. A. K., and Taylor, J. D.: Amyloidosis in rheumatoid arthritis. *J Pathol Bacteriol, 71:*179-192, 1956.

Missmahl, H.-P.: Reticulin and collagen as important factors for the localization of amyloid: the use of polarization microscopy as a tool in the detection of the composition of amyloid. In Mandema, E., Ruinen, L., Scholten, J. H., and Cohen, A. S. (Eds.): *Symposium on Amyloidosis,* Amsterdam, Excerpta Medica Foundation, 1968, pp. 22-33.

Mitchell, D. N., Rees, R. J. W., and Salsbury, A. J.: Possible transmissibility of human myelomatosis in immunologically deficient mice. *Lancet, 2:* 1009-1012, 1971.

Mitchell, D. N., Rees, R. J. W., and Salsbury, A. J.: Human myeloma marrow cells in immunologically deficient mice. *Br J Cancer, 30:*33-41, 1974.

Mitrou, P., Schubert, J. C. F., and Martin, H.: Die Behandlung der Makroglobulinämie Waldenström mit Procarbazin. *Dtsch Med Wochenschr, 97:* 1864-1869, 1972.

Miturzyńska, H.: Niedoczynność przedniego płata przysadki w przebiegu szpiczaka mnogiego. *Pol Tyg Lek, 17*:224-226, 1962.

Moazzenzadeh, A., Potter, R. T., Castellaneta, C., Westring, D., Son, Y. H., and Perfetto, J. A.: Solitary plasmacytoma of sternum. *NY State J Med, 73*:275-277, 1973.

Moeschlin, S.: Macroglobulinemia Waldenström with miliary lunginfiltrations and terminal plasmacell-leukemia: chlorambucil induced clinical remission despite autoradiographically persistent DNA- and RNA-synthesis. *Acta Med Scand 179* Suppl *445*:154-162, 1966.

Moesner, J., Birkeland, S. A., and Ebbesen, P.: *In vitro* transformation of mouse spleen cells by casein, phytohaemagglutinin and allogeneic cells in casein-induced amyloidosis. *Acta Pathol Microbiol Scand* [B], *82*:287-293, 1974.

Moldow, R. E., Bearman, S., and Edelman, M. H.: Pulmonary amyloidosis simulating tuberculosis. *Am Rev Respir Dis, 105*:114-117, 1972.

Mole, J. E., and Bennett, J. C.: J-chain: amino acid sequence of the C-terminal cyanogen bromide fragment (abstract). *Fed Proc, 33*:747, 1974.

Mole, J. E., Bhown, A. S., and Bennett, J. C.: The primary structure of J chain: sequence analyses of the major proteolytic fragments (abstract). *Fed Proc, 34*:953, 1975.

Montie, J. E., and Stewart, B. H.: Massive bladder hemorrhage after cystoscopy in a patient with secondary systemic amyloidosis. *J Urol, 109*:49-50, 1973.

Moon, J. H., and Edmonson, J. H.: Procarbazine (NSC-77213) and multiple myeloma. *Cancer Chemother Rep, 54*:245-262, 1970.

Moore, D. F., Migliore, P. J., Shullenberger, C. C., and Alexanian, R.: Monoclonal macroglobulinemia in malignant lymphoma. *Ann Intern Med, 72*:43-47, 1970.

Morell, A., Skvaril, F., Hijmans, W., and Scherz, R.: Cytoplasmic immunofluorescence of bone marrow plasma cells producing immunoglobulins of the four IgG subclasses. *J Immunol, 115*:579-583, 1975.

Morell, A., Skvaril, F., Noseda, G., and Barandun, S.: Metabolic properties of human IgA subclasses. *Clin Exp Immunol, 13*:521-528, 1973.

Morell, A., Skvaril, F., Steinberg, A. G., van Loghem, E., and Terry, W. D.: Correlations between the concentrations of the four subclasses of IgG and Gm allotypes in normal human sera. *J Immunol, 108*:195-206, 1972.

Morell, A., Terry, W. D., and Waldmann, T. A.: Metabolic properties of IgG subclasses in man. *J Clin Invest, 49*:673-680, 1970.

Morel-Maroger, L., Basch, A., Danon, F., Verroust, P., and Richet, G.: Pathology of the kidney in Waldenström's macroglobulinemia: study of sixteen cases. *N Engl J Med, 283*:123-129, 1970.

Morgan, C., Jr., and Hammack, W. J.: Intravenous urography in multiple myeloma. *N Engl J Med, 275*:77-79, 1966.

Mork, J. N., Johnson, J. R., Zinneman, H. H., and Bjorgen, J.: Pulmonary alveolar proteinosis associated with IgG monoclonal gammopathy. *Arch Intern Med, 121:*278-283, 1968.

Morley, J. B., and Schwieger, A. C.: The relation between chronic polyneuropathy and osteosclerotic myeloma. *J Neurol Neurosurg Psychiatry, 30:* 432-442, 1967.

Morris, W. T., and Pead, J. L.: Myeloma of the oesophagus. *J Clin Pathol, 25:*537-538, 1972.

Morse, D., Dailey, R. C., and Bunn, J.: Prehistoric multiple myeloma. *Bull NY Acad Med, 50:*447-458, 1974.

Moschella, S. L.: Plane xanthomatosis associated with myelomatosis. *Arch Dermatol, 101:*683-687, 1970.

Muggia, F. M., Heinemann, H. O., Farhangi, M., and Osserman, E. F.: Lysozymuria and renal tubular dysfunction in monocytic and myelomonocytic leukemia. *Am J Med, 47:*351-366, 1969.

Muir, W. A., and Steinberg, A. G.: On the genetics of the human allotypes, Gm and Inv. *Semin Hematol, 4:*156-173, 1967.

Muller, S. A., Sams, W. M., Jr., and Dobson, R. L.: Amyloidosis masquerading as epidermolysis bullosa acquisita. *Arch Dermatol, 99:*739-747, 1969.

Mullinax, F., Himrod, B., and Berry, E. R.: Myeloma protein with specific binding of choline (abstract). *Clin Res, 18:*83, 1970.

Mundy, G. R., and Baikie, A. G.: Myeloma treated with cyclophosphamide and terminating in reticulum cell sarcoma. *Med J Aust, 1:*1240-1241, 1973.

Murphy, W. M., and Deodhar, S. D.: Studies in multiple myeloma. I. Characteristics by immunoglobulin class. *Cleve Clin Q, 40:*1-7, 1973.

Myers, G. H., Jr., and Witten, D. M.: Acute renal failure after excretory urography in multiple myeloma (editorial). *Am J Roentgenol Radium Ther Nucl Med, 113:*583-588, 1971.

Naqvi, M. A., Roach, J. A., and Gyorfi, A. W.: Plasmacytoma of the caecum: case report and review of the literature. *NS Med Bull, 49:*183-188, 1970.

Narasimhan, P., Jagathambal, K., Elizalde, A. M., and Rosner, F.: Chronic lymphocytic leukemia and lymphosarcoma associated with multiple myeloma: report of three cases. *Arch Intern Med, 135:*729-732, 1975.

Nashel, D. J., Widerlite, L. W., and Pekin, T. J., Jr.: IgD myeloma with amyloid arthropathy. *Am J Med, 55:*426-430, 1973.

Natelson, E. A., Duncan, W. C., Macossay, C. R., and Fred, H. L.: Amyloidosis palpebrarum. *Arch Intern Med, 125:*304-307, 1970.

Natvig, J. B., and Kunkel, H. G.: Human immunoglobulins: classes, subclasses, genetic variants, and idiotypes. *Adv Immunol, 16:*1-59, 1973.

Neiman, H. L., Wolson, A. H., and Berenson, J. E.: Pulmonary and pleural manifestations of Waldenström's macroglobulinemia: a case report with a review of the literature. *Radiology, 107:*301-302, 1973.

Neuberg, R.: Immunosuppression and plasmocytoma of the cervix. *J Obstet Gynaecol Br Commonw, 81*:165-167, 1974.

Newell, G. R., Krementz, E. T., Roberts, J. D., and Kinnear, B. K.: Multiple primary neoplasms in blacks compared to whites. I. Further cancers in patients with Hodgkin's disease, leukemia, and myeloma. *J Natl Cancer Inst, 52*:635-638, 1974.

Newmark, S. R., and Himathongkam, T.: Hypercalcemic and hypocalcemic crises. *JAMA, 230*:1438-1439, 1974.

Nielsen, S. M., Schenken, J. R., and Cawley, L. P.: Primary colonic plasmacytoma. *Cancer, 30*:261-267, 1972.

Nishiyama, H., Anderson, R. E., Ishimaru, T., Ishida, K., Ii, Y., and Okabe, N.: The incidence of malignant lymphoma and multiple myeloma in Hiroshima and Nagasaki atomic bomb survivors, 1945-1965. *Cancer, 32*: 1301-1309, 1973.

Nixon, R. K.: The relation of mastocytosis and lymphomatous disease. *Ann Intern Med, 64*:856-860, 1966.

Nomenclature Committee of the IUIS: Notation for human immunoglobulin subclasses. *Bull WHO, 35*:953, 1966.

Nomenclature Committee of the IUIS: Recommendations for the nomenclature of human immunoglobulins. *J Immunol, 108*:1733-1734, 1972.

Noojin, R. O., and Arrington, T. S.: Unusual cutaneous findings in primary systemic amyloidosis: report of a case. *Arch Dermatol, 92*:157-159, 1965.

Noorani, M. A.: Plasmacytoma of middle ear and upper respiratory tract. *J Laryngol Otol, 89*:105-113, 1975.

Nørgaard, O.: Three cases of multiple myeloma in which the preclinical asymptomatic phases persisted throughout 15 to 24 years. *Br J Cancer, 25*: 417-422, 1971.

Northover, J. M. A., Pickard, J. D., Murray-Lyon, M., Presbury, D. G. C., Haskell, R., and Keith, D. A.: Bullous lesions of the skin and mucous membranes in primary amyloidosis. *Postgrad Med J, 48*:351-353, 1972.

Nossal, G. J. V., Warner, N. L., and Lewis, H.: Incidence of cells simultaneously secreting IgM and IgG antibody to sheep erythrocytes. *Cell Immunol, 2*:41-53, 1971.

Oberkircher, P. E., Miller, W. T., and Arger, P. H.: Nonosseous presentation of plasma-cell myeloma. *Radiology, 104*:515-520, 1972.

O'Bryan, R. M., Luce, J. K., Talley, R. W., Gottlieb, J. A., Baker, L. H., and Bonadonna, G.: Phase II evaluation of Adriamycin in human neoplasia. *Cancer, 32*:1-8, 1973.

Odeberg, H., Johansson, B. G., and Berlin, S.-O.: Immunoglobulin analysis in families of myeloma patients. *Acta Med Scand, 196*:361-367, 1974.

Odelberg-Johnson, O.: Osteosclerotic changes in myelomatosis: report of a case. *Acta Radiol* (Stockh), *52*:139-144, 1959.

Österberg, G., and Rausing, A.: Reticulum cell sarcoma in Waldenström's macroglobulinemia after chlorambucil treatment. *Acta Med Scand, 188:* 497-504, 1970.

Özer, F. L., Telatar, H., Telatar, F., and Müftüoğlu, E.: Monoclonal gammopathy with hyperlipidemia. *Am J Med, 49:*841-844, 1970.

Ogawa, M., Kochwa, S., Smith, C., Ishizaka, K., and McIntyre, O. R.: Clinical aspects of IgE myeloma. *N Engl J Med, 281:*1217-1220, 1969.

Ogawa, M., McIntyre, O. R., Ishizaka, K., Ishizaka, T., Terry, W. D., and Waldmann, T. A.: Biologic properties of E myeloma proteins. *Am J Med, 51:*193-199, 1971.

Ogawa, M., Wurster, D. H., and McIntyre, O. R.: Multiple myeloma in one of a pair of monozygotic twins. *Acta Haematol* (Basel), *44:*295-304, 1970.

O'Grady, J. F., and O'Connell, T. C. J.: Primary systemic amyloidosis presenting with severe intestinal haemorrhage. *Ir J Med Sci, 1:*445-448, 1968.

Okano, H., Azar, H. A., and Osserman, E. F.: Plasmacytic reticulum cell sarcoma: case report with electron microscopic studies. *Am J Clin Pathol, 46:* 546-555, 1966.

Oldham, R. K., and Polmar, S. H.: Extramedullary plasmacytomas following successful radiotherapy of Hodgkin's disease: clinical and immunologic aspects. *Am J Med, 54:*761-767, 1973.

Oliai, A., and Koff, R. S.: Primary amyloidosis presenting as "sicca complex" and severe intrahepatic cholestasis. *Am J Dig Dis,* ns, *17:*1033-1036, 1972.

Ooi, B. S., Pesce, A. J., Pollak, V. E., and Mandalenakis, N.: Multiple myeloma with massive proteinuria and terminal renal failure. *Am J Med, 52:* 538-546,1972.

Oriol, R., Huerta, J., Bouvet, J. P., and Liacopoulos, P.: Two myeloma globulins, IgGl-κ and IgGl-λ, from a single patient (Im). I. Purification and immunochemical characterization. *Immunology, 27:*1081-1093, 1974.

Osgood, E. E.: The survival time of patients with plasmocytic myeloma. *Cancer Chemother Rep, 9:*1-10, 1960.

Osserman, E. F.: Amyloidosis and plasma cell dyscrasia. In Grabar, P., and Miescher, P. A. (Eds.): *Immunopathology* (IVth International Symposium). New York, Grune & Stratton, 1965a, pp. 283-293.

Osserman, E. F.: Melphalan and antigenic type of Bence Jones proteins in myeloma. *Science, 149:*564, 1965b.

Osserman, E. F., and Isobe, T.: Lymphoreticular disorders—malignant proliferative response and/or abnormal immunoglobin synthesis—plasma cell dyscrasias. In Williams, W. J., Beutler, E., Erslev, A. J., and Rundles, R. W. (Eds.): *Hematology,* McGraw-Hill Book Company, 1972, pp. 950-956; 977-984.

Osserman, E. F., and Takatsuki, K.: Plasma cell myeloma: gamma globulin synthesis and structure: a review of biochemical and clinical data, with the description of a newly-recognized and related syndrome, "Hγ-2 chain (Franklin's) disease." *Medicine* (Baltimore), *42:*357-384, 1963.

Osserman, E. F., and Takatsuki, K.: Clinical and immunochemical studies of four cases of heavy (Hγ^{-2}) chain disease. *Am J Med, 37*:351-373, 1964.

Osserman, E. F., Takatsuki, K., and Talal, N.: The pathogenesis of "amyloidosis": studies on the role of abnormal gamma globulins and gamma globulin fragments of the Bence Jones (L-polypeptide) type in the pathogenesis of "primary" and "secondary amyloidosis," and the "amyloidosis" associated with plasma cell myeloma. *Semin Hematol, 1*:3-86, 1964.

Osterland, C. K., and Espinoza, L. R.: Biological properties of myeloma proteins. *Arch Intern Med, 135*:32-36, 1975.

Ottó, S., Puskás, É., Medgyesi, G. A., and Gergely, J.: Diclonal and multiple gammopathies. *Haematologia* (Budap), *6*:471-487, 1972.

Ouchterlony, Ö.: Antigen-antibody reactions in gels. IV. Types of reactions in coordinated systems of diffusion. *Acta Pathol Microbiol Scand, 32*:231-240, 1953.

Oxelius, V.-A.: Alternating apperance of IgD and IgG myeloma protein during treatment. *Scand J Haematol, 8*:439-445, 1971.

Ozdemir, A. I., Wright, J. R., and Calkins, E.: Influence of rheumatoid arthritis on amyloidosis of aging: comparison of 47 rheumatoid patients with 47 controls matched for age and sex. *N Engl J Med, 285*:534-538, 1971.

Page, D. L., Isersky, C., Harada, M., and Glenner, G. G.: Immunoglobulin origin of localized nodular pulmonary amyloidosis. *Res Exp Med* (Berl), *159*:75-86, 1972.

Palutke, M., and McDonald, J. M.: Monoclonal gammopathies associated with malignant lymphomas. *Am J Clin Pathol, 60*:157-165, 1973.

Pankovich, A. M., and Griem, M. L.: Plasma-cell myeloma: a thirty-year follow-up. *Radiology, 104*:521-522, 1972.

Paraf, A., Coste, T., Rautureau, J., and Texier, J.: La régression de l'amylose: disparition d'une amylose hépatique massive après nephrectomie pour cancer. *Presse Med, 78*:547-548, 1970.

Paraskevas, F., Heremans, J., and Waldenström, J.: Cytology and electrophoretic pattern in γ_{1A} (β_{2A}) myeloma. *Acta Med Scand, 170*:575-589, 1961.

Park, B. H., and Good, R. A.: *Principles of Modern Immunobiology: Basic and Clinical*. Philadelphia, Lea & Febiger, 1974, pp. 91-107.

Parker, A. C.: A case of acute myelomonocytic leukaemia associated with myelomatosis. *Scand J Haematol, 11*:257-260, 1973.

Parkhouse, R. M. E.: Assembly and secretion of immunoglobulin M (IgM) by plasma cells and lymphocytes. *Transplant Rev, 14*:131-144, 1973.

Parkhouse, R. M. E.: Non-covalent association of IgM subunits produced by reduction and alkylation. *Immunology, 27*:1063-1071, 1974.

Parr, D. M., Connell, G. E., Powell, A. J., and Pruzanski, W.: A pathologic IgM occurring in serum as pentamer, dimer, and monomer. *J Immunol, 113*:2020-2026, 1974.

Parr, D. M., Pruzanski, W., Scott, J. G., and Mills, D. M.: Primary amyloidosis with plasmacytic dyscrasia and a tetramer of Bence Jones type lambda globulin in the serum and urine. *Blood, 37*:473-484, 1971.

Pascoe, H. R., and Dorfman, R. F.: Extramedullary plasmacytoma of the submaxillary gland. *Am J Clin Pathol, 51*:501-507, 1969.

Pasmantier, M. W., and Azar, H. A.: Extraskeletal spread in multiple plasma cell myeloma: a review of 57 autopsied cases. *Cancer, 23*:167-174, 1969.

Patterson, R., Weiszer, I., Rambach, W., Roberts, M., and Suszko, I. M.: Comparative cellular and immunochemical studies of two cases of pyroglobulinemia. *Am J Med, 44*:147-153, 1968.

Paulsen, S.: Multinodular stenosing cardiovascular amyloidosis with involvement of the conductive tissue. *Acta Pathol Microbiol Scand* [A], *82*:514-518, 1974.

Payne, R. B.: A red herring in the detection of Bence-Jones protein (letter to the editor). *J Clin Pathol, 25*:183, 1972.

Payne, R. B., Little, A. J., Williams, R. B., and Milner, J. R.: Interpretation of serum calcium in patients with abnormal serum proteins. *Br Med J, 4*: 643-646, 1973.

Pengelly, C. D. R., Mondal, B. K., and Barua, A. R.: Haemolytic anaemia in myelomatosis. *Postgrad Med J, 49*:279-281, 1973.

Penman, H. G., and Thomson, K. J.: Amyloidosis and renal adenocarcinoma: a post-mortem study. *J Pathol, 107*:45-47, 1972.

Penn, G. M., Cawley, L. P., and O'Grady, J.: Antigenic differences between monoclonal IgA proteins: IgA subclass or deletion. *Am J Clin Pathol, 62*: 143, 1974.

Penn, I., Halgrimson, C. G., and Starzl, T. E.: De novo malignant tumors in organ transplant recipients. *Transplant Proc, 3*:773-778, 1971.

Penny, R., Castaldi, P. A., and Whitsed, H. M.: Inflammation and haemostasis in paraproteinaemias. *Br J Haematol, 20*:35-44, 1971.

Penny, R., and Hughes, S.: Repeated stimulation of the reticuloendothelial system and the development of plasma-cell dyscrasias. *Lancet, 1*:77-78, 1970.

Perkins, H. A., MacKenzie, M. R., and Fudenberg, H. H.: Hemostatic defects in dysproteinemias. *Blood, 35*:695-707, 1970.

Perlman, M., and Walker, R.: Acute leukemia following cytotoxic chemotherapy (letter to the editor). *JAMA, 224*:250, 1973.

Perlzweig, W. A., Delrue, G., and Geschickter, C.: Hyperproteinemia associated with multiple myelomas: report of an unusual case. *JAMA, 90*:755-757, 1928.

Pernis, B., and Chiappino, G.: Identification in human lymphoid tissues of cells that produce group 1 or group 2 gamma-globulins. *Immunology, 7*: 500-506, 1964.

Perry, H. O., Montgomery, H., and Stickney, J. M.: Further observations on lichen myxedematosus. *Ann Intern Med, 53*:955-969, 1960.

Perry, M. C.: Personal communication.

Perry, M. C., and Kyle, R. A.: The clinical significance of Bence Jones proteinuria. *Mayo Clin Proc, 50:*234-238, 1975.

Peters, H. A., and Clatanoff, D. V.: Spinal muscular atrophy secondary to macroglobulinemia: reversal of symptoms with chlorambucil therapy. *Neurology* (Minneap), *18:*101-108, 1968.

Petersen, H. S.: Erythroleukaemia in a melphalan-treated patient with primary macroglobulinaemia. *Scand J Haematol, 10:*5-11, 1973a.

Petersen, H. S.: Waldenström's macroglobulinaemia with xanthomatosis and hypercholesterolaemia: report of a case. *Acta Med Scand, 193:*573-576, 1973b.

Pettersson, T., and Wegelius, O.: Biopsy diagnosis of amyloidosis in rheumatoid arthritis: malabsorption caused by intestinal amyloid deposits. *Gastroenterology, 62:*22-27, 1972.

Philips, E. D., El-Mahdi, A. M., Humphrey, R. L., and Furlong, M. B., Jr.: The effect of the radiation treatment on the polyneuropathy of multiple myeloma. *J Can Assoc Radiol, 23:*103-106, 1972.

Pike, I. M., Yount, W. J., Puritz, E. M., and Roberts, H. R.: Immunochemical characterization of a monoclonal γG4, λ human antibody to Factor IX. *Blood, 40:*1-10, 1972.

Pindyck, J., Lichtman, H. C., and Kohl, S. G.: Cryofibrinogenaemia in women using oral contraceptives. *Lancet, 1:*51-53, 1970.

Pinkhas, J., Djaldetti, M., and Yaron, M.: Coincidence of multiple myeloma with Gaucher's disease. *Isr J Med Sci, 1:*537-540, 1965.

Pirofsky, B.: *Autoimmunization and the Autoimmune Hemolytic Anemias.* Baltimore, Williams & Wilkins Company, 1969, pp. 127-131.

Pittman, F. E., Tripathy, K., Isobe, T., Bolaños, O. M., Osserman, E. F., Pittman, J. C., Lotero, H. R., and Duque, E. E.: IgA heavy chain disease: a case detected in the western hemisphere. *Am J Med, 58:*424-430, 1975.

Pitts, N. C., and McDuffie, F. C.: Defective synthesis of IgM antibodies in macroglobulinemia. *Blood, 30:*767-771, 1967.

Plaut, A. G., Wistar, R., Jr., and Capra, J. D.: Differential susceptibility of human IgA immunoglobulins to streptococcal IgA protease. *J Clin Invest, 54:*1295-1300, 1974.

Poger, M. E., and Lamm, M. E.: Localization of free and bound secretory component in human intestinal epithelial cells: a model for the assembly of secretory IgA. *J Exp Med, 139:*629-642, 1974.

Polliack, A., and Hershko, C.: Spontaneous rupture of the spleen in amyloidosis. *Isr J Med Sci, 8:*57-60, 1972.

Polliack, A., Laufer, A., George, R., and Fields, M.: The effect of cortisone on the formation and resorption of experimental amyloid. *Br J Exp Pathol, 54:*6-12, 1973.

Polliack, A., Rachmilewitz, D., and Zlotnick, A.: Plasma cell leukemia: unassembled light and heavy chains in the urine. *Arch Intern Med, 134*:131-134, 1974.

Pope, R. M., Fletcher, M. A., Mamby, A., and Shapiro, C. M.: Rheumatoid arthritis associated with hyperviscosity syndrome and intermediate complex formation. *Arch Intern Med, 135*:281-285, 1975.

Porter, D. D., Dixon, F. J., and Larsen, A. E.: The development of a myeloma-like condition in mink with Aleutian disease. *Blood, 25*:736-742, 1965.

Porter, F. S., Jr.: Multiple myeloma in a child. *J Pediatr, 62*:602-604, 1963.

Porter, R. R.: The structure of antibodies. *Sci Am, 217*:81-90, 1967.

Porter, R. R.: Structural studies of immunoglobulins. *Science, 180*:713-716, 1973.

Poth, J. L., and George, R. P.: Hemorrhagic ascites: an unusual complication of multiple myeloma. *Calif Med, 115*:61-64, Sept. 1971.

Potter, M.: Myeloma proteins (M-components) with antibody-like activity. *N Engl J Med, 284*:831-838, 1971.

Potter, M.: Experimental plasma cell tumors and other immunoglobin-producing lymphoreticular neoplasms in mice. In Azar, H. A., and Potter, M. (Eds.) : *Multiple Myeloma and Related Disorders,* Vol 1. Hagerstown, Maryland, Harper & Row, Publishers, 1973a, pp. 153-194.

Potter, M.: The developmental history of the neoplastic plasma cell in mice: a brief review of recent developments. *Semin Hematol, 10*:19-32, 1973b.

Potter, M., Sklar, M. D., and Rowe, W. P.: Rapid viral induction of plasmacytomas in pristane-primed BALB/c mice. *Science, 182*:592-594, 1973.

Poulik, M. D., Berman, L., and Prasad, A. S.: "Myeloma protein" in a patient with monocytic leukemia. *Blood, 33*:746-758, 1969.

Powles, R., Smith, C., Kohn, J., and Fairley, G. H.: Method of removing abnormal protein rapidly from patients with malignant paraproteinaemias. *Br Med J, 3*:664-667, 1971.

Pratt, P. W., Estren, S., and Kochwa, S.: Immunoglobulin abnormalities in Gaucher's disease: report of 16 cases. *Blood, 31*:633-640, 1968.

Prentice, C. R. M., Izatt, M. M., Adams, J. F., McNicol, G. P., and Douglas, A. S.: Amyloidosis associated with the nephrotic syndrome and transfusion reactions in a haemophiliac. *Br J Haematol, 21*:305-311, 1971.

Preud'homme, J.-L., Buxbaum, J., and Scharff, M. D.: Mutagenesis of mouse myeloma cells with "melphalan." *Nature, 245*:320-322, 1973.

Preuss, H. G., Weiss, F. R., Iammarino, R. M., Hammack, W. J., and Murdaugh, H. V., Jr.: Effects on rat kidney slice function *in vitro* of proteins from the urines of patients with myelomatosis and nephrosis. *Clin Sci Mol Med, 46*:283-294, 1974.

Priester, W. A., and Mason, T. J.: Human cancer mortality in relation to poultry population, by county, in 10 southeastern states. *J Natl Cancer Inst, 53*:45-49, 1974.

Pringle, J. P., Graham, R. C., and Bernier, G. M.: Detection of myeloma cells in the urine sediment. *Blood, 43*:137-143, 1974.

Prowse, C. B.: Amyloidosis of the lower respiratory tract. *Thorax, 13*:308-320, 1958.

Pruzanski, W., Katz, A., Nyburg, S. C., and Freedman, M. H.: *In vitro* production of an amyloid-like substance from γ_3 heavy chain disease protein. *Immunol Commun, 3*:469-476, 1974a.

Pruzanski, W., Platts, M. E., and Ogryzlo, M. A.: Leukemic form of immunocytic dyscrasia (plasma cell leukemia): a study of ten cases and a review of the literature. *Am J Med, 47*:60-74, 1969.

Pruzanski, W., Underdown, B., Silver, E. H., and Katz, A.: Macroglobulinemia-myeloma double gammopathy: a study of four cases and a review of the literature. *Am J Med, 57*:259-266, 1974b.

Pruzanski, W., Warren, R. E., Goldie, J. H., and Katz, A.: Malabsorption syndrome with infiltration of the intestinal wall by extracellular monoclonal macroglobulin. *Am J Med, 54*:811-818, 1973.

Pruzanski, W., and Watt, J. G.: Serum viscosity and hyperviscosity syndrome in IgG multiple myeloma: report on 10 patients and a review of the literature. *Ann Intern Med, 77*:853-860, 1972.

Putnam, F. W.: Immunoglobulin structure: variability and homology. *Science, 163*:633-644, 1969.

Putnam, F. W., Easley, C. W., Lynn, L. T., Ritchie, A. E., and Phelps, R. A.: The heat precipitation of Bence-Jones proteins. I. Optimum conditions. *Arch Biochem Biophys, 83*:115-130, 1959.

Putnam, F. W., Florent, G., Paul, C., Shinoda, T., and Shimizu, A.: Complete amino acid sequence of the mu heavy chain of a human IgM immunoglobulin. *Science, 182*:287-291, 1973.

Putnam, F. W., and Hardy, S.: Proteins in multiple myeloma. III. Origin of Bence-Jones protein. *J Biol Chem, 212*:361-369, 1955.

Queisser, W., Hoelzer, D., and Queisser, U.: Cytophotometrisch-autoradiographische Untersuchung der Zellproliferation bei paraproteinämischen Hämoblastosen mit leukämischen Blutbildveränderungen. *Klin Wochenschr, 51*:230-234, 1973.

Raab, E. L.: Intraorbital amyloid. *Br J Ophthalmol, 54*:445-449, 1970.

Rabiner, S. F., Aprill, S. N., and Radner, D. B.: Waldenström's macroglobulinemia: report of a case with pulmonary involvement and improvement in pulmonary symptoms only following chlorambucil therapy. *Am J Med, 53*:685-689, 1972.

Rachmilewitz, E. A., Sacks, M. I., and Zlotnick, A.: Essential cryofibrinogenemia: clinical, pathological and immunological studies. *Isr J Med Sci, 6*:32-43, 1970.

Rádl, J., and Hollander, C. F.: Homogeneous immunoglobulins in sera of mice during aging. *J Immunol, 112*:2271-2273, 1974.

Rádl, J., and Masopust, J.: Idiopathische Paraproteinämie. *Schweiz Med Wochenschr, 94*:961-967, 1964.

Rajan, V. T., and Kikkawa, Y.: Alveolar septal amyloidosis in primary amyloidosis: an electron microscopic study. *Arch Pathol, 89*:521-525, 1970.

Ramot, B., and Salomi, M.: Myelomatosis (letter to the editor). *Lancet, 2*: 725, 1961.

Randall, R. E., Jr., Still, W. J. S., Tung, M. Y., Jain, U., Lomvardias, S., Bear, E. S., and Moncure, C. W.: Multiple organ disease from light-chain deposition (abstract). *J Clin Invest, 54*:77a, 1972.

Rebuck, J. W., and Crowley, J. H.: A method of studying leukocytic functions *in vivo*. *Ann NY Acad Sci, 59*:757-794, 1955.

Redleaf, P. D., Davis, R. B., Kucinski, C., Hoilund, L., and Gans, H.: Amyloidosis with an unusual bleeding diathesis: observations on the use of epsilon amino caproic acid. *Ann Intern Med, 58*:347-354, 1963.

Rees, E. D., and Waugh, W. H.: Factors in the renal failure of multiple myeloma. *Arch Intern Med, 116*:400-405, 1965.

Reimann, H. A., Koucky, R. F., and Eklund, C. M.: Primary amyloidosis limited to tissue of mesodermal origin. *Am J Pathol, 11*:977-988, 1935.

Remigio, P. A., and Klaum, A.: Extramedullary plasmacytoma of stomach. *Cancer, 27*:562-568, 1971.

Renal Transplant Registry: Renal transplantation in congenital and metabolic diseases: a report from the ASC/NIH renal transplant registry. *JAMA, 232*:148-153, 1975.

Renner, R. R., and Smith, J. R.: Plasma cell dyscrasias (except myeloma). *Semin Roentgenol, 9*:209-218, 1974.

Richards, A. I., and Hines, J. D.: Recovery from acute renal failure in plasma cell leukemia: case report. *Am J Med Sci, 266*:293-297, 1973.

Richards, F. F., Konigsberg, W. H., Rosenstein, R. W., and Varga, J. M.: On the specificity of antibodies. *Science, 187*:130-137, 1975.

Ricks, J., Robinson, J. D., Sachs, D. H., and Terry, W. D.: Radioimmunoassay for myeloma idiotype (abstract). *Clin Res, 23*:281A, 1975.

Ritzmann, S. E., Loukas, D., Sakai, H., Daniels, J. C., and Levin, W. C.: Idiopathic (asymptomatic) monoclonal gammopathies. *Arch Intern Med, 135*: 95-106, 1975.

Ritzmann, S. E., Stoufflet, E. J., Houston, E. W., and Levin, W. C.: Coexistent chronic myelocytic leukemia, monoclonal gammopathy and multiple chromosomal abnormalities. *Am J Med, 41*:981-989, 1966.

Ritzmann, S. E., Thurm, R. H., Truax, W. E., and Levin, W. C.: The syndrome of macroglobulinemia: review of the literature and a report of two cases of macrocryogelglobulinemia. *Arch Intern Med, 105*:939-965, 1960.

Ritzmann, S. E., Wolf, R. E., Lawrence, M. C., Hart, J. S., and Levin, W. C.:

The Sia euglobulin test: a re-evaluation. *J Lab Clin Med, 73*:698-705, 1969.

Rivat, C., Ropartz, C., and Rowe, D. S.: Antigenic heterogeneity of human IgD immunoglobulins (letter to the editor). *Nature* [New Biol], *231:* 279-280, 1971.

River, G. L., and Schorr, W. F.: Malignant skin tumors in multiple myeloma. *Arch Dermatol, 93*:432-438, 1966.

Rivers, S. L., and Patno, M. E.: Cyclophosphamide vs melphalan in treatment of plasma cell myeloma. *JAMA, 207*:1328-1334, 1969.

Robboy, S. J., Lewis, E. J., Schur, P. H., and Colman, R. W.: Circulating anticoagulants to Factor VIII: immunochemical studies and clinical response to Factor VIII concentrates. *Am J Med, 49*:742-752, 1970.

Roberts, M., Rinaudo, P. A., Vilinskas, J., and Owens, G.: Solitary sclerosing plasma-cell myeloma of the spine: case report. *J Neurosurg, 40*:125-129, 1974.

Rodman, H. I., and Font, R. L.: Orbital involvement in multiple myeloma: review of the literature and report of three cases. *Arch Ophthalmol, 87:* 30-35, 1972.

Rodriguez, L. H., Finkelstein, J. B., Shullenberger, C. C., and Alexanian, R.: Bone healing in multiple myeloma with melphalan chemotherapy. *Ann Intern Med, 76*:551-556, 1972.

Rogers, D. R.: Screening for amyloid with the thioflavin-T fluorescent method. *Am J Clin Pathol, 44*:59-61, 1965.

Romhányi, G.: Selective differentiation between amyloid and connective tissue structures based on the collagen specific topo-optical staining reaction with Congo red. *Virchows Arch* [Pathol Anat], *354*:209-222, 1971.

Romhányi, G.: Differences in ultrastructural organization of amyloid as revealed by sensitivity or resistance to induced proteolysis. *Virchows Arch* [Pathol Anat], *357*:29-52, 1972.

Ronis, M. L., Rojer, C. L., and Ronis, B. J.: Otologic manifestations of Waldenström's macroglobulinemia. *Laryngoscope, 76*:513-523, 1966.

Ropars, C., Doinel, C., and Saleun, J. P.: Fixation of albumin to the hinge region of a macroglobulin. *Biomedicine* [Express], *19*:228-230, 1973.

Ropars, C., Saleun, J. P., Bergeret, G., and Doinel, C.: Dissociable IgM-albumin interaction in a case of Waldenström's macroglobulinemia. *Rev Eur Etud Clin Biol, 17*:854-859, 1972.

Rosen, B. J., Smith, T. W., and Bloch, K. J.: Multiple myeloma associated with two serum M components, γG type K and γA type L. *N Engl J Med, 277*:902-907, 1967a.

Rosen, F. S.: The macroglobulins. *N Engl J Med, 267*:491-497; 546-550, 1962.

Rosen, S., Cortell, S., Adner, M. M., Papadopoulos, N. M., and Barry, K. G.: Multiple myeloma and the nephrotic syndrome: a biochemical and morphologic study. *Am J Clin Pathol, 47*:567-579, 1967b.

Rosenbaum, A. E., Zingesser, L. H., Reiss, J. H., Schechter, M. M., and Sanders, C. D.: Myeloma: unusual cause of exophthalmos: an angioarchitectural study. *Radiology, 94*:379-386, 1970

Rosenberg, B., Attie, J. N., and Mandelbaum, H. L.: Breast tumor as the presenting sign of multiple myeloma. *N Engl J Med, 269*:359-361, 1963.

Rosenbloom, J.: An appreciation of Henry Bence Jones (1814-1873). *Ann Med Hist, 2*:262-264, 1919.

Rosenblum, W. I.: Vasoconstriction, blood viscosity, and erythrocyte aggregation in macroglobulinemic and polycythemic mice. *J Lab Clin Med, 73:* 359-365, 1969.

Rosenblum, W. I., and Asofsky, R. M.: Factors affecting blood viscosity in macroglobulinemic mice. *J Lab Clin Med, 71*:201-211, 1968.

Rosenthal, C. J., and Franklin, E. C.: Variation with age and disease of an amyloid A protein-related serum component. *J Clin Invest 55*:746-753, 1975.

Rosenthal, T., Bank, H., Aladjem, M., David, R., and Gafni, J.: Systemic amyloidosis in Behçet's disease. *Ann Intern Med, 83*:220-223, 1975.

Rosner, F., and Grünwald, H. (For Acute Leukemia Group B) : Multiple myeloma terminating in acute leukemia: report of 12 cases and review of the literature. *Am J Med, 57*:927-939, 1974.

Rosner, F., Soong, B. C., Krim, M., and Miller, S. P.: Normal pregnancy in a patient with multiple myeloma. *Obstet Gynecol, 31*:811-820, 1968.

Rowe, D. S., and Fahey, J. L.: A new class of human immunoglobulins. I. A unique myeloma protein. *J Exp Med, 121*:171-184, 1965.

Rowland, L. P., Osserman, E. F., Scharfman, W. B., Balsam, R. F., and Ball, S.: Myasthenia gravis with a myeloma-type, gamma-G (IgG) immunoglobulin abnormality. *Am J Med, 46*:599-605, 1969.

Ruben, R. J., Distenfeld, A., Berg, P., and Carr, R.: Sudden sequential deafness as the presenting symptom of macroglobulinemia. *JAMA, 209*:1364-1365, 1969.

Rubies-Prat, J., Gallart, M. T., Frison, J. C., Caralps, A., Schwartz, S., and Bacardi, R.: IgG myeloma, Sia test, and serum hyperviscosity. *Acta Haematol* (Basel), *52*:107-111, 1974.

Rudders, R. A., and Bloch, K. J.: Myeloma renal disease: evaluation of the role of muramidase (lysozyme). *Am J Med Sci, 262*:79-85, 1971.

Rukavina, J. G., Block, W. D., Jackson, C. E., Falls, H. F., Carey, J. H., and Curtis, A. C.: Primary systemic amyloidosis: a review and an experimental, genetic, and clinical study of 29 cases with particular emphasis on the familial form. *Medicine* (Baltimore), *35*:239-334, 1956.

Rustizky, J.: Multiples myelom. *Dtsch Z Chir, 3*:162-172, 1873.

Rywlin, A. M., Civantos, F., Ortega, R. S., and Dominguez, C. J.: Bone marrow histology in monoclonal macroglobulinemia. *Am J Clin Pathol, 63:* 769-778, 1975.

Sadeghee, S. A., and Moore, S. W.: Rheumatoid arthritis, bilateral amyloid tumors of the breast, and multiple cutaneous amyloid nodules. *Am J Clin Pathol, 62:*472-476, 1974.

Safa, A. M., and Van Ordstrand, H. S.: Pleural effusion due to multiple myeloma. *Chest, 64:*246-248, 1973.

Saidi, P., Uhlman, W. E., and Goldberg, I.: Herpes zoster and multiple myeloma. *J Med Soc NJ, 70:*836-838, 1973.

Sakalová, A., Gažová, S., Hrubiško, M., and Gáliková, J.: Clinical utilization of plasmapheresis and cyclophosphamide in the treatment of malignant lymphoproliferative processes. *Neoplasma, 20:*335-339, 1973.

Salmon, S. E.: Immunoglobulin synthesis and tumor kinetics of multiple myeloma. *Semin Hematol, 10:*135-147, 1973.

Salmon, S. E.: Expansion of the growth fraction in multiple myeloma with alkylating agents. *Blood, 45:*119-129, 1975.

Salmon, S. E., and Durie, B. G. M.: Cellular kinetics in multiple myeloma: a new approach to staging and treatment. *Arch Intern Med, 135:*131-138, 1975.

Salmon, S. E., and Fudenberg, H. H.: Abnormal nucleic acid metabolism of lymphocytes in plasma cell myeloma and macroglobulinemia. *Blood, 33:* 300-312, 1969.

Salmon, S. E., Samal, B. A., Hayes, D. M., Hosley, H., Miller, S. P., and Schilling, A.: Role of gamma globulin for immunoprophylaxis in multiple myeloma. *N Engl J Med, 277:*1336-1340, 1967.

Salmon, S. E., and Seligmann, M.: B-cell neoplasia in man. *Lancet, 2:*1230-1233, 1974.

Salmon, S. E., and Smith, B. A.: Immunoglobulin synthesis and total body tumor cell number in IgG multiple myeloma. *J Clin Invest, 49:*1114-1121, 1970.

Sanchez-Avalos, J., Soong, B. C. F., and Miller, S. P.: Coagulation disorders in cancer. II. Multiple myeloma. *Cancer, 23:*1388-1398, 1969.

Sander, S.: Whipple's disease associated with amyloidosis. *Acta Pathol Microbiol Scand, 61:*530-536, 1964.

Sanders, J. H., Fahey, J. L., Finegold, I., Ein, D., Reisfeld, R., and Berard, C.: Multiple anomalous immunoglobulins: clinical, structural and cellular studies in three patients. *Am J Med, 47:*43-59, 1969.

Sanders, T. E., Podos, S. M., and Rosenbaum, L. J.: Intraocular manifestations of multiple myeloma. *Arch Ophthalmol, 77:*789-794, 1967.

Santos, G. W.: Immunosuppressive drugs. *Fed Proc, 26:*907-913, 1967.

Satyanarayana, B. V., Raju, P. S., Kumari, K. R., and Reddy, C. R. R. M.: Amyloidosis in leprosy. *Int J Lepr, 40:*278-280, 1972.

Sawkar, L. A.: Familial xanthelasma, hyperlipidemia and multiple myeloma. *J Assoc Physicians India, 19:*329-334, 1971.

Sawkar, L. A.: Hyperviscosity syndrome in acute plasma cell leukaemia. *J Assoc Physicians India, 20:*397-402, 1972.

Scheinberg, M., Cathcart, E. S., and Goldstein, A. L.: Suppression of amyloid disease in the mouse by thymosin treatment (abstract). *Clin Res, 23:*296A, 1975.

Scheinberg, M. A., and Cathcart, E. S.: Casein-induced experimental amyloidosis. III. Response to mitogens, allogeneic cells, and graft-versus-host reactions in the murine model. *Immunology, 27:*953-963, 1974.

Scheinberg, M. A., and Cathcart, E . S.: Amyloid disease and polyclonal B cell activation (abstract). *Clin Res, 23:*342A, 1975.

Schilling, A., and Finkel, H. E.: Ancillary measures in treatment of myeloma: use of immune serum globulin, fluoride, or androgen. *Arch Intern Med, 135:*193-196, 1975.

Schimke, R. N., Hartmann, W. H., Prout, T. E., and Rimoin, D. L.: Syndrome of bilateral pheochromocytoma, medullary thyroid carcinoma and multiple neuromas: a possible regulatory defect in the differentiation of chromaffin tissue. *N Engl J Med, 279:*1-7, 1968.

Schlenker, J. D., Vega, G., and Heiple, K. G.: Clostridium pyoarthritis of the shoulder associated with multiple myeloma. *Clin Orthop, 88:*89-91, 1972.

Schmidt, H. W., McDonald, J. R., and Clagett, O. T.: Amyloid tumors of the lower part of the respiratory tract and mediastinum. *Ann Otol Rhinol Laryngol, 62:*880-891, 1953.

Schneck, S. A., and Penn, I.: De-novo brain tumours in renal-transplant recipients. *Lancet, 1:*983-986, 1971.

Schroeder, J. S., Billingham, M. E., and Rider, A. K.: Cardiac amyloidosis: diagnosis by transvenous endomyocardial biopsy. *Am J Med, 59:*269-273, 1975.

Schubert, G. E., and Adam, A.: Glomerular nodules and long-spacing collagen in kidneys of patients with multiple myeloma. *J Clin Pathol, 27:*800-805, 1974.

Schubert, G. E., Veigel, J., and Lennert, K.: Structure and function of the kidney in multiple myeloma. *Virchows Arch* [Pathol Anat], *355:*135-157, 1972.

Schur, P. H.: Human gamma-G subclasses. *Prog Clin Immunol, 1:*71-104, 1972.

Schur, P. H., and Appel, L.: Waldenström's macroglobulinemia with pleural effusion. *NY State J Med, 61:*2431-2439, 1961.

Schur, P. H., Kyle, R. A., Bloch, K. J., Hammack, W. J., Rivers, S. L., Sargent, A., Ritchie, R. F., McIntyre, O. R., Moloney, W. C., and Wolfson, L.: IgG subclasses: relationship to clinical aspects of multiple myeloma and frequency distribution among M-components. *Scand J Haematol, 12:* 60-68, 1974.

Schwartz, H. C., and Olson, D. J.: Amyloidosis: a rational approach to diagnosis by intraoral biopsy. *Oral Surg, 39:*837-843, 1975.

Schwartz, P.: Senile cerebral, pancreatic insular and cardiac amyloidosis. *Trans NY Acad Sci, 27:*393-413, 1965.

Schwartz, P.: *Amyloidosis: Cause and Manifestation of Senile Deterioration.* Springfield, Illinois, Charles C Thomas, Publisher, 1970.

Scott, R. B., Elmore, S. M., Brackett, N. C., Jr., Harris, W. O., Jr., and Still, W. J. S.: Neuropathic joint disease (Charcot joints) in Waldenström's macroglobulinemia with amyloidosis. *Am J Med, 54:*535-538, 1973.

Scurr, J. A.: Myeloma occurring in Paget's disease. *Proc R Soc Med, 65:*725, 1972.

Sebastian, A., McSherry, E., Ueki, I., and Morris, R. C., Jr.: Renal amyloidosis, nephrotic syndrome, and impaired renal tubular reabsorption of bicarbonate. *Ann Intern Med, 69:*541-548, 1968.

Seibert, D. J., Hayes, D. M., Cooper, T., Blom, J., and Ebaugh, F. G., Jr.: Intravenous urethane (ethyl carbamate) therapy of multiple myeloma: from the Acute Leukemia Group B. *Cancer, 19:*710-712, 1966.

Seligmann, M.: Alpha chain disease: immunoglobulin abnormalities, pathogenesis and current concepts. *Br J Cancer 31* Suppl *2:*356-361, 1975a.

Seligmann, M.: Immunochemical, clinical, and pathological features of α-chain disease. *Arch Intern Med, 135:*78-82, 1975b.

Seligmann, M., and Basch, A.: The clinical significance of pathological immunoglobulins. In *XII Congress of the International Society of Hematology,* New York, 1968, pp. 21-31.

Seligmann, M., and Brouet, J. C.: Antibody activity of human myeloma globulins. *Semin Hematol, 10:*163-177, 1973.

Seligmann, M., Danon, F., Hurez, D., Mihaesco, E., and Preud'homme, J.-L.: Alpha-chain disease: a new immunoglobulin abnormality. *Science, 162:* 1396-1397, 1968.

Seligmann, M., Danon, F., Mihaesco, C., and Fudenberg, H. H.: Immunoglobulin abnormalities in families of patients with Waldenström's macroglobulinemia. *Am J Med, 43:*66-83, 1967.

Seligmann, M., Mihaesco, E., and Frangione, B.: Studies on alpha chain disease. *Ann NY Acad Sci, 190:*487-500, 1971.

Seligmann, M., Sassy, C., and Chevalier, A.: A human IgG myeloma protein with anti-$\alpha 2$ macroglobulin antibody activity. *J Immunol, 110:*85-90, 1973.

Selroos, O.: Thrombocytosis. *Acta Med Scand, 193:*431-436, 1973.

Selroos, O., Brander, L., and Virolainen, M.: Sarcoidosis and myeloma of lambda-type IgG. *Acta Med Scand, 195:*59-63, 1974.

Selroos, O., and von Knorring, J.: Immunoglobulins in pernicious anaemia: including a report on a patient with pernicious anaemia, IgA deficiency and an M component of kappa-type IgG. *Acta Med Scand, 194:*571-574, 1973.

Seon, B.-K., Yagi, Y., and Pressman, D.: Comparative chemical study of α- and μ-chains from a single patient (SC). *J Immunol, 111*:1285-1287, 1973.

Shaheen, N. A., Salman, S. D., and Nassar, V. H.: Fatal bronchopulmonary hemorrhage due to unrecognized amyloidosis. *Arch Otolaryngol, 101*:259-261, 1975.

Shahid, M. J., Alami, S. Y., Nassar, V. H., Balikian, J. B., and Salem, A. A.: Primary intestinal lymphoma with paraproteinemia. *Cancer, 35*:848-858, 1975.

Shanbrom, E.: Multiple myeloma and coexistent carcinoma of the sigmoid colon: a review of the literature and report of four cases. *Am J Clin Pathol, 40*:67-71, 1963.

Shanbrom, E., Miller, S., and Haar, H.: Herpes zoster in hematologic neoplasias: some unusual manifestations. *Ann Intern Med, 53*:523-533, 1960.

Shapiro, S. S.: Characterization of Factor VIII antibodies. *Ann NY Acad Sci, 240*:350-360, 1975.

Shapiro, S. T., Kohut, R. I., and Potter, J. M.: Amyloid goiter: new associations and surgical treatment. *Arch Otolaryngol, 93*:203-208, 1971.

Sharma, H. M., and Geer, J. C.: Multiple transfusions with sensitization associated with amyloidosis: report of a case. *Arch Pathol, 89*:473-476, 1970.

Shaw, M. T., Twele, T. W., and Nordquist, R. E.: Plasma cell leukemia: detailed studies and response to therapy. *Cancer, 33*:619-625, 1974.

Shearn, M. A., Epstein, W. V., and Engleman, E. P.: Serum viscosity in rheumatic diseases and macroglobulinemia. *Arch Intern Med, 112*:684-687, 1963.

Shirahama, T., Benson, M. D., Cohen, A. S., and Tanaka, A.: Fibrillar assemblage of variable segments of immunoglobulin light chains: an electron microscopic study. *J Immunol, 110*:21-30, 1973.

Shuster, J., Gutkowski, A., and Silverman, M.: Renal metabolism of Bence-Jones protein (abstract). *Clin Res, 18*:733, 1970.

Shuster, M., Causing, W. C., Young, A., Gerard, A., Ramirez, G., and Dinio, R.: Chronic lymphatic leukemia and lymphosarcoma: terminating in multiple myeloma. *J Med Soc NJ, 68*:365-368, 1971.

Silva, J., Jr., Newell, G. R., and Schlott, D. W.: Macroglobulinemia associated with subcutaneous tumors: report of two cases. *Johns Hopkins Med J, 125*:84-91, 1969.

Silverstein, A., and Doniger, D. E.: Neurologic complications of myelomatosis. *Arch Neurol, 9*:534-544, 1963.

Skagseth, E., Jr., and Normann, T.: Localized amyloid tumour of the lung. *Scand J Thorac Cardiovasc Surg, 4*:135-138, 1970.

Skinner, M., Cohen, A. S., Shirahama, T., and Cathcart, E. S.: P-component (pentagonal unit) of amyloid: isolation, characterization, and sequence analysis. *J Lab Clin Med, 84*:604-614, 1974.

Skvarvil, F., Juricic, D., Spengler, G. A., and Morell, A.: The IgG subclass distribution in double M-component sera. In Peeters, H. (Ed.) : *Colloquium on the Protides of the Biological Fluids.* Oxford, Pergamon Press, 1973, pp. 273-277.

Skvarvil, F., and Morell, A.: Distribution of IgA subclasses in sera and bone marrow plasma cells of 21 normal individuals. In Mestecky, J., and Lawton, A. R. (Eds.): *International Symposium on the Immunoglobin A System. Volume 45: Advances in Experimental Medicine and Biology.* New York, Plenum Pr. Plenum Pub., 1974, pp. 433-435.

Skvaril, F., Morell, A., and Barandun, S.: The IgG subclass distribution in 659 myeloma sera. *Vox Sang, 23:*546-551, 1972.

Slavens, J. J.: Multiple myeloma in a child. *Am J Dis Child, 47:*821-835, 1934.

Slavin, R. G., Suriano, J. R., and Dreesman, G.: Studies on cryogelglobulinemia associated with IgA myeloma protein. *Int Arch Allergy Appl Immunol, 40:*739-748, 1971.

Sleeper, C. A., and Cawley, L. P.: Detection and diagnosis of monoclonal gammopathy. *Am J Clin Pathol, 51:*395-400, 1969.

Smetana, K., Gyorkey, F., Gyorkey, P., and Busch, H.: Ultrastructural studies on human myeloma plasmacytes. *Cancer Res, 33:*2300-2309, 1973.

Smit, C. G. S., and Meyler, L.: Acute myeloid leukaemia after treatment with cytostatic agents (letter to the editor). *Lancet, 2:*671-672, 1970.

Smith, C.: Clinicopathologic conference: hepatomegaly for 17 years in a 65-year-old white man. *Med Ann DC, 40:*380-383, 1971

Smith, E., Kochwa, S., and Wasserman, L. R.: Aggregation of IgG globulin *in vivo.* I. The hyperviscosity syndrome in multiple myeloma. *Am J Med, 39:*35-48, 1965.

Smith, J. R., and Phelps, P.: Septic arthritis, gout, pseudogout and osteoarthritis in the knee of a patient with multiple myeloma. *Arthritis Rheum, 15:*89-94, 1972.

Smith, S. B., and Arkin, C.: Cryofibrinogenemia: incidence, clinical correlations, and a review of the literature. *Am J Clin Pathol, 58:*524-530, 1972.

Snapper, I., and Kahn, A.: *Myelomatosis: Fundamentals and Features.* Baltimore, University Park Press, 1971.

Sølling, K., and Askjaer, S. A.: Multiple myeloma with urinary excretion of heavy chain components of IgG and nodular glomerulosclerosis. *Acta Med Scand, 194:*23-30, 1973.

Solly, S.: Remarks on the pathology of mollities ossium: with cases. *Med Chir Trans* (Lond), *27:*435-461, 1844.

Solomon, A., and Fahey, J. L.: Plasmapheresis therapy in macroglobulinemia. *Ann Intern Med, 58:*789-800, 1963.

Solomon, A., and Kunkel, H. G.: A "monoclonal" type, low molecular weight protein related to γM-macroglobulins. *Am J Med, 42:*958-967, 1967.

Solomon, A., and McLaughlin, C. L.: Immunoglobulin structure determined from products of plasma cell neoplasms. *Semin Hematol, 10:*3-17, 1973.

Solomon, J., and Steinfeld, J. L.: Pyroglobulinemia: report of a case, with protein turnover studies. *Am J Med, 38:*937-942, 1965.

Somer, T.: The viscosity of blood, plasma and serum in dys- and parapro-teinemias. *Acta Med Scand, 180* Suppl *456:*1-97, 1966.

Somer, T.: Hyperviscosity syndrome in plasma cell dyscrasias. *Adv Microcirc, 6:*1-55, 1975.

Someren, A., Osgood, C. P., Jr., and Brylski, J.: Solitary posterior fossa plasmacytoma: case report. *J Neurosurg, 35:*223-228, 1971.

Sorenson, G. D.: Electron microscopic observations of viral particles within myeloma cells of man. *Exp Cell Res, 25:*219-221, 1961.

Sorenson, G. D.: Virus-like particles in myeloma cells of man. *Proc Soc Exp Biol Med, 118:*250-252, 1965.

Southeastern Cancer Study Group: Treatment of myeloma: comparison of melphalan, chlorambucil, and azathioprine. *Arch Intern Med, 135:*157-162, 1975.

Southwest Oncology Group Study: Remission maintenance therapy for mul-tiple myeloma. *Arch Intern Med, 135:*147-152, 1975.

Sparagana, M.: Multiple myeloma with pulmonary lesions. *Postgrad Med, 47:* 209-213, 1970.

Speed, D. E., Galton, D. A. G., and Swan, A.: Melphalan in the treatment of myelomatosis. *Br Med J, 1:*1664-1669, 1964

Spengler, G. A., Siebner, H., and Riva, G.: Chromosomal abnormalities in macroglobulinemia Waldenström: discordant findings in uniovular twins. *Acta Med Scand* [Suppl], *445:*132-139, 1966.

Spengler, G. A., Steinberg, A. G., and Skvaril, F.: Development of a second monoclonal immunoglobulin G in a patient with late manifestation of myeloma. *Acta Med Scand, 192:*309-314, 1972.

Spiegelberg, H. L.: Biological activities of immunoglobulins of different classes and subclasses. *Adv Immunol, 19:*259-294, 1974.

Spiegelberg, H. L., Fishkin, B. G., and Grey, H. M.: Catabolism of human γG-immunoglobulins of different heavy chain subclasses. I. Catabolism of γG-myeloma proteins in man. *J Clin Invest, 47:*2323-2330, 1968.

Spiegelberg, H. L., Heath, V. C., and Lang, J. E.: IgG half-molecules: clinical and immunologic features in a patient with plasma cell leukemia. *Blood, 45:*305-313, 1975.

Spiegelberg, H. L., and Weigle, W. O.: The production of antisera to human γG subclasses in rabbits using immunological unresponsiveness. *J Immunol, 101:*377-380, 1968.

Stamp, T. C. B., Child, J. A., and Walker, P. G.: Treatment of osteolytic myelomatosis with mithramycin. *Lancet, 1:*719-722, 1975.

Stankler, L., and Davidson, J. F.: Multiple extra-medullary plasmacytomas of the skin: case report with a note on prognosis. *Br J Dermatol, 90:*217-221, 1974.

Stanley, P., Baker, S. L., and Byers, P. D.: Unusual bone trabeculation in a patient with macroglobulinaemia simulating fibrogenesis imperfecta ossium. *Br J Radiol, 44*:305-313, 1971.

Stavem, P., and Harboe, M.: Acute erythroleukaemia in a patient treated with melphalan for the cold agglutinin syndrome. *Scand J Haematol, 8*:375-379, 1971.

Stavem, P., Hjort, P. F., Elgjo, K., and Sommerschild, H.: Solitary plasmocytoma of the spleen with marked polyclonal increase of gamma G, normalized after splenectomy. *Acta Med Scand, 188*:115-118, 1970.

Stavem, P., Hovig, T., Frøland, S., and Skrede, S.: Immunoglobulin-containing intranuclear inclusions in plasma cells in a case of IgG myeloma. *Scand J Haematol, 13*:266-275, 1974.

Stavem, P., Vandvik, B., Skrede, S., and Hovig, T.: Needle-like crystals in plasma cells in a patient with a plasma cell proliferative disorder. *Scand J Haematol, 14*:24-34, 1975.

Stefani, D. V., Gusev, A. I., and Mokeeva, R. A.: Isolation of immunochemically pure IgE from serum of E-myeloma patient Yu. *Immunochemistry, 10*:559-561, 1973.

Stefanini, M., McDonnell, E. E., Andracki, E. G., Swansbro, W. J., and Durr, P.: Macropyroglobulinemia: immunochemical studies in three cases. *Am J Clin Pathol, 54*:94-101, 1970.

Stein, H., and Kaiserling, E.: Myeloma producing nonsecretory IgM and secretory IgG. *Scand J Haematol, 12*:274-283, 1974.

Stein, R. S., Ellman, L., and Bloch, K. J.: The clinical correlates of IgM M-components: an analysis of thirty-four patients. *Am J Med Sci, 269*:209-216, 1975.

Stein, S. F., Terry, W. D., and Woods, R.: Method for the determination of light chain type of Waldenström macroglobulins in unfractionated serum using radial immunodiffusion (abstract). *Clin Res, 21*:589, 1973.

Steinberg, A. G.: Globulin polymorphisms in man. *Annu Rev Genet, 3*:25-52, 1969.

Stevens, A. R., Jr.: Evolution of multiple myeloma. *Arch Intern Med, 115*:90-93, 1965.

Stites, D. P., and Whitehouse, M. J.: Evolution of multiple myeloma with nonsecreted paraproteins (abstract). *Clin Res, 23*:283A, 1975.

Stone, M. J., and Frenkel, E. P.: The clinical spectrum of light chain myeloma: a study of 35 patients with special reference to the occurrence of amyloidosis. *Am J Med, 58*:601-619, 1975.

Stoop, J. W., Zegers, B. J. M., van der Heiden, C., and Ballieux, R. E.: Monoclonal gammopathy in a child with leukemia. *Blood, 32*:774-786, 1968.

Strauss, R. G., Schubert, W. K., and McAdams, A. J.: Amyloidosis in childhood. *J Pediatr, 74*:272-282, 1969.

Strisower, E. H., and Galleto, A. T.: Waldenström's macroglobulinemia: differential diagnosis, lipoprotein study, and case report. *Am J Med, 32:* 304-312, 1962.

Strong, G. H., Kelsey, D., and Hoch, W.: Primary amyloid disease of the bladder. *J Urol, 112:*463-466, 1974.

Strunge, P.: Waldenström's macroglobulinaemia: an unusual case having only pleuropulmonary manifestations. *Acta Med Scand, 185:*83-87, 1969.

Sugai, S.: IgA pyroglobulin, hyperviscosity syndrome and coagulation abnormality in a patient with multiple myeloma. *Blood, 39:*224-237, 1972.

Sugai, S., Pillarisetty, R., and Talal, N.: Monoclonal macroglobulinemia in NZB/NZW F_1 mice. *J Exp Med, 138:*989-1002, 1973.

Suissa, L., LaRosa, J., and Linn, B.: Plasmacytoma of lymph nodes: a case report. *JAMA, 197:*294-296, 1966.

Sullivan, P. W., and Salmon, S. E.: Kinetics of growth and regression in IgG multiple myeloma. *J Clin Invest, 51:*1697-1708, 1972.

Svien, H. J., Price, R. D., and Bayrd, E. D.: Neurosurgical treatment of compression of the spinal cord caused by myeloma. *JAMA, 153:*784-786, 1953.

Symmers, W. St. C.: Primary amyloidosis: a review. *J Clin Pathol, 9:*187-211, 1956.

Taddeini, L., and Schrader, W.: Concomitant myelomonocytic leukemia and multiple myeloma. *Minn Med, 55:*446-448, 1972.

Talal, N., Sokoloff, L., and Barth, W. F.: Extrasalivary lymphoid abnormalities in Sjögren's syndrome (reticulum cell sarcoma, "pseudolymphoma," macroglobulinemia). *Am J Med, 43:*50-65, 1967.

Talerman, A., and Haije, W. G.: The frequency of M-components in sera of patients with solid malignant neoplasms. *Br J Cancer, 27:*276-282, 1973.

Talerman, A., Serjeant, G. R., and Milner, P. F.: Normal pregnancy in a patient with multiple myeloma and sickle cell anaemia. *West Indian Med J, 20:*97-100, 1971.

Tan, M., and Epstein, W.: Polymer formation during the degradation of human light chain and Bence-Jones proteins by an extract of the lysosomal fraction of normal human kidney. *Immunochemistry, 9:*9-16, 1972.

Tavassoli, M., and Baughan, M.: Virus-like particles in human myeloma without paraproteinemia. *Arch Pathol, 96:*347-349, 1973.

Terry, W. D., and Fahey, J. L.: Subclasses of human γ_2-globulin based on differences in the heavy polypeptide chains. *Science, 146:*400-401, 1964.

Terry, W. D., Page, D. L., Kimura, S., Isobe, T., Osserman, E. F., and Glenner, G. G.: Structural identity of Bence Jones and amyloid fibril proteins in a patient with plasma cell dyscrasia and amyloidosis. *J Clin Invest, 52:* 1276-1281, 1973.

Theologides, A., Osterberg, K., and Kennedy, B. J.: Cerebral toxoplasmosis in multiple myeloma. *Ann Intern Med, 64:*1071-1074, 1966.

Thijs, L. G., Hijmans, W., Leene, W., Muntinghe, O. G., Pietersz, R. N. I., and Ploem, J. E.: Blast cell leukaemia associated with IgA paraproteinaemia and Bence Jones protein. *Br J Haematol, 19*:485-492, 1970.

Thomas, F. B., Clausen, K. P., and Greenberger, N. J.: Liver disease in multiple myeloma. *Arch Intern Med, 132*:195-202, 1973.

Thomas, P. K., and King, R. H. M.: Peripheral nerve changes in amyloid neuropathy. *Brain, 97*:395-406, 1974.

Tiselius, A.: Electrophoresis of serum globulin. II. Electrophoretic analysis of normal and immune sera. *Biochem J, 31*:1464-1477, 1937.

Tiselius, A., and Kabat, E. A.: An electrophoretic study of immune sera and purified antibody preparations. *J Exp Med, 69*:119-131, 1939.

Tomasi, T. B., Jr.: Human immunoglobulin A. *N Engl J Med, 279*:1327-1330, 1968.

Tomasi, T. B., Jr.: Secretory immunoglobulins. *N Engl J Med, 287*:500-506, 1972.

Tranchida, L., Palutke, M., Poulik, M. D., and Prasad, A. S.: Primary acquired sideroblastic anemia preceding monoclonal gammopathy and malignant lymphoma. *Am J Med, 55*:559-564, 1973.

Triger, D. R., and Joekes, A. M.: Renal amyloidosis: a fourteen-year follow-up. *Q J Med*, ns, *42*:15-40, 1973.

Tuddenham, E. G. D., Whittaker, J. A., Bradley, J., Lilleyman, J. S., and James, D. R.: Hyperviscosity syndrome in IgA multiple myeloma. *Br J Haematol, 27*:65-76, 1974.

Tulliez, M., Ricard, M. F., Jan, F., and Sultan, C.: Preleukaemic abnormal myelopoiesis induced by chlorambucil: a case study. *Scand J Haematol, 13*:179-183, 1974.

Turesson, I.: Nucleolar size in benign and malignant plasma cell proliferation. *Acta Med Scand, 197*:7-14, 1975.

Tursz, T., Flandrin, G., Brouet, J.-C., Briere, J., and Seligmann, M.: Simultaneous occurrence of acute myeloblastic leukaemia and multiple myeloma without previous chemotherapy. *Br Med J, 2*:642-643, 1974.

Twomey, J. J., and Douglass, C. C.: An in vitro study of lymphocyte and macrophage function with lymphoproliferative neoplasms. *Cancer, 33*:1034-1038, 1974.

Twomey, J. J., Laughter, A. H., Villanueva, N. D., Kao, Y. S., Lidsky, M. D., and Jordan, P. H., Jr.: Gastric secretory and serologic studies on patients with neoplastic and immunologic disorders. *Arch Intern Med, 128*:746-749, 1971.

Ullmann, A. S.: Primary amyloidosis of the renal pelvis: a case report and review of literature. *Mich Med, 72*:29-33, 1973.

Underdown, B. J., and Dorrington, K. J.: Studies on the structural and conformational basis for the relative resistance of serum and secretory immunoglobulin A to proteolysis. *J Immunol, 112*:949-959, 1974.

Upstate Medical Center: Left thigh mass. *NY State J Med, 74*:1798-1801, 1974.

Vaerman, J.-P., and Heremans, J. F.: Subclasses of human immunoglobulin A based on differences in the alpha polypeptide chains. *Science, 153:*647-649, 1966.

Vaerman, J.-P., Heremans, J. F., and Laurell, C.-B.: Distribution of α-chain subclasses in normal and pathological IgA-globulins. *Immunology, 14:*425-432, 1968.

Vaerman, J.-P., Johnson, L. B., Mandy, W., and Fudenberg, H. H.: Multiple myeloma with two paraprotein peaks: an instructive case. *J Lab Clin Med, 65:*18-25, 1965.

Van Boxel, J. A., Paul, W. E., Terry, W. D., and Green, I.: IgD-bearing human lymphocytes. *J Immunol, 109:*648-651, 1972.

Vander, J. B., and Johnson, H. A.: Chronic lymphatic leukemia and multiple myeloma in the same patient. *Ann Intern Med, 53:*1052-1059, 1960.

Van der Waal, I., Fehmers, M. C. O., and Kraal, E. R.: Amyloidosis: its significance in oral surgery; review of the literature and report of a case. *Oral Surg, 36:*469-481, 1973.

Vermess, M., Pearson, K. D., Einstein, A. B., and Fahey, J. L.: Osseous manifestations of Waldenström's macroglobulinemia. *Radiology, 102:*497-504, 1972.

Victor, M., Banker, B. Q., and Adams, R. D.: The neuropathy of multiple myeloma. *J Neurol Neurosurg Psychiatry, 21:*73-88, 1958.

Videbaek, A., Mansa, B., and Kjems, E.: A human IgA-myeloma protein with anti-streptococcal hyaluronidase (ASH) activity. *Scand J Haematol, 10:* 181-185, 1973.

Virella, G., and Hobbs, J. R.: Heavy chain typing in IgG monoclonal gammopathies with special reference to cases of serum hyperviscosity and cryoglobulinaemia. *Clin Exp Immunol, 8:*973-980, 1971.

Virella, G., and Parkhouse, R. M. E.: Determination of the molecular weight of human gamma-3 chains by polyacrylamide gel electrophoresis in the presence of sodium dodecyl sulphate. *Immunology, 23:*857-860, 1972.

Virella, G., Preto, R. V., and Graça, F.: Polymerized monoclonal IgA in two patients with myelomatosis and hyperviscosity syndrome. *Br J Haematol, 30:*479-487, 1975.

Vladutiu, A., and Sielski, L.: Macroglobulinaemia or multiple myeloma? (Letter to the editor.) *Lancet, 1:*1122-1123, 1973.

Vodopick, H., Chaskes, S. J., Solomon, A., and Stewart, J. A.: Transient monoclonal gammopathy associated with cytomegalovirus infection. *Blood, 44:* 189-195, 1974.

Wager, O., Mustakallio, K. K., and Räsänen, J. A.: Mixed IgA-IgG cryoglobulinemia: immunological studies and case reports of three patients. *Am J Med, 44:*179-187, 1968.

Wahner, H. W., Kyle, R. A., and Beabout, J. W.: Unpublished data.

Waldenström, J.: Incipient myelomatosis or "essential" hyperglobulinemia with fibrogenopenia: a new syndrome? *Acta Med Scand, 117:*216-247, 1944.

Waldenström, J.: Abnormal proteins in myeloma. *Adv Intern Med, 5*:398-440, 1952.

Waldenström, J.: Studies on conditions associated with disturbed gamma globulin formation (gammopathies). *Harvey Lect, 56*:211-231, 1961.

Waldenström, J.: Hypergammaglobulinemia as a clinical hematological problem: a study in the gammopathies. *Prog Hematol, 3*:266-293, 1962.

Waldenström, J. G.: *Monoclonal and Polyclonal Hypergammaglobulinemia: Clinical and Biological Significance.* Nashville, Vanderbilt University Press, 1968.

Waldenström, J. G.: *Diagnosis and Treatment of Multiple Myeloma.* New York, Grune & Stratton, 1970.

Waldeyer, W.: Ueber Bindegewebszellen. *Arch Mikrosk Anat, 11*:176-194, 1875.

Waldmann, T. A.: Disorders of immunoglobulin metabolism. *N Engl J Med, 281*:1170-1177, 1969.

Waldmann, T. A., Bull, J. M., Bruce, R. M., Broder, S., Jost, M. C., Balestra, S. T., and Suer, M. E.: Serum immunoglobulin E levels in patients with neoplastic disease. *J Immunol, 113*:379-386, 1974.

Wall, R. L., and Clausen, K. P.: Carcinoma of the urinary bladder in patients receiving cyclophosphamide. *N Engl J Med, 293*:271-273, 1975.

Walsh, J. C.: The neuropathy of multiple myeloma: an electrophysiological and histological study. *Arch Neurol, 25*:404-414, 1971.

Wanebo, H. J., and Clarkson, B. D.: Essential macroglobulinemia: report of a case including immunofluorescent and electron microscopic studies. *Ann Intern Med, 62*:1025-1045, 1965.

Wang, A. C., Fudenberg, H. H., and Wells, J. V.: A new subgroup of the kappa chain variable region associated with anti-Pr cold agglutinins (letter to the editor). *Nature* [New Biol], *243*:126-128, 1973.

Ward, A. M., and Preston, F. E.: The kidney and intravascular coagulation in myelomatosis. *Br Med J, 2*:529-531, 1974.

Ward, A. M., Shortland, J. R., and Darke, C. S.: Lymphosarcoma of the lung with monoclonal (IgM) gammopathy: a clinicopathologic, histochemical, immunologic, and ultrastructural study. *Cancer, 27*:1009-1028, 1971.

Warne, G. L., Fairley, K. F., Hobbs, J. B., and Martin, F. I. R.: Cyclophosphamide-induced ovarian failure. *N Engl J Med, 289*:1159-1162, 1973.

Warner, N. L., Potter, M., and Metcalf, D.: *Multiple Myeloma and Related Immunoglobulin-Producing Neoplasms* (UICC Technical Report Series). Vol. 13. Geneva, International Union Against Cancer, 1974.

Watanabe, A., Kitamura, M., and Shimizu, M.: Immunoglobulin A (IgA) with properties of both cryoglobulin and pyroglobulin. *Clin Chim Acta, 52*:231-237, 1974.

Watkins, J., and Tee, D. E. H.: Catabolism of γG-globulin and myeloma proteins of the subclasses γG$_1$ and γG$_2$ in a healthy volunteer. *Immunology, 18*:537-543, 1970.

Waxman, S., and Dove, J. T.: Cryofibrinogenemia aggravated during hypothermia. *N Engl J Med, 281*:1291-1292, 1969.

Webb, H. E., Harrison, E. G., Jr., Masson, J. K., and ReMine, W. H.: Solitary extramedullary myeloma (plasmacytoma) of the upper part of the respiratory tract and oropharynx. *Cancer, 15*:1142-1155, 1962.

Weber, F. P.: A case of multiple myeloma (myelomatosis) with Bence-Jones proteid in the urine (myelopathic albumosuria of Bradshaw, Kahler's disease) and a summary of Bence-Jones albumosuria: with a report on the chemical pathology by R. Hutchison and J. J. R. Macleod). *Med Chir Trans* (Lond), *86*:395-470, 1903.

Wegelius, O., Skrifvars, B., and Andersson, L.: Rheumatoid arthritis terminating in plasmocytoma. *Acta Med Scand, 187*:133-138, 1970.

Weiss, A. H., Smith, E., Christoff, N., and Kochwa, S.: Cerebrospinal fluid paraproteins in multiple myeloma. *J Lab Clin Med, 66*:280-293, 1965.

Weiss, H. J., and Kochwa, S.: Antihaemophilic globulin (AHG) in multiple myeloma and macroglobulinaemia. *Br J Haematol, 14*:205-214, 1968.

Welton, J., Walker, S. R., Sharp, G. C., Herzenberg, L. A., Wistar, R., Jr., and Creger, W. P.: Macroglobulinemia with bone destruction. *Am J Med, 44*: 280-288, 1968.

Wernet, P., Kickhöfen B., and Westerhausen, M.: A monoclonal immunoglobulin with combining specificity for transferrin in a case of hemochromatosis of the liver (abstract). *Clin Res, 20*:521, 1972.

Werther, J. L., Schapira, A., Rubinstein, O., and Janowitz, H. D.: Amyloidosis in regional enteritis: a report of five cases. *Am J Med, 29*:416-423, 1960.

Westermark, P., and Stenkvist, B.: A new method for the diagnosis of systemic amyloidosis. *Arch Intern Med, 132*:522-523, 1973.

Western Cancer Study Group: Sequential therapy compared with combination therapy in multiple myeloma. *Arch Intern Med, 135*:163-171, 1975.

Westin, J., Eyrich, R., Falsen, E., Lindholm, L., Lundin, P., Lonnroth, I., and Weinfeld, A.: Gamma heavy chain disease: reports of three patients. *Acta Med Scand, 192*:281-292, 1972.

Whitehouse, G. H., Bottomley, J. P., and Bradley, J.: Lymphographic appearances in Waldenström's macroglobulinaemia. *Br J Radiol, 47*:226-229, 1974.

Wiernik, P. H.: Amyloid joint disease. *Medicine* (Baltimore), *51*:465-479, 1972.

Wild, C.: Beitrag zur Kenntnis der amyloiden und der hyalinen Degeneration des Bindegewebes. *Beitr Pathol Anat, 1*:175-200, 1886.

Wilks, S.: Cases of lardaceous disease and some allied affections: with remarks. *Guys Hosp Rep, 2*:103-132, 1856.

Williams, H. M., Diamond, H. D., Craver, L. F., and Parsons, H.: *Neurological Complications of Lymphomas and Leukemias.* Springfield, Illinois, Charles C Thomas, Publisher, 1959.

Williams, R. C., and Gibbons, R. J.: Inhibition of bacterial adherence by secretory immunoglobin A: a mechanism of antigen disposal. *Science, 177:* 697-699, 1972.

Williams, R. C., Jr., Bailly, R. C., and Howe, R. B.: Studies of "benign" serum M-components. *Am J Med Sci, 257:*275-293, 1969.

Williams, R. C., Jr., Brunning, R. D., and Wollheim, F. A.: Light-chain disease: an abortive variant of multiple myeloma. *Ann Intern Med, 65:*471-486, 1966.

Williams, R. C., Jr., Cathcart, E. S., Calkins, E., Fite, G. L., Rubio, J. B., and Cohen, A. S.: Secondary amyloidosis in lepromatous leprosy: possible relationships of diet and environment. *Ann Intern Med, 62:*1000-1007, 1965.

Williams, R. C., Jr., Erickson, J. L., Polesky, H. F., and Swaim, W. R.: Studies of monoclonal immunoglobulins (M-components) in various kindreds. *Ann Intern Med, 67:*309-327, 1967.

Williamson, R. C. N.: Primary amyloidosis of the rectum. *Proc R Soc Med, 65:*74, 1972.

Wilson, S. K., Buchanan, R. D., Stone, W. J., and Rhamy, R. K.: Amyloid deposition in the prostate. *J Urol, 110:*322-323, 1973.

Winterbauer, R. H., Riggins, R. C. K., Griesman, F. A., and Bauermeister, D. E.: Pleuropulmonary manifestations of Waldenstrom's macroglobulinemia. *Chest, 66:*368-375, 1974.

Wintrobe, M. M., and Buell, M. V.: Hyperproteinemia associated with multiple myeloma: with report of a case in which an extraordinary hyperproteinemia was associated with thrombosis of the retinal veins and symptoms suggesting Raynaud's disease. *Bull Johns Hopkins Hosp, 52:*156-165, 1933.

Wochner, R. D., Strober, W., and Waldmann, T. A.: The role of the kidney in the catabolism of Bence Jones proteins and immunoglobulin fragments. *J Exp Med, 126:*207-221, 1967.

Wolf, R. E., Riedel, L. O., Levin, W. C., and Ritzmann, S. E.: Remission of macroglobulinemia coincident with hepatitis: report of case and review of literature. *Arch Intern Med, 130:*392-395, 1972.

Wolfe, J. A.: Panhypopituitarism due to multiple myeloma. *South Med J, 63:* 32-33, 1970.

Wolfenstein-Todel, C., Franklin, E. C., and Rudders, R. A.: Similarities of the light chains and the variable regions of the heavy chains of the IgG$_2$ λ and IgA$_1$ λ myeloma proteins from a single patient. *J Immunol, 112:* 871-876, 1974.

Wong, C.-K.: Lichen amyloidosus: a relatively common skin disorder in Taiwan. *Arch Dermatol, 110:*438-440, 1974.

Wood, T. A., and Frenkel, E. P.: An unusual case of macroglobulinemia. *Arch Intern Med, 119:*631-637, 1967.

Wright, C. J. E.: Long survival in solitary plasmacytoma of bone. *J Bone Joint Surg* [Br] *43:*767-771, 1961.

Wright, J. H.: A case of multiple myeloma. *Johns Hopkins Hosp Rep, 9*:359-366, 1900.

Wright, J. R., Calkins, E., Breen, W. J., Stolte, G., and Schultz, R. T.: Relationship of amyloid to aging: review of the literature and systematic study of 83 patients derived from a general hospital population. *Medicine* (Baltimore), *48*:39-60, 1969.

Wu, T. T., and Kabat, E. A.: An analysis of the sequences of the variable regions of Bence Jones proteins and myeloma light chains and their implications for antibody complementarity. *J Exp Med, 132*:211-250, 1970.

Yamaguchi, K.: Pathology of macroglobulinemia: a review of Japanese cases. *Acta Pathol Jap, 23*:917-952, 1973.

Yentis, I.: The so-called solitary plasmocytoma of bone. *J Faculty Radiologists, 8*:132-144, 1956.

Yount, W. J., Dorner, M. M., Kunkel, H. G., and Kabat, E. A.: Studies on human antibodies. VI. Selective variations in subgroup composition and genetic markers. *J Exp Med, 127*:633-646, 1968.

Yuill, G. M.: Amyloidosis complicated by intractable postural hypotension. *Postgrad Med J, 49*:52-56, 1974.

Yunginger, J. W., and Gleich, G. J.: Seasonal changes in IgE antibodies and their relationship to IgG antibodies during immunotherapy for ragweed hay fever. *J Clin Invest, 52*:1268-1275, 1973.

Zawadzki, Z. A., and Benedek, T. G.: Rheumatoid arthritis, dysproteinemic arthropathy, and paraproteinemia. *Arthritis Rheum, 12*:555-568, 1969.

Zawadzki, Z. A., Benedek, T. G., Ein, D., and Easton, J. M.: Rheumatoid arthritis terminating in heavy-chain disease. *Ann Intern Med, 70*:335-347, 1969.

Zawadzki, Z. A., and Edwards, G. A.: Dysimmunoglobulinemia associated with hepatobiliary disorders. *Am J Med, 48*:196-202, 1970a.

Zawadzki, Z. A., and Edwards, G. A.: Pseudoparaproteinemia due to hypertransferrinemia. *Am J Clin Pathol, 54*:802-809, 1970b.

Zawadzki, Z. A., and Edwards, G. A.: Nonmyelomatous monoclonal immunoglobulinemia. *Prog Clin Immunol, 1*:105-156, 1972.

Zelis, R., Mason, D. T., and Barth, W.: Abnormal peripheral vascular dynamics in systemic amyloidosis. *Ann Intern Med, 70*:1167-1172, 1969.

Zimelman, A. P.: Thrombocytosis in multiple myeloma (letter to the editor). *Ann Intern Med, 78*:970-971, 1973.

Zinneman, H. H., and Seal, U. S.: Double spike in myeloma serum due to retention of light chains. *Arch Intern Med, 124*:77-80, 1969.

Zlotnick, A., and Landau, S.: Immunoelectrophoretic studies in patients with cryofibrinogenemia. *J Lab Clin Med, 68*:70-80, 1966.

Zlotnick, A., and Robinson, E.: Chronic lymphatic leukemia associated with macroglobulinemia. *Isr J Med Sci, 6*:365-372, 1970.

Zlotnick, A., and Rosenmann, E.: Renal pathologic findings associated with monoclonal gammopathies. *Arch Intern Med, 135:*40-45, 1975.

Zucker-Franklin, D., and Franklin, E. C.: Ultrastructural and immunofluorescence studies of the cells associated with μ-chain disease. *Blood, 37:*257-271, 1971.

Zucker-Franklin, D., Franklin, E. C., and Cooper, N. S.: Production of macroglobulins in vitro and a study of their cellular origin. *Blood, 20:*56-64, 1962.

Author Index

Subject Index